Approach to Lower Limb Oedema

Satyendra K. Tiwary
Editor

Approach to Lower Limb Oedema

Springer

Editor
Satyendra K. Tiwary
Department of General Surgery
Institute of Medical Sciences, Banaras Hindu University
Varanasi, India

ISBN 978-981-16-6208-9 ISBN 978-981-16-6206-5 (eBook)
https://doi.org/10.1007/978-981-16-6206-5

This Springer imprint is published by the registered company Springer Nature Singapore Pte Ltd.
The registered company address is: 152 Beach Road, #21-01/04 Gateway East, Singapore 189721, Singapore

Foreword

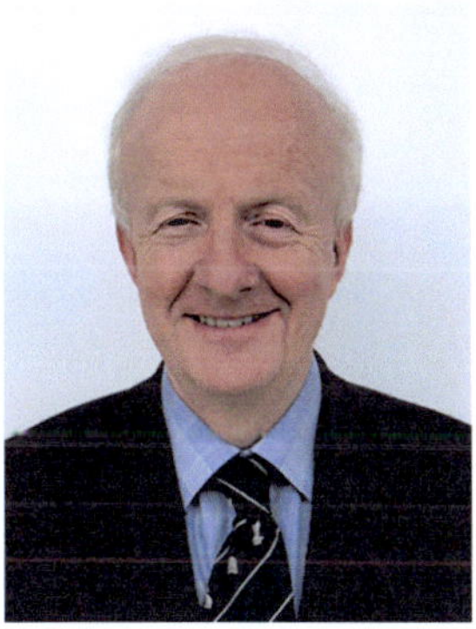

It gives me great pleasure to write the foreword for this text that has been put together by the hard work of Dr. Satyendra Kumar Tiwary from the Banaras Hindu University of Varanasi.

Many of us, as treating clinicians, are often confronted with how to manage a patient with lower limb edema. This text very much reviews the issues of lower limb edema, looking at not only the anatomy and physiology but also those issues that confront the clinician looking after these patients. There is a worldwide group of experts who have contributed to this text and looking at all the various investigations and potential treatment pathways for this cohort of patients. I very much hope that many practising physicians will be able to find information in this excellent text that will allow them to benefit the large number of patients worldwide who suffer from swelling in their lower legs.

Academic Department of Vascular Surgery
Imperial College London
London, UK

Alun H. Davies

Foreword

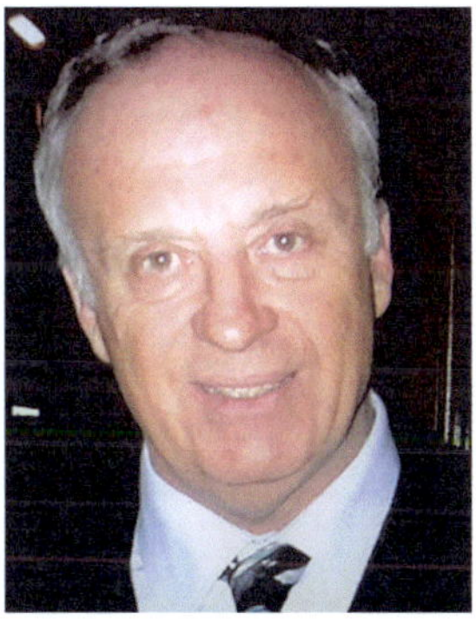

Edema of the lower limbs is a very common clinical picture: people of every age, from childhood to the elderly complain of it.

Edema has several causes and the origin is not always clearly and immediately understood. For example, slight swelling in young teenagers, which disappear spontaneously, or local, limited, painful swelling of a foot, maybe sometimes of unclear origin.

Commonly, edema is discussed as a clinical sign in a paper or in a chapter dedicated to a specific disease, like venous insufficiency, but is not a single argument itself.

However, as the symptom is common, alternative diagnoses need to be considered if the cause is not clear. Several diseases, related to different specialties, maybe the cause of limb swelling, requiring to have a multispecialty overview to find out the origin of edema. Moreover, some rare diseases, like vascular malformations, or genetic disorders may be difficult to be considered as causes of swelling.

The result is that the patient is sent to different specialists, wasting time and money, to get a correct diagnosis.

This book, which collects all the pathologies that may be the cause of lower limb edema, is an important aid for the correct diagnosis and treatment of limb swelling. It will help the physician not only to understand and update his own knowledge about physiopathology of fluid accumulation in the limbs but also to have available, in a single book, a series of chapters regarding all the diseases that may create edema, including rare one which may be difficult to consider in unclear cases.

For these reasons, this book is an original and helpful publication that each physician, involved in lower limb diseases, should have in his library.

Center for Vascular Malformations
Clinical Institute Humanitas "Mater Domini"
Castellanza (Varese), Italy

Raul E. Mattassi

Preface

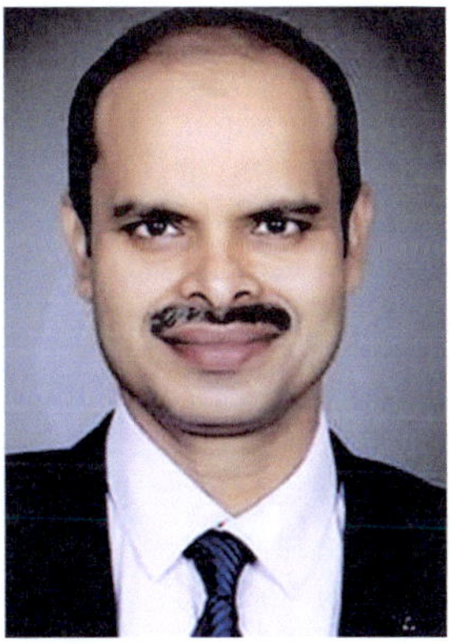

Lower limb oedema is the commonest peripheral oedema affecting legs, ankle, and foot. The cause may be simple, sometimes like sitting for a long time in a plane or standing for too long in journey or work. Sometimes, it may be a result of more serious underlying disease like systemic diseases in the form of cardiac failure, liver disease, or renal impairment, etc. It is a manifestation leading to consultation from so many specialists like Surgery, Plastic Surgery, Orthopaedics, Neurology, Vascular Surgery, Cardiology, Nephrology, Medicine, Radiotherapy, Physical Medicine and Rehabilitation. Despite patients consulting in so many specialties, I have observed in my surgical practice of 20 years in university teaching hospital that it is a complex clinical scenario for which the cause, cure, and complications need very careful work up from the clinician as results and outcome may be difficult, unpredictable, and limited sometimes amidst uncertainties.

Lower limb oedema may be trivial, temporary, transient, or terrible not responding to treatment. Cellular fluid balance disruption and accumulation in interstitial space with gravitational pull effect driving fluid in dependent part is the culprit in lower limb oedema. Peripheral oedema is common in older adults and pregnant women, but it can occur at any age group including children. It may affect one or both legs and may be acute or chronic.

With so many disciplines needed with overlapping and myriad manifestations of many underlying pathology in different patients, makes it difficult to work up and treat lower limb oedema systematically and honestly by consultants of every discipline. Dedicated book as well focus on specific limb oedema during teaching and training is lacking in literature as well as custom. Considering so many patients of all age group, children, middle aged, old, pregnant affected and lack of very lucid clinical approach with targeted treatment in lower limb oedema led me to the concept and completion of this book. With 23 chapters contributed by competent consultants in their field covering every aspect of lower limb oedema comprising anatomy, physiology, aetiology, pathogenesis, investigations, differential diagnosis, clinical manifestations, genetics, local causes, systemic causes, acute oedema, chronic oedema, compression therapy and quality of life. A lot of flow charts, figures, tables, and diagrams have been included in chapters as per requirement to clear the clouds of confusion and construct a complete clinical concept for consultants.

This book has been framed with contents to answer the queries in lower limb oedema whether that is acute or chronic, unilateral or bilateral, local or systemic, trivial or terrible, persistent or progressive. It fulfils the gap in scientific knowledge helping General Surgeon, Plastic Surgeon, Orthopaedician, Neurologist, Vascular surgeon, Cardiologist, Nephrologist, Family physician, and helping trainee and fellows in different disciplines once they come through a case of lower limb oedema.

I acknowledge the help of Dr Naren Agarwal, Ms. Jagjit Kaur Saini, and Ms. Beauty Christobel Gunasekaran from Springer Nature to bring out the book in present form with their valuable inputs and suggestions till the finishing of the project. I am highly indebted to Mrs. Sangita Yadav (Chandrapur) for continuous and valuable suggestions in English, grammar, and corrections to shape the book finally in publication. I am indebted to my family Hema, Apoorva, and Advaita who provided me all the moral support and will forgive me for any negligence which was unavoidable.

I dedicate this book to all the patients managed during my entire career who were the resource as well as inspiration in the management of this complex manifestation of lower limb oedema.

It is my earnest desire that this book becomes a valuable source of understanding and management of common to complex clinical condition of lower limb oedema to the students, trainees, fellows as well as clinicians who may have difficulty at any point getting corrected with aid of this resource.

I conclude my words here with a quote from most ancient scientific literature of the world, Rigveda told about 5000 years back. Have you ever wondered—what did the seers (ऋषि) of the Vedas yearn for?

In a hymn addressed to the Visvedevas (विश्वेदेवा:) in the Rig Veda, they prayed for noble thoughts from all directions.

आनो भद्राः क्रतवो यन्तु विश्वत: | – ऋग्वेद – 1.89.1

(āno bhadrāḥ kratavo yantu viśvato)

कल्याणकारक विचार चारों ओर से हमारे पास आयें|

Let noble thoughts come to us from all directions.

—Rig Veda 1.89.1

Varanasi, India Satyendra K. Tiwary

Contents

1 Introduction of Lower Limb Edema

Satyendra K. Tiwary, Vivek Kumar Katiyar, and Ankush

1.1 Background

Lower limb edema is the commonest peripheral edema affecting legs, ankle, and foot. The cause may be simple, sometimes like sitting for a long time on a plane or standing for too long or it may be a result of more serious underlying diseases such as systemic diseases in the form of cardiac failure, liver disease, or renal impairment. It is a manifestation leading to consultation from so many specialists like surgery, plastic surgery, orthopedics, neurology, vascular surgery, cardiology, nephrology, medicine, radiotherapy, physical medicine, and rehabilitation. Lower limb edema may be trivial, temporary, transient, or terrible sometimes not responding to treatment. Cellular fluid balance disruption and accumulation in the interstitial space with gravitational pull effect driving fluid in dependent parts is the culprit in lower limb edema. Peripheral edema is common in older adults and pregnant women, but it can occur in any age group including children. It may affect one or both legs and may be acute or chronic.

Swelling of the lower limb is a frequent finding in clinical practice and often harmless, but the cause should always be identified to avoid irreversible changes over the skin and subcutaneous tissue of lower extremity. Apart from harmless causes manifesting as edema, sometimes underlying serious systemic diseases need immediate attention. The pathophysiology of edema is mainly based on disturbances in the microcirculation. However, the differential diagnosis for lower limb

S. K. Tiwary (✉)
Institute of Medical Sciences, Banaras Hindu University, Varanasi, India

V. K. Katiyar
Trauma Centre, Institute of Medical Sciences, Banaras Hindu University, Varanasi, India

Ankush
Department of General Surgery, Institute of Medical Sciences, Banaras Hindu University, Varanasi, India

S. K. Tiwary (ed.), *Approach to Lower Limb Oedema*,
https://doi.org/10.1007/978-981-16-6206-5_1

swelling is always broader, and it may be multifactorial in etiology. In systemic disorders, medications of the underlying pathology are central in the management while localized underlying causes such as chronic venous disorder, lymphedema, deep vein thrombosis, cellulitis, and trauma may need intervention and meticulous follow-up from time to time. Patients with lower limb swelling may suffer from functional as well as cosmetic compromises requiring lifelong treatment and psychological support.

1.2 Introduction

Edema can be described as accumulation of fluid in tissues caused by an expanded interstitial fluid compartment due to vascular leakage with or without decreased lymphatic drainage [1].Water accounts for approximately 60% of the body weight in an adult out of which the intracellular fluid occupies three-fourths and the rest is extracellular fluid. Extracellular fluid is further constituted by three-fourths of the interstitial compartment while only one-fourth comprises the plasma which accounts for about 5% of the lean body weight. This microcirculatory homeostasis is meticulously maintained by the Starling forces which include capillary hydrostatic pressure, interstitial hydrostatic pressure, capillary oncotic pressure, and interstitial oncotic pressure. Any alternation or disturbance in this mechanism either due to local causes or systemic diseases can lead to edema which can cause clinical symptoms and signs. Edema can be exudative with high protein content and transudative with decreased protein content. Albumin makes up for most of the protein content in the body and any level below 2 g/dl can precipitate edema [1, 2].

1.3 Etiology and Classification

Multifactorial association in lower limb edema always needs evaluation locally as well as systemically, but as a rule unilateral edema is mostly due to underlying local causes such as chronic venous disease, deep vein thrombosis, cellulitis, lymphedema, and trauma while systemic diseases such as cardiac failure, renal failure, hepatic failure or pulmonary hypertension, anemia, and myxedema manifest as bilateral and generalized swelling of the body. Impaired activity of either cardiac muscle or calf muscle may manifest ultimately in edema. Both venous and lymphatic systems must act to prevent accumulation of fluid in extracellular space. The basic mechanism in edema is either underperformance of the venous system and lymphatic system in local pathological conditions such as chronic venous disease, lymphedema, and deep vein thrombosis or overload of the fluid not returned by the normal veno-lymphatic system in systemic diseases leading to fluid overload.

RISK FACTORS [3, 4]

1. Physiological	(i) Age	Incidence increases with increasing age due to incompetent vessels
	(ii) Pregnancy	• Increased plasma volume and retention of fluid • Pressure on the venous system causing decreased return to the heart
	(iii) Menstrual hormonal changes	• Impaired venous return and retention of fluids • Increased plasma volume leading to increased capillary hydrostatic pressure
2. Lifestyle related	(i) Immobility	• In the absence of normal muscle function, venous and lymphatic drainage is hampered • Stasis leads to edema in dependent parts owing to gravity
	(ii) Obesity	Pressure on vessels in the groin leads to decreased lymphatic and venous return
	(iii) High sodium intake	Edema due to water retention
3. Drugs	(i) Vasodilators	Increased capillary hydrostatic pressure
	(ii) Calcium channel blockers	Selective arteriolar vasodilation leading to increased capillary hydrostatic pressure
	(iii) Estrogen-based drugs	Fluid retention
	(iv) Steroids	Sodium retention
	(v) NSAIDs	PGE2 inhibition causing increased sodium reabsorption
4. Systemic diseases	(i) Congestive cardiac failure	• Increased capillary hydrostatic pressure • Decreased renal blood flow
	(ii) Cirrhosis	Decreased protein synthesis leading to decreased plasma oncotic pressure
	(iii) Renal failure	Sodium water retention
	(iv) Malnutrition	Decreased protein in the body leading to decreased plasma oncotic pressure
	(v) Chronic venous insufficiency	Regional venous hypertension causing increased capillary hydrostatic pressure
	(vi) Deep vein thrombosis	
5. Lymphatic obstruction	(i) Filariasis	
	(ii) Cancer surgeries	
	(iii) Radiotherapy	
6. Others	(i) Cellulitis	Increased capillary permeability
	(ii) Burns	
	(iii) Trauma	

CLASSIFICATION:

(I) BASED ON SITE OF INVOLVEMENT

1. UNILATERAL: involving only one limb
2. BILATERAL: involving both the limbs

(II) **BASED ON THE VESSEL INVOLVED**
   1. VENOUS: Increased capillary filtration that cannot be drained by normal lymphatic drainage results in a low viscosity, transudative collection.
   2. LYMPHATIC: Lymphatic dysfunction leads to exudative edematous fluid within the skin and subcutaneous tissue. It is of two types.
      (i) Primary—Present at birth
      (ii) Secondary—Acquired due to lymphatic system abnormality
   3. LIPEDEMA: A fat-rich collection; it is sometimes considered as a form of fat maldistribution rather than a true edema.

(III) **BASED ON DURATION OF SYMPTOMS**
   1. ACUTE: less than 72 h
   2. CHRONIC: more than 72 h

(IV) **BASED ON ETIOLOGY**
   1. LOCAL CAUSES: Trauma, infections, etc.
   2. SYSTEMIC CAUSES: Heart failure, renal failure, liver failure, diabetes, etc.
   3. POST-SURGERY: Cancer surgeries and lymph node dissections often lead to lymphedema.

(V) **BASED ON REACTION TO PRESSURE**
   1. PITTING: Fluid drains to the surrounding areas on application of pressure, thus leaving a depression that can be visualized even after the pressure is released.
   2. NON-PITTING: Fluid is pushed along the lymphatic vessels when pressure is applied and fills up rapidly as soon as the pressure is removed.

1.4 Pathophysiology

The basic physiological forces responsible for maintaining fluid balance between the capillaries and interstitium are defined by Starling. The basic mechanisms involved in the production of edema include:

1. Difference between intracapillary blood pressure and extravascular hydrostatic pressure (ΔP)
2. Differences in oncotic (colloid osmotic) pressure ($\Delta\pi$)
3. The permeability of the blood vessel wall (K_f)

According to Starling, net fluid movement (F_M) across a semipermeable membrane is $\mathbf{F_M = K_f (\Delta P - \Delta\pi)}$.

Hence the factors causing pedal edema are:

1. Increased intravascular/intracapillary hydrostatic pressure
2. Decreased plasma oncotic (colloid osmotic) pressure
3. Increased vascular permeability
4. Increased osmotic pressure in the interstitial space

Along with this, other factors causing pedal edema are:

- Impairment of lymphatic drainage in congenital or inflammatory diseases of lymphatics
- Local injury and infection causing damage to capillary endothelial barrier (causing increased permeability)
- Drugs leading to bilateral edema mostly

1.5 Diagnosis

Diagnosis of limb swelling includes the history, examination, and radiological imaging.

History includes the duration of the edema whether acute or chronic. Acute presentation is when the edema has appeared in less than 72 h. Deep vein thrombosis and cellulitis are strongly considered if the onset is acute [5].

However, even after 72 h, DVT cannot be ruled out merely on the basis of the history of duration of symptoms and concomitant examination and imaging must be carried out. History related to trauma and post-surgery edema is also essential for the diagnosis. Painful swelling is usually seen in deep vein thrombosis and reflex sympathetic dystrophy [6].

It may also be present in cellulitis. Pain will be low grade in chronic venous insufficiency. Lymphedema is usually painless [7].

History related to systemic diseases like heart, liver, or kidney disease, etc., and drugs like calcium channel blockers, prednisone, and anti-inflammatory should be taken as they are common causes of leg edema [8, 9].

History related to pelvic/abdominal neoplasm or radiation can also cause lower limb edema. Sleep apnea history should also be elicited as it can cause pulmonary hypertension, which is a cause of leg edema. Sleep apnea includes snoring or apnea during sleep, daytime somnolence, or a neck circumference of more than 17 inches. Obesity is also a risk factor for swelling and lipedema.

Venous edema improves overnight as compared to lymphedema due to elevation of the leg at the level of the heart [10].

The elicitation of history is very important to approach a patient with edema. The duration of edema will point out about acute (<72 h) or chronic onset. If acute onset, the most likely diagnosis is deep vein thrombosis, but it may be considered even in chronic onset edema if clinical findings are compatible. The presence of pain favors diagnosis of deep vein thrombosis and reflex sympathetic dystrophy. Low grade pain in the presence of edema points toward chronic venous insufficiency, while lymphedema is usually painless. The history of the presence of systemic diseases such as cardiac, renal, and hepatobiliary system should be ruled out by clinical examinations and investigations. Any history of radiation exposure and abdominal surgery for malignant disease again favors deep vein thrombosis. If edema of legs improves during night, it is most likely venous in origin.

In determining the cause of swelling, a thorough physical examination is just as important as a thorough clinical history. Even though the complaint may be unilateral, it is critical to evaluate both lower limbs for complete diagnosis and further management.

The other limb is frequently swollen, and this can reveal information about the reasons of swelling in the more affected limb. It is important to pay attention to how the swelling is distributed.

Despite the fact that the primary symptom is in the lower limbs, a thorough examination of the heart, lungs, and abdomen is necessary to rule out any systemic etiologies or contributing factors. Heart failure, a bloated belly with ascitic fluid, or crackles in the lungs may cause increased jugular venous distension or crackles in the lungs.

The skin of the lower extremities should be inspected extensively. Erythema and increased temperature can accompany infection and thrombophlebitis.

Varicose veins (Fig. 1.1), particularly those with a gaiter distribution of hemosiderin staining, eczematous dermatitis, or atrophy blanche, are all signs of venous insufficiency[11]. Systemic illness evaluation is required, especially in older

Fig. 1.1 This patient presented with swelling of the right lower limb and after evaluation was diagnosed as varicose veins

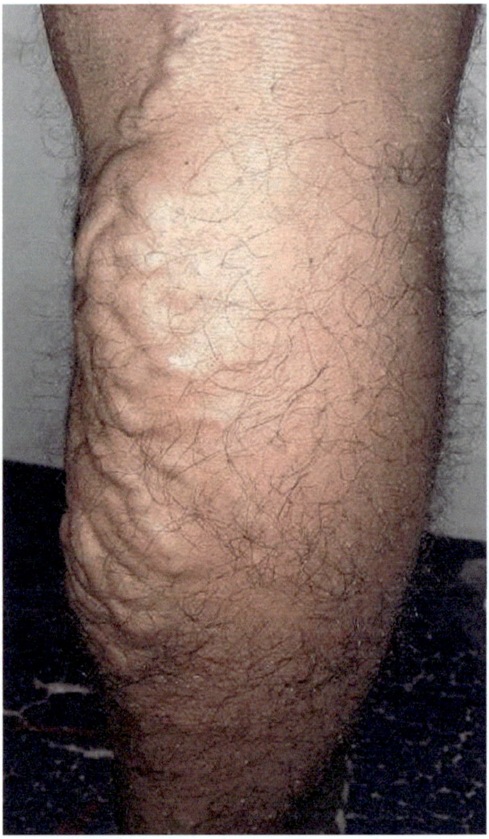

Table 1.1 Clinical findings and possible diagnosis

Clinical findings	Possible diseases
BMI > 35(obesity)	Venous insufficiency
Unilateral leg edema	Deep vein thrombosis, venous insufficiency, lymphedema
Bilateral leg edema	Systemic diseases (cardiac, renal, and hepatic) Local: Abdominal malignancy compressing both femoral veins
Generalized without involvement of the dorsum of feet	Lipedema
Predominant edema of the dorsum of feet	Lymphedema
Tender edema	Deep vein thrombosis, lipedema
Nontender edema	Lymphedema
Edema with periorbital puffiness	Renal diseases
Pitting edema	Deep vein thrombosis, venous insufficiency, early phase of lymphedema
Non-pitting edema	Myxedema, late phase of lymphedema
Varicose vein	Chronic venous insufficiency
Positive Kaposi-Stemmer sign	Lymphedema
Brownish induration of skin with papillomatosis	Chronic lymphedema
Brown hemosiderin deposits of legs and ankles	Venous insufficiency
Warm tender skin with profuse sweating initially followed by thin shiny and cool skin	Reflex sympathetic dystrophy
Dry atrophic skin with flexion contracture	Reflex sympathetic dystrophy
Raised JVP, bilateral basal crackles, significant murmur/rub over the pericardium, and tender hepatomegaly	Cardiac diseases
Clubbing, gynecomastia, spider nevi, jaundice, and ascites	Chronic liver disease

individuals with several concomitant disorders that may be contributing to their largely bilateral leg edema. An underlying cause may be the onset or aggravation of cardiac, renal, hematological, hepatic, or endocrine problems.

Malignant venous compression can be diagnosed by a history of unexplained weight loss or adenopathy.

The relevant findings of clinical examination with their interpretation are mentioned in Table 1.1.

1.6 Management and Outcome

Depending on the underlying suspected cause, a complete blood count, a metabolic panel including creatinine, urinalysis, thyroid function test, atrial natriuretic peptide, and liver function tests be done first in cases of acute edema which may detect the underlying abnormalities [11]. In some circumstances, a D-dimer level can be useful in suggesting DVT which can be confirmed with Duplex scan [12, 13].

Table 1.2 Investigations in patients with edema

First line	Second line
• CBC • Serum electrolytes, creatinine • Blood sugar • Serum total protein/albumin • Thyroid function tests • Routine urine and microscopy	• Deep vein thrombosis: D-dimer and color Doppler study • Heart failure: ECG, 2D echocardiogram, chest X-ray, NT-proBNP • Liver failure: ALT, AST, albumin, bilirubin total and direct, PT, APTT • Renal failure: Complete urine analysis, blood urea, serum creatinine, and electrolytes, USG-KUB • Serum lipid profile: Useful in nephrotic syndrome • Malignancy: Abdominal/pelvic CT • Lymphedema: Abdominal/pelvic CT • Lymphoscintigraphy: To distinguish lymphedema from venous edema

The recommended investigations with their interpretations are mentioned in Table 1.2.

Patients should weigh themselves nude and with an empty bladder before food or fluids in the morning and at bedtime. A mean weight gain >0.7 kg is consistent with idiopathic edema. Water load test is another way to detect idiopathic patients with idiopathic edema; less than 55% of water load is excreted in the upright position and more than 65% in the recumbent position.

The most commonly advised initial imaging modality in edema of the lower extremity is Duplex scan (DUS) [11] to detect deep vein thrombosis which needs immediate attention and proper treatment to prevent progression and pulmonary thromboembolism which has a high mortality rate. With the Duplex ultrasound, the vein diameters are measured which is important for further deciding the modality of intervention, and reflux times are assessed in every case with the patient examined in reverse Trendelenburg using Valsalva maneuver. Distal compression of the vein helps in detecting the reflux. The severity of the reflux is classified as follows: 0.5 to 2 s is mild, 2 to 5 s is moderate, and >5 s or continuous flow with Valsalva is severe [14].

If additional abdominal or pelvic imaging is required after DUS, contrast-enhanced venous phase computed tomography (CT) or magnetic resonance (MR) imaging are options. It is simple to see the mass effect of a tumor or larger lymph nodes, iliocaval compression/obstruction, and overall venous architecture.

Additional benefits of MR imaging can also be utilized to assess musculoskeletal or neurologic causes where no venous, arterial, or lymphatic disorder is identified.

Investigating is not only to confirm the diagnosis but also to exclude a potentially lethal condition, such as DVT. Diagnosis of lower limb edema is a clinical diagnosis but history is most important to detect the underlying cause. Chronic venous insufficiency is the commonest cause of lower limb edema in the age group of above 50 years. In female patients, it is quite common in the age group of below 50 years age group observe premenstrual edema and pregnancy induced edema but a group of females also have idiopathic edema which is managed with conservative treatment [15].

Most individuals with primary lymphedema and lipedema have normal venous imaging. Both disorders are often diagnosed based on a patient's medical history and physical exam findings. It is crucial to note, however, that these basic signs do not appear in all cases. When the normal appearance of lymphedema is not apparent or when surgical therapy is being considered, lymphatic imaging may be useful to plan further intervention. By excluding substantial venous illness in cases with subcutaneous fluid or excessive adipose tissue accumulation, DUS can help identify patients with lymphedema and lipedema.

1.7 Deep Vein Thrombosis

Deep vein thrombosis is an acute emergency and if undiagnosed leads to pulmonary embolism, superior vena cava syndrome, and sudden death. It is a common cause of unilateral leg edema but may be bilateral. The edematous limb may be warm, erythematous, painful, and tender (Fig. 1.2). Homan's sign may be positive. The risk factors of deep vein thrombosis are congenital deficiency of protein C, S, and antithrombin III, homocystinuria, factor V laden mutation, dysfibrinogenemia, prolonged immobilization of limbs (hemiplegia or paraplegia), polycythemia, SLE, anti-phospholipid antibody syndrome, indwelling catheter in femoral vein, septicemia, paroxysmal nocturnal hemoglobinuria, nephrotic syndrome, and pelvic malignancy. Wells score is used to predict the probability of DVT.

The increased level of D-dimer indicates high probability of deep vein thrombosis but not diagnostic in patients with intermediate or high risk [16]. Patients with

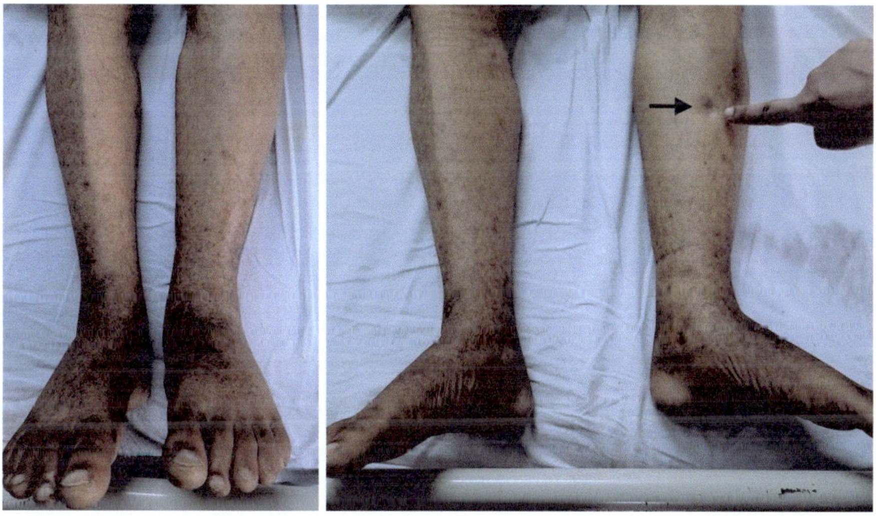

Fig. 1.2 Unilateral (left lower limb) pitting pedal oedema. A case of deep vein thrombosis of left lower limb

high probability of DVT should be immediately subjected to Doppler flow study. If the D-dimer is positive and Doppler flow study is negative, phlebography should be done in 3–7 days.

1.8 Lymphedema

The diagnosis is suggested by clinical manifestations e.g. increase in the girth of limbs, USG of affected parts, lymphangiography, computed tomography (CT), and magnetic resonance imaging (MRI) [7].

The primary objective of management is to halt the progression of disease, reduce the size of the affected extremities, alleviate the symptoms, and reduce the risk of infection. The brief outline of approach to such patients is mentioned below.

1. Conservative: skincare, lymph drainage, compressive stocks.
2. Drugs: flavonoids (effective in the venous stasis).
3. Surgery: Debulking or bypass procedures should be considered if other modalities of therapies are ineffective, effective provided the venous system is patent, continent, and the lymphatic system is functioning properly [7].

The treatment of lymphedema should be decided by a physician who is having knowledge in the field concerned. The above conservative approach may be helpful, but some form of treatment is always necessary to mobilize the excess fluid present in the tissues. The most acceptable approach to lymphedema treatment is called complex decongestive physiotherapy (CDPT), which is focused over reducing the size of the affected limb. Essential components of CDPT comprise manual lymphatic drainage with multilayer bandage to decrease the size and volume of the limb. The treatment is prolonged, time-consuming, and labor intensive but effective [17, 18].

Manual lymphatic drainage (MLD) increases the contraction of lymphatic channels. Light-touch skin stimulation in MLD opens the lymphatic capillaries. MLD should be performed by a trained lymphedema team with a trained therapist. CDPT is then followed by application of compression garments to augment the effect of MLD. Another option is an intermittent pneumatic compression device that can also be a helpful adjunct to compression garments.

1.9 Conclusion

Edema is common in all ages and presents several different pathologies.

Bilateral leg swelling is often related to systemic diseases (heart, liver, and/or renal), but venous insufficiency in the elderly or idiopathic edema in young women should be ruled out.

In case of rapid onset edema, either unilateral or bilateral, and if soft tissue infections have been ruled out, deep vein thrombosis should be considered.

USG with Doppler flow study (Duplex Ultrasongram) is useful in localized edema as well as in detecting DVT and inferior vena cava obstruction.

References

1. Kumar V, Abbas AK, Aster JC, Perkins JA. Robbins basic pathology. 10th ed. Philadelphia: Elsevier; 2018.
2. Kimura G. Pathogenesis of edema and its classification. Nihon Rinsho. 2005 Jan;63(1):11–6. Japanese. PMID: 15675311.
3. Moffatt C, Keeley V, Franks P, Rich A, Pinnington L, Chronic oedema; A prevalent health care problem for UK health services. Int Wound J, 4 December 2016.
4. Goyal A, Cusick AS, Bansal P. Peripheral Edema. [Updated 2020 Nov 20]. In: StatPearls [Internet]. Treasure Island (FL): StatPearls Publishing; 2021.
5. Gorman WP, Davis KR, Donnelly R. ABC of arterial and venous disease. Swollen lower limb-1: general assessment and deep vein thrombosis. BMJ. 2000;320:1453–6.
6. Yale SH, Mazza JJ. Approach to diagnosing lower extremity edema. Compr Ther. 2001;27:242–52.
7. Tiwari A, Cheng KS, Button M, Myint F, Hamilton G. Differential diagnosis, investigation, and current treatment of lower limb lymphedema. Arch Surg. 2003;138:152–61.
8. Messerli FH. Vasodilatory oedema: a common side effect of antihypertensive therapy. Curr Cardiol Rep. 2002;4:479–82.
9. Freshman WH. Effects of nonsteroidal anti-inflammatory drug therapy on blood pressure and peripheral oedema. Am J Cardiol. 2002;89:18D–25D.
10. Topsham EJ, Mortimer PS. Chronic lower limb oedema. Clin Med. 2002;2:28–31.
11. Gasparis AP, Kim PS, Dean SM, Kailanni NM, Markopoulos N. Diagnostic approach to lower limb oedema. Phlebology 2020 Oct;35(9):650–55. https://doi.org/10.1177/0268355520938283. Pub 2020 July 6.
12. Ely JW, Sheriff JA, Chambliss ML, Abell MH. Approach to leg oedema of unclear aetiology [published correction appears in J Am Board Fam Med. 2008 Jan-Feb;21(1):86]. J Am Board Fam Med 2006;19(2):148–60. https://doi.org/10.3122/jabfm.19.2.148.
13. Trays KP, Studio JS, Pickle S, Tully AS. oedema: diagnosis and management. Am Fam Physician. 2013;88(2):102–10.
14. Eberhardt RT, Raffetto JD. Chronic venous insufficiency. Circulation. 2014;130(4):333–46.
15. Garcia R, Markopoulos N. Duplex ultrasound for the diagnosis of acute and chronic venous diseases. Surg Clin North Am. 2018;98(2):201–18. https://doi.org/10.1016/j.suc.2017.11.007.
16. Wells PS, Owen C, Doucette S, Fergusson D, Tran H. Does this patient have deep vein thrombosis? JAMA. 2006;295(2):199–207. https://doi.org/10.1001/jama.295.2.199.
17. Rickson SG. Lymphedema. Vasco Med. 2016;21(1):77–81. https://doi.org/10.1177/1358863X15620852.
18. Rickson SG. Current concepts and future directions in the diagnosis and management of lymphatic vascular disease. Vasco Med. 2010;15(3):223–31. https://doi.org/10.1177/1358863X10364553.

Anatomy of Lower Limb

2

Marian Simka

2.1 Anatomy of Venous System of the Lower Extremity

Veins of the lower extremity can be categorized into three hierarchically ordered groups: the superficial veins, interfascial veins, and deep veins. Under normal conditions, superficial veins empty into interfascial veins and also directly into the deep ones, while interfascial veins empty into the deep veins. Such a flow direction is preferred, even if reverse flow (still, of a low volume) is regarded as physiological. Furthermore, the deep and interfascial veins, and sometimes the deep and superficial ones, are interconnected by the perforating veins, which are defined as veins penetrating the muscular fascia. These perforating veins form the so-called connecting venous system. There are about 150 perforators in the lower extremity, but only a few are of clinical relevance. Currently, eponyms (such as the Dodd's or Cockett's perforators) should no longer be used to describe these veins. Instead, their terminology should designate their location, for example the foot, leg, knee, or thigh perforators, and the medial, posterior, or lateral ones.

Each of these three groups of veins, the superficial, interfascial, and deep one, is located inside a specific fascial compartment (Fig. 2.1). Superficial veins of the lower extremity are defined as veins located above the superficial fascia (anatomically: the membranous layer of subcutaneous tissue). Deep veins are located below the muscular fascia of the extremity. These two fibrous layers—the superficial and muscular ones—fuse with each other, except for small areas surrounding the saphenous veins. Here, these fascias are not fused and form a separate fascial compartment enclosing the vein, and usually also small artery, lymphatic vessels, adipose tissue, and sometimes the accompanying nerve. In an ultrasonographic transverse scan, the interfascial compartment with vein located in its center forms the so-called Egyptian eye. Doctors take advantage of this specific anatomy of interfascial veins

M. Simka (✉)
Department of Anatomy, University of Opole, Opole, Poland

S. K. Tiwary (ed.), *Approach to Lower Limb Oedema*,
https://doi.org/10.1007/978-981-16-6206-5_2

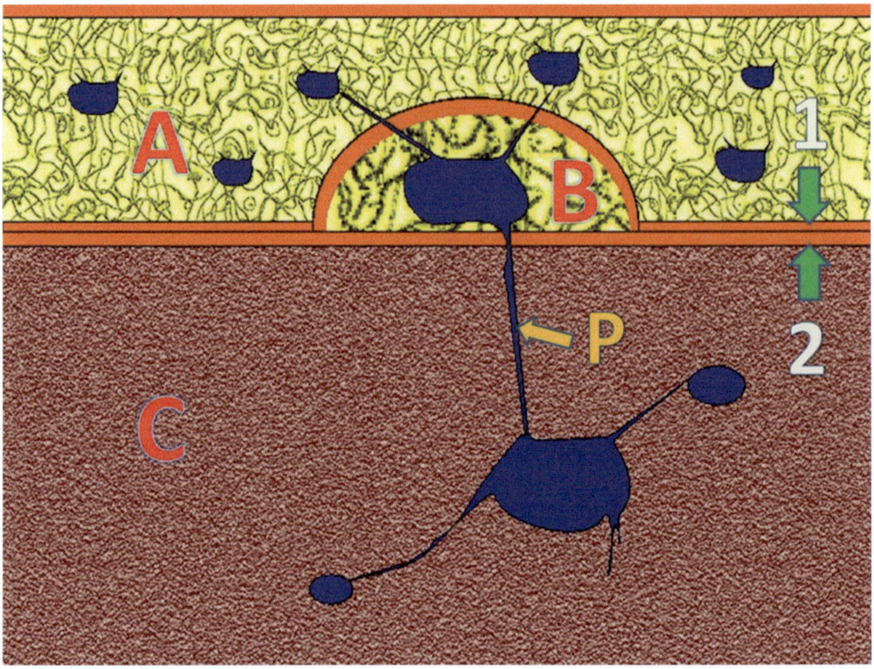

Fig. 2.1 Schematic representation of the lower limb veins: 1—superficial (saphenous) fascia, 2—muscular fascia, A—superficial compartment with superficial veins, B—interfascial (saphenous) compartment, C—deep compartment with deep veins, P—perforating vein

during endovascular treatments for varicose veins; a relatively low volume of anesthetic fluid injected into the interfascial compartment compresses the vein and separates it from adjacent anatomical structures, such as skin and nerves. This is not possible in the case of "true" superficial veins, which are not enclosed by fibrous sheaths; here, a much higher volume of anesthetic fluid is needed.

In the past, the interfascial veins—for example, the great or small saphenous vein—were categorized as superficial veins. But nowadays expert panels of vascular scientific societies recommend to regard these veins as a separate group, because of their unique topography, physiology, and clinical relevance. The group of interfascial veins of the lower limb comprises four veins: the great saphenous vein, the small saphenous vein, the anterior accessory saphenous vein, and the Giacomini's vein. These veins are superficially covered by the membranous layer of subcutaneous tissue (the so-called saphenous fascia) and deeply by the muscular fascia. The great and small saphenous veins are present in the majority of people. On the contrary, the anterior accessory saphenous vein, which is a vein that runs laterally to the great saphenous vein and typically drains into the femoral vein, and the Giacomini's vein, which is the vein joining the great and small saphenous veins, are present only in some individuals, while in the majority of people these veins are either hypoplastic or absent. Still, the anterior accessory saphenous vein and the Giacomini's vein are clinically relevant, since in patients presenting with varicose veins they are quite often the main source of pathological reflux. Anatomical variants of the small saphenous vein represent another clinical problem related to the treatment of varicose veins. Embryologically, this vein develops from the primitive fibular vein. The sapheno-popliteal junction, the most proximal part of the small saphenous vein, where it merges with the popliteal vein, is a remnant of the popliteal crossroad found in embryo; consequently, anatomically this area is highly variable. In some individuals, the small saphenous vein is doubled; there are some people presenting with the junction between the small saphenous vein and the popliteal vein located above the level of the knee joint, with continuation of the small saphenous vein located at the posterior aspect of the thigh in the interfascial compartment (this anatomic variant, the cranial extension of the small saphenous vein, resembles venous anatomy of an embryo), or with a continuation of the small saphenous vein toward the great saphenous vein (this anatomic variant is referred to as the Giacomini's vein). Besides, at the level of the knee joint, in some patients there is a connection between superficially located vein and the popliteal vein. Since this superficial vein is not situated in the interfascial compartment, as the small saphenous vein is, this vein is referred to as the perforator of popliteal fossa. Varicose veins associated with this perforator should be managed differently than those resulting from small saphenous vein incompetence. Topographically, the deep veins accompany their corresponding arteries. Below the knee, deep veins of the lower extremity are usually doubled or tripled; beginning from the popliteal vein there is usually a single vein, although in many individuals paired popliteal or femoral veins are present. The main deep veins of the lower leg comprise the posterior tibial veins that drain the posterior fascial compartment of the lower leg, the anterior tibial veins that drain the anterior fascial compartment, and the fibular veins that primarily drain the deep posterior fascial compartment. Besides, the posterior tibial veins receive venous blood from the plantar part of the foot. The anterior tibial veins receive venous outflow coming from this part of the dorsal aspect of the foot, which is not drained by saphenous veins. The popliteal vein is the main deep vein of the lower leg. This vein is a continuation of the merged posterior and anterior tibial veins. The popliteal vein receives several clinically relevant muscular tributaries, particularly the soleal and gastrocnemius veins. These veins, which drain the triceps surae muscle, constitute the most important component of the so-called calf muscle pump. Morphologically, these muscular veins significantly differ from each other. While the gastrocnemius veins are paired and are equipped with typical bicuspid valves that are located in the main venous trunks and branches, the soleal veins exhibit very irregular course, with some portions of veins that are not paired, their merging is repeated, there are only a few valves in the main trunks, and their venous valves are incomplete. The soleal veins build up rather a venous plexus, and not typical venous tree. All these features of the soleal veins promote venous stasis inside the soleal muscle, which can result in venous thrombosis. Usually, at the level of the knee joint, the popliteal vein merges with the small saphenous vein that belongs to the interfascial veins. Yet, in some individuals this junction is situated above the knee level or even missing.

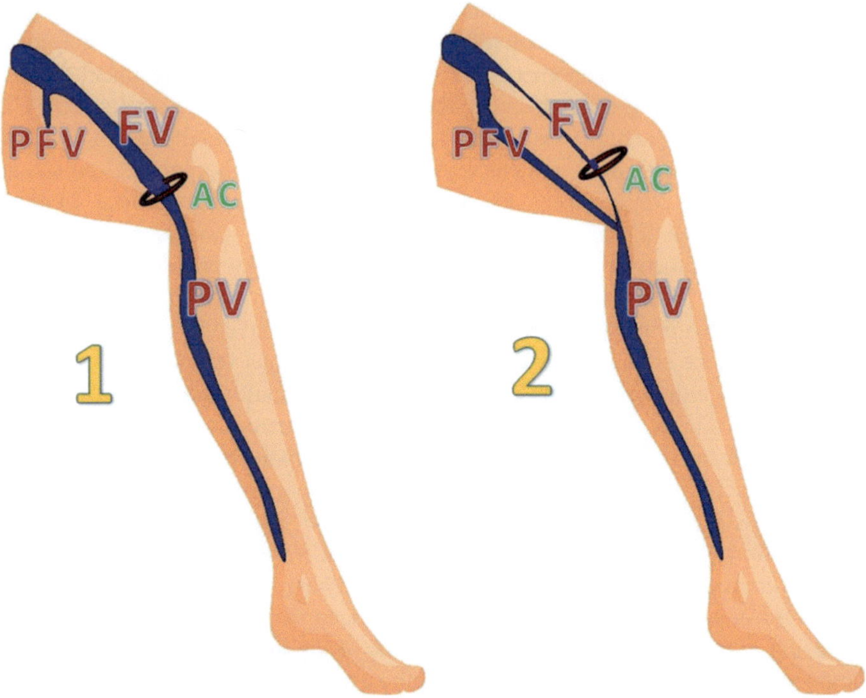

Fig. 2.2 1—Typical anatomy of deep veins of the thigh; 2—Anatomical variant with hypoplastic femoral vein and main outflow through the profunda femoris vein. *PV* popliteal vein, *FV* femoral vein, *PFV* profunda femoris vein, *AC* adductor canal

At the hiatus adductorius (opening in the adductor magnus muscle) the popliteal vein continues proximally as the femoral vein. The femoral vein is typically the main deep vein of the thigh. However, in about 3% of people, the main outflow from the lower leg does not go through the hiatus adductorius, but continues proximally within the posterior fascial compartment of the thigh (Fig. 2.2). In these individuals, venous outflow is finally directed toward the profunda femoris vein (synonym: the deep vein of thigh), either through the axiofemoral trunk (a wide vein developed from the merged axial and profunda femoris veins) or the deep femoral trunk (an elongated distally profunda femoris vein). These anatomical variants are a consequence of abnormal embryological development of veins of the lower limb (see the next subchapter).

In the majority of people, the profunda femoris vein is a short wide vein that drains the posterior and medial fascial compartments of the thigh and empties into the femoral vein. This vein can constitute a primary outflow route from the distal parts of the lower extremity in case of femoral vein occlusion or hypoplasia. Just below the inguinal ligament the femoral vein merges with the main vein of the interfascial system, the great saphenous vein. In some individuals, the femoral vein also communicates with another interfascial vein, the anterior accessory saphenous vein. Above the inguinal ligament the femoral vein continues proximally as the external iliac vein.

The segment of the great saphenous vein in the proximity of its connection with the femoral vein is referred to as the saphenofemoral junction. This part of the great saphenous vein is typically equipped with two valves: the terminal valve that is located close (1–2 mm) to the estuary of this vein and the pre-terminal valve that is located 3–5 cm distally from connection with the femoral vein. These two valves play an important role in the pathogenesis of varicose veins in the draining area of the great saphenous vein. They are also of particular importance during endovascular procedures for the incompetent great saphenous vein. In the area of the saphenofemoral junction, the great saphenous vein receives several tributaries that can be of clinical relevance during the treatment for varicose veins, especially if venous reflux originates in the perineum or pelvis (see subchapter on venous connections between the pelvis and lower limb). These tributaries of clinical interest comprise the superficial epigastric vein, the superficial circumflex iliac vein, the superficial external pudendal vein, and the anterior circumflex femoral vein. In some individuals, any of these tributaries can empty directly into the femoral vein, instead of the great saphenous vein [1–9].

2.2 Embryological Development of Veins of the Lower Extremity: Clinical Aspects of Atypical Anatomy

In order to better understand abnormal venous outflows from the lower limbs, one should comprehend embryological development of the lower extremity veins. It should be remembered that typical adult anatomical pattern of these veins is very different from that seen in the embryos and fetuses, and that in some adult individuals this embryonic or fetal venous anatomy is still present. It should also be emphasized that anatomical terms of embryonic veins do not always correspond to such terms of veins found in adult humans; therefore, a descriptor "primitive" is often used. For example, the "primitive" posterior tibial vein in embryo is not the same blood vessel as the posterior tibial vein found in an adult. Reader of this subchapter should be careful with these "overlapping" anatomical terms. Besides, it should be noted that current knowledge on venous embryogenesis in humans is primarily based on the research performed in animal embryos (particularly rabbits) and also on detailed anatomical observations in adult humans and thus should be extrapolated to human embryos and fetuses with caution.

In humans at an early stage of embryogenesis, between the 5th and 6th weeks of embryo's life, the lower (caudal) part of the embryo receives oxygenated blood from the umbilical vein that connects to the paired posterior cardinal veins (synonym: the postcardinal veins). The first vein that develops in the primitive bud of the lower limb is the primitive fibular vein, with its distal extension, the primitive lateral marginal vein, and proximal extension, the primitive axial (sciatic) vein that receives blood from the umbilical vein. At this stage of embryogenesis, the limb receives blood through the veins and is drained by arteries.

Later, the primitive fibular vein develops two branches: the primitive anterior tibial vein and the connecting branch. At this stage of organogenesis, the primitive anterior tibial vein becomes the main vein of the lower limb, while the primitive fibular vein evolutes to become the small saphenous vein. The primitive anterior tibial vein and the primitive fibular vein merge cranially to form the axial (sciatic) vein, which is the main venous channel draining the limb at this stage of embryogenesis. Thereafter, the connecting branch (a tributary of the primitive fibular vein) evolves into the femoral vein, which connects to the postcardinal vein anteriorly from the axial (sciatic) vein, while at this stage of embryogenesis the sciatic vein begins to involute. In this way, an adult anatomical pattern of lower extremity veins develops, with the femoral vein being the main venous channel draining the limb.

This stage of venous embryogenesis, which takes place between the 7th and 8th week of embryo's life, is regulated by so-called angio-guiding nerves. The newly developed nerves secrete several agents, such as vascular endothelial growth factor (VEGF) and ephrins. These substances trigger the growth of venous blood vessels. There are three main such angio-guiding nerves in the bud of the lower extremity: the axial nerve (it will become the sciatic nerve), the pre-axial nerve (it will transform into the femoral nerve), and the post-axial nerve (precursor of the posterior femoral cutaneous nerve). These nerves are responsible for the growth of the sciatic vein, the femoral vein, and the cranial extension of the small saphenous vein, respectively (Fig. 2.3).

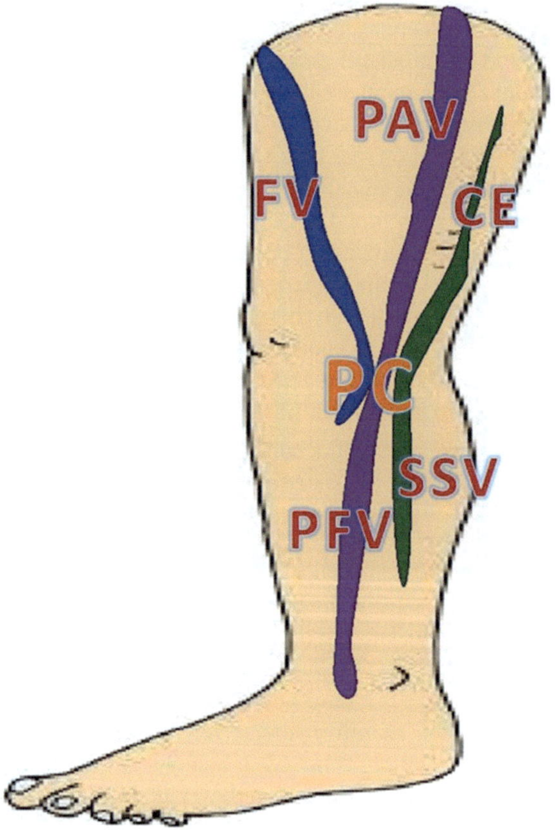

Fig. 2.3 Scheme of the venous system in an 8 weeks-old embryo: *FV* femoral vein, *PAV* primitive axial vein, *CE* cranial extension of the small saphenous vein, *PC* popliteal crossroad, *PFV* primitive fibular vein, *SSV* small saphenous vein

As the primitive femoral vein grows distally, it forms the primitive posterior tibial vein, which is the precursor of the great saphenous vein. Importantly, at this stage of venous embryogenesis, the limb of human embryo rotates and its cranial aspect becomes medial (tibial), while the caudal aspect becomes lateral (fibular). At the end of the 12th week, the development of lower extremity veins is almost completed, except for the femoral and sciatic veins. Initially, the sciatic vein is the dominant one. As it involutes, the femoral vein becomes the main vein draining the lower limb, as it is seen in the majority of adult humans. Small veins accompanying the sciatic vein in adults are referred to as the sciatic nerve veins. If a large vein is present in the proximity of this nerve, it is then called the persistent sciatic vein.

There are many connections between three main embryonic venous channels (axial, pre-, and post-axial). Some of these connections are still seen in adult humans, while others in the majority of individuals involute. At the level of the popliteal fossa, all these three venous channels are connected. It is the so-called embryonic popliteal crossroad. The sapheno-popliteal junction is the remnant of this crossroad, but it should be emphasized that in some adult humans venous anatomy in this area is more complex (present Giacomini's vein, connection between the small saphenous vein with the veins of the sciatic nerve, etc.), which is related to the anatomical topography of this part of the lower limb in embryo.

In general, venous embryogenesis of the lower limb consists of three stages. During the first stage, the primitive fibular vein is the main vein of the extremity. During the second stage, it is replaced by the axial vein, and finally by the femoral vein. In some patients, an embryonic pattern of venous drainage persists. If the second stage does not occur correctly, as it is seen in Klippel-Trenaunay syndrome patients, the primitive fibular vein is still the main vein of the limb, and is then referred to as the marginal vein. Since the marginal vein is an embryonic vein, hence is valveless, its presence is associated with severe venous reflux and venous stasis. If the passage from the second to third stage is not complete, the sciatic vein remains an important and in some individuals the only outflow route from the lower extremity. Such an atypical anatomy can make proper ultrasonographic assessment of the limb difficult, for example in patients presenting with deep vein thrombosis associated with hypoplastic femoral vein, or in patients with unusual varicose veins associated with persistent marginal or axial veins [10–14].

2.3 Anatomical Routes Connecting Pelvic Veins with Those of the Lower Extremity

Stenosis or occlusion of the common iliac vein leads to an overload of venous system in the draining area of the internal iliac veins. Although in these cases venous outflow from the lower extremity is shifted, either toward the azygos veins through the ascending lumbar veins, or toward veins of the anterior wall of the abdomen through the inferior epigastric vein, in the majority of patients these outflow routes cannot prevent from venous stasis in the pelvis. Similarly, a venous stasis is seen in patients presenting with refluxing ovarian veins and also in pregnant women. It should be remembered that although the ovarian veins drain to the left renal vein and the inferior vena cava, they are connected to the draining area of the internal iliac veins through venous plexuses surrounding the uterus. Thus, an incompetence of the ovarian veins results in venous stasis in the uterine venous plexus and adjacent veins.

Venous hypertension in the pelvis may lead to the development of varicose veins in the lower extremity. Still, these varicosities are anatomically different from those associated with incompetence of the saphenous veins. It should be emphasized that anatomically the pelvis is separated from the lower extremity by bones, muscles, ligaments, and fibrous membranes, and that there are only a few routes through which pelvic veins can communicate with the veins of the lower limb. Besides, at normal conditions valves situated in these small connecting veins protect the limb from venous reflux originating in the pelvis. Yet, in the settings of venous stasis, these veins dilate and are no longer competent. There are four important connections between the pelvic and lower extremity veins. A majority of varicose veins that emerge due to pelvic venous stasis have their origins in these points (Fig. 2.4).

- Point “I” (inguinal)—This leakage point is situated at the superficial inguinal ring (external opening of the inguinal canal). In women in this area the veins of the round ligament of uterus, which communicate through the veins of the broad

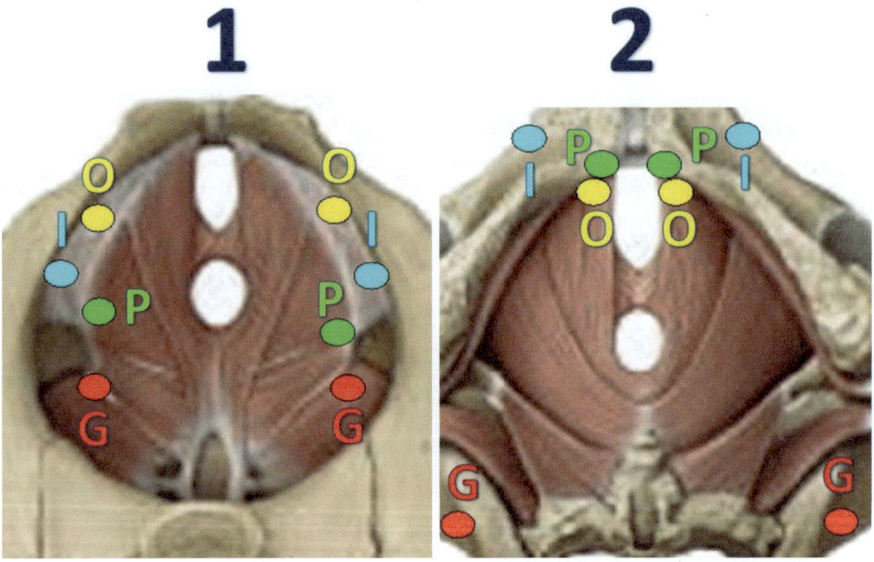

Fig. 2.4 Connections between pelvic and lower extremity veins; 1—view from above, entry points of reflux; 2—view from below, leaving points of reflux. I—inguinal communication running alongside the inguinal canal, O—obturator communication beginning at the obturator foramen and running toward superficial veins of the perineum, P—perineal communication that begins at the lesser sciatic foramen together with the internal pudendal vessels and running toward superficial veins of the perineum, G—gluteal communication originating at the greater sciatic foramen and running to the subcutaneous tissue below the buttocks

ligament of the uterus with the uterine venous plexus, connect to the superficial veins of the anterior wall of the abdomen and also to the tributaries of the great saphenous vein.

- Point "O" (obturator)—This communication route begins at the obturator canal, through which the obturatory vein passes. This vein, which is a tributary of the internal iliac vein, has communication with the venous system of the medial compartment of the thigh, and also with other parts of the thigh through the circumflex femoral veins. Besides, there are connections of the obturatory vein with the pudendal veins and also with the inferior epigastric vein. Reflux through the obturatory vein is typically associated with varicose veins in the perineum.
- Point "P" (perineal)—This pathway originates at the lesser sciatic foramen where the pudendal blood vessels enter the pudendal canal. The leakage point is situated in the area where the perineal veins traverse the anterior part of the perineal membrane (fibrous sheath separating pelvic cavity from the perineum). These veins provide a communication between the pudendal venous plexus, which is located behind the pubic symphysis and the inferior pubic ligament, and the subcutaneous venous plexus in the urogenital area that comprises the anterior and posterior labial (scrotal, in males) veins and other subcutaneous veins in this area. The veins of the labia majora (scrotum, in males) have connections with tributaries of the great saphenous vein and also communicate with the veins of the contralateral labium. Therefore, there is a possibility of transmission of reflux not only to the ipsilateral great saphenous vein, but also contralaterally, through the labio-labial venous anastomoses.
- Point "G" (gluteal)—This leakage point is situated in the region of buttocks. In this area the veins of sciatic vein, which in adult humans are of variable size (see subchapter on venous embryology), connect to the inferior gluteal veins. The inferior gluteal veins enter the pelvis through the infrapiriform part of the greater sciatic foramen, together with the sciatic nerve, and finally drain into the internal iliac vein. The veins of sciatic vein have connections with the profunda femoris vein. In case of venous stasis in the pelvis or a persistent sciatic vein, these veins provide communication between the draining areas of the thigh and pelvis. Besides, the inferior gluteal veins communicate with a number of superficial veins in the gluteal region, primarily the gluteal perforating veins and their subcutaneous tributaries [15–17].

2.4 Anatomy of Lymphatic System of Lower Extremity

Current knowledge on the anatomy of the lymphatic system of the lower extremity is primarily based on investigations performed in the nineteenth century. This body of evidence has been augmented in the twentieth century by lymphoscintigraphic studies, which are—unfortunately—two-dimensional and of low resolution. Also, CT and MR lymphographies that are used for diagnostic purposes in the living subjects are of low resolution and cannot be used during anatomical studies in cadavers, since they require active lymphatics that propel the contrast. This has changed recently with the use of novel contrasts that enable a novel method of three-dimensional presentation of lymphatics in the cadaver specimens. Anatomical studies on the lymphatic system in the lower extremities, which utilized zinc oxide contrast injected into the foot lymphatics in fresh cadavers, have revealed that there are 2 outflow routes of lymph from the lower extremity. The first one begins in the medial and dorsal aspects of foot and runs superficially at the middle aspect of the lower leg and thigh, alongside the great saphenous vein, toward the superficial inguinal lymph nodes. The other outflow pathway originates in the calcaneal region of the foot and runs toward the popliteal lymph nodes, alongside the small saphenous vein. The efferent lymphatics leaving the popliteal lymph nodes run subfascially, along the femoral artery and vein, toward the deep inguinal nodes. Outflow from the popliteal lymph nodes can also be differently directed, since some efferent lymphatic vessels coming out of the popliteal lymph nodes leave the deep compartment and go superficially, toward the great saphenous vein compartment, finally joining the superficial inguinal lymph nodes. Interestingly, in some individuals the efferent lymphatics coming from the popliteal lymph nodes bypass all inguinal lymph nodes and outflow directly into the external iliac ones (Fig. 2.5).

Lymph nodes in the inguinal region are the most important lymph nodes of the lower extremity. These lymph nodes are categorized into the superficial and deep ones. Superficial inguinal lymph nodes are situated above the muscular fascia, while the deep nodes are located below this fibrous sheath, in the proximity of femoral vein. The deep inguinal lymph nodes primarily receive lymph coming from the popliteal lymph nodes. Superficial inguinal lymph nodes are further divided into the

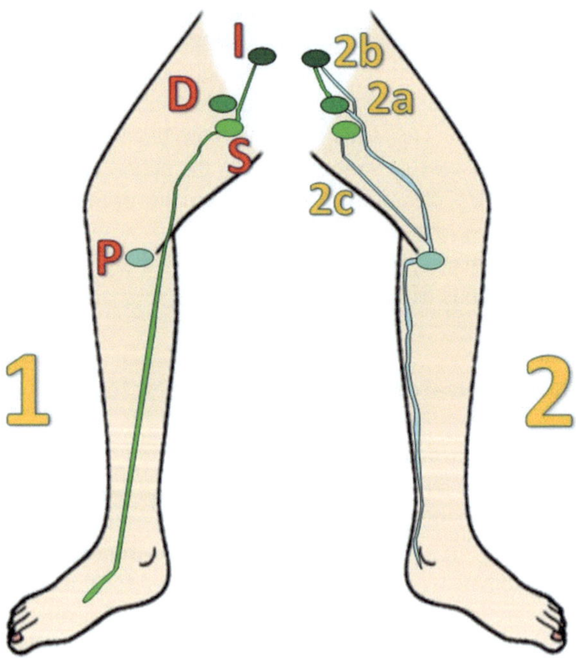

Fig. 2.5 Lymphatic outflow routes from the lower extremities. 1—superficial outflow route alongside the great saphenous vein toward the superficial inguinal lymph nodes; 2—outflow through the popliteal lymph nodes to the deep inguinal lymph nodes (2a), directly to the iliac lymph nodes (2b), or joining the superficial route to the superficial inguinal lymph nodes (2c). P—popliteal lymph nodes, S—superficial inguinal lymph nodes, D—deep inguinal lymph nodes, I—iliac lymph nodes

horizontal and vertical groups. The horizontal group is located along the lower border of the inguinal ligament. Medially situated lymph nodes of this group primarily drain the lower part of the anterior wall of the abdomen and also external genitals. Those situated laterally drain the gluteal region. The vertical group of the superficial inguinal lymph nodes is located next to the proximal part of the great saphenous vein. These lymph nodes drain the majority of the lower extremity. Recent studies have revealed that this group of lymph nodes comprises two functionally separated groups (the so-called lymphosomes). Lymph nodes located medially (there is usually 2–3 of such lymph nodes) receive afferent lymphatics running along the great saphenous vein. Efferent lymphatic vessels coming out of these lymph nodes typically bypass the deep inguinal lymph nodes and run along the femoral and external iliac arteries toward the iliac lymph nodes. Lymph nodes of the vertical group that are located laterally receive afferent lymphatics draining the lateral part of the thigh. In conclusion, lymphatic outflow from particular parts of the lower extremity is associated with distinct lymph nodes (Fig. 2.6).

Anatomically, these draining areas are separated (lymphosomes), which explains why an injury to a few such nodes (surgery, irradiation) can result in lymphedema.

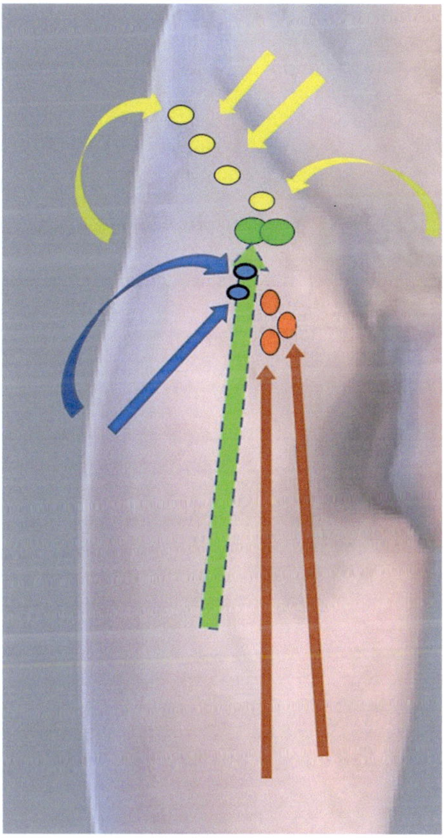

Fig. 2.6 Inguinal lymph nodes and their draining areas. Yellow—horizontal group of the superficial inguinal lymph nodes; Blue—lateral part of vertical group of the superficial inguinal lymph nodes; Orange—medial part of vertical group of the superficial inguinal lymph nodes; Green—the deep inguinal lymph nodes that receive lymph from the popliteal nodes

Besides, the only lymphatic outflow route from the lower extremity is located under the inguinal ligament, in the femoral canal, and alongside the external iliac blood vessels. There are no alternative pathways for lymph flowing out of the lower extremity, neither toward the abdominal wall nor the perineum or buttocks [18–20].

References

1. Caggiati A, Bergan JJ, Gloviczki P, et al. Nomenclature of the veins of the lower limbs: an international interdisciplinary consensus statement. J Vasc Surg. 2002;36:416–22.
2. Caggiati A. The saphenous compartment: the saphenous veins are not real superficial veins. Ital J Anat Embryol. 2013;118:40.
3. De Maeseneer M, Kakkos SK. What's in a mane?... ten years after publication of the VEIN-TERM. Eur J Vasc Endovasc Surg. 2019;58:3–4
4. Kachlik D, Pechacek V, Baca V, et al. The superficial venous system of the lower extremity: new nomenclature. Phlebology. 2010;25:113–23.
5. Kachlik D, Pechacek V, Musil V, et al. Information on the changes in the revised anatomical nomenclature of the lower limb veins. Biomed Pap Med Fac Univ Palacky Olomouc Czech Repub. 2010;154:93–8.
6. Kachlik D, Pechacek V, Musil V, et al. The deep venous system of the lower extremity: new nomenclature. Phlebology. 2012;27:48–58.
7. Oğuzkurt L. Ultrasonographic anatomy of the lower extremity superficial veins. Diagn Interv Radiol. 2012;18:423–30.
8. Perrin M, Eklöf B, Maleti O, et al. The vein glossary. 2018; Institut la Conférence Hippocrate, Suresnes Cedex, France.
9. Reich-Schupke S, Stücker M. Nomenclature of the veins of the lower limbs – current standards. J Dtsch Dermatol Ges. 2011;9:189–94.
10. Koç T, Gilan IY, Külekçi GD, et al. Bilateral persistent sciatic vein: report of a case with developmental, histological and clinical aspects. Surg Radiol Anat. 2014;36:189–94.
11. Lee BB. Venous embryology: the key to understanding anomalous venous conditions. Phlebolymphology. 2012;19:170–81.
12. Uhl JF, Gillot C, Chahim M. Anatomical variations of the femoral vein. J Vasc Surg. 2010;52:714–9.
13. Uhl JF, Gillot C. Anatomy and embryology of the small saphenous vein: nerve relationships and implications for treatment. Phlebology. 2012;28:4–15.
14. Uhl JF. Focus on venous embryogenesis of the human lower limbs. Phlebolymphology. 2015;22:55–63.
15. Balian E, Lasry JL, Coppé G, et al. Pelviperineal venous insufficiency and varicose veins of the lower limbs. Phlebolymphology. 2008;15:17–26.
16. Francheschi C, Bahnini A. Treatment of lower extremity venous insufficiency due to pelvic leak points in women. Ann Vasc Surg. 2005;19:1–6.
17. Kachlik D, Pechacek V, Musil V, et al. The venous system of the pelvis: new nomenclature. Phlebology. 2010;25:162–73.
18. Scaglioni MF, Suami H. Lymphatic anatomy of the inguinal region in aid of vascularized lymph node flap. J Plast Recontr Aesthet Surg. 2015;68:419–27.
19. Suami H, Scaglioni MF. Anatomy of the lymphatic system and the lymphosome concept with reference to lymphedema. Semin Plast Surg. 2018;32:5–11.
20. Yamazaki S, Suami H, Imanishi N, et al. Three-dimensional demonstration of the lymphatic system in the lower extremities with multi-detector-row computed tomography: a study in a cadaver model. Clin Anat. 2013;26:258–66.

Physiological Basis of Lower Limb Edema

3

Sanjeev K. Singh and Ravindran Revand

3.1 Introduction

The human body is bestowed with the circulatory system which acts as a conduit for supplying nutrients and oxygen to different organs and for collecting back carbon dioxide and metabolic waste products for excretion through the kidneys and lungs. The **capillary microcirculation** acts as the major platform for exchange of various materials like water, gases, ions, and solutes between the intravascular and interstitial compartments. This microcirculation unit consists of arterioles and venules that load and unload, respectively, the intermediary tiny capillary network of the blood that has to be filtered or whose components have to be exchanged through the thin capillary wall made up of a single layer of endothelium. Capillaries are named as "**exchange vessels**" owing to their major role in interchange of materials between fluid compartments, thereby maintaining their compositions within physiological limits. These functions of the capillaries are in fact regulated and controlled by several intrinsic and extrinsic factors, i.e., myogenic autoregulation and autonomic controls, respectively.

3.2 Architecture of Microcirculation Unit

The larger arteries serially divide and finally end in an arteriole (50–100 μm diameter) that are feeder vessels to the capillaries (5–10 μm diameter) either directly or through the meta-arterioles (10–20 μm diameter). The meta arterioles also act as "**thoroughfare channels**" for the blood in arterioles to reach venules unfiltered,

S. K. Singh (✉) · R. Revand
Department of Physiology, Institute of Medical Sciences, Banaras Hindu University, Varanasi, India
e mail: drsks07@bhu.ac.in

S. K. Tiwary (ed.), *Approach to Lower Limb Oedema*,
https://doi.org/10.1007/978-981-16-6206-5_3

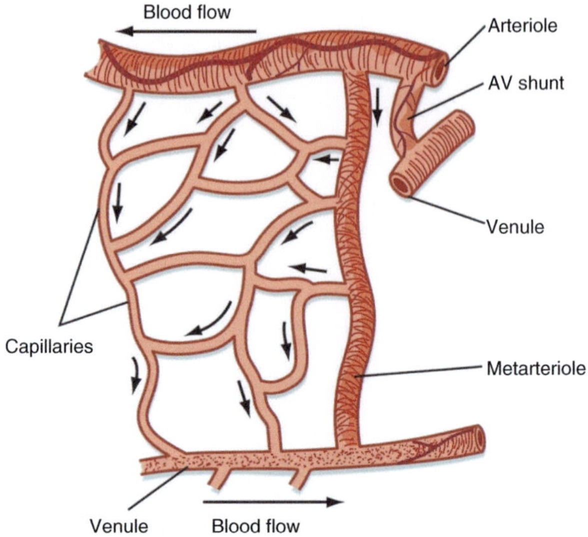

Fig. 3.1 Schematic diagram of microcirculation unit showing the nutritional flow through the capillary meshwork and non-nutritional flow through the meta-arterioles. Arrows indicate the direction of blood flow

bypassing the capillary mesh. As the flow in the physiological meta-arteriole shunts are not useful in exchange of materials, it can be described as **non-nutritional flow** (Fig. 3.1), while that flow through the capillary network is called **nutritional flow**. The walls of the arterioles and meta-arterioles are innervated by sympathetic nerve fibers that contribute to extrinsic regulation of capillary circulation. The distribution of capillaries in different tissues depends on their metabolic states. Metabolically active tissues like skeletal muscles and glands have a higher **capillary density** while subcutaneous tissue and cartilage have a lower capillary density [1].

3.3 Myogenic Autoregulation of Capillary Microcirculation

Transmural pressure (difference between intravascular and extravascular pressures) is the pressure exerted on the walls of blood vessels. Whenever flow in the precapillary vessels (arterioles) increases the intravascular pressure, the arteriolar transmural pressure increases. This increases the flow in the cognate capillaries leading to greater volume to be filtered. To avoid the capillaries being overburdened with fluid volume, the capillary intravascular volume is autoregulated at the myogenic level in the arterioles itself. When the transmural pressure increases, the arteriolar smooth muscles respond by contraction leading to narrowing of precapillary vascular diameter (Fig. 3.2). This reduces the blood flow and the filtration load in the capillaries. Stretch-induced calcium ion channels are implicated in this process of arteriolar smooth muscle contraction [2].

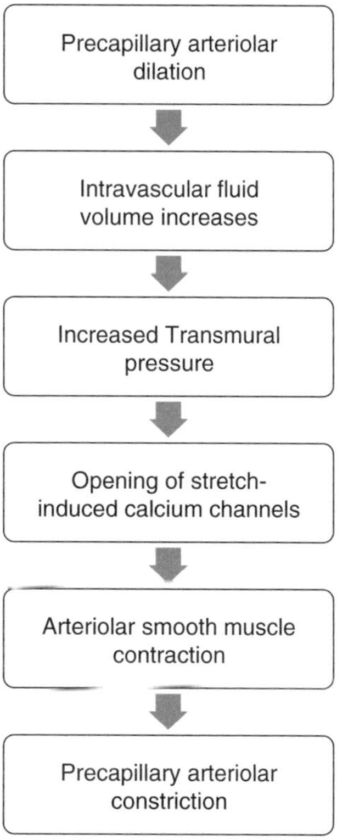

Fig. 3.2 Flowchart showing the mechanism of myogenic autoregulation of capillary microcirculation

The random or rhythmic oscillatory behavior caused by contraction and relaxation of precapillary vessels is called "**vasomotion**." Vasomotion or myogenic autoregulation plays an important role in maintaining the intravascular fluid volume by preventing excessive fluid shift into the interstitial compartment during posture change from supine to standing [3]. Arteriolar constriction and venular dilation reduce the capillary fluid load while arteriolar dilation and venular constriction increase the same. Thus, the diameter of the capillaries and hence the capillary blood flow are passively regulated by the changes in the precapillary and postcapillary resistances [2, 4, 5].

3.4 Capillary Endothelium as Regulator of Microcirculation

The thin single-layered walls of the capillaries are highly flexible and elastic. This facilitates the capillaries to withstand very high transmural pressure without getting ruptured as explained by Laplace law. **Prostacyclin** (PGI_2) is produced in the endothelial cells from arachidonic acid by cyclooxygenase and PGI_2 synthase and **nitric oxide** (NO) or **endothelium-derived relaxing factor** (EDRF) is produced from arginine by NO synthase. The principal stimulus is known to be sheer stress on the vessel wall due to the blood flow, which causes production and release of PGI_2 and NO, thereby causing cAMP- and cGMP-mediated smooth muscle relaxation and subsequent vasodilation, respectively, to ease the blood flow through the vessel. **Endothelin**, a potent vasoconstrictor, affects the vascular tone and blood pressure in pathological states such as atherosclerosis, but its role in physiological regulation of microcirculation is not established [6–8].

3.5 Transcapillary Exchange Across Endothelium

Solutes and solvents move across the capillary endothelium by one of the three processes: diffusion, filtration, and pinocytosis. Electron microscopic studies revealed the presence of pores and fenestrations of varying sizes in between the capillary endothelial cells. Capillaries can possess **pores or clefts** (4 nm width) as in cardiac and skeletal muscles or **fenestrations** (20 to 100 nm width) as in renal glomeruli, choroid plexus, glands, and intestinal villi or **discontinuous epithelium** (600 to 3000 nm width) as in the liver, bone marrow, and spleen. Capillaries that are not densely fenestrated are called **continuous capillaries** (Fig. 3.3). In brain, tight junctions between endothelial cells constitute the blood–brain barrier. Clefts or pores allow passage of smaller molecules across the endothelium while large molecules can pass only through fenestrations or discontinuous epithelium. Still larger molecules need special mechanisms of transport using endothelial vesicles like pinocytosis [9].

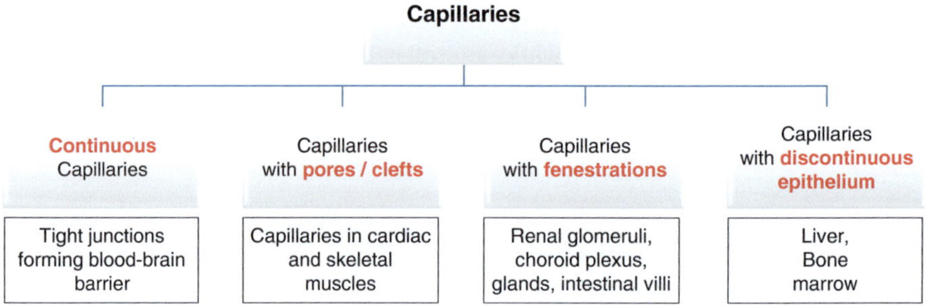

Fig. 3.3 Types of capillaries based on the endothelial structure and communications

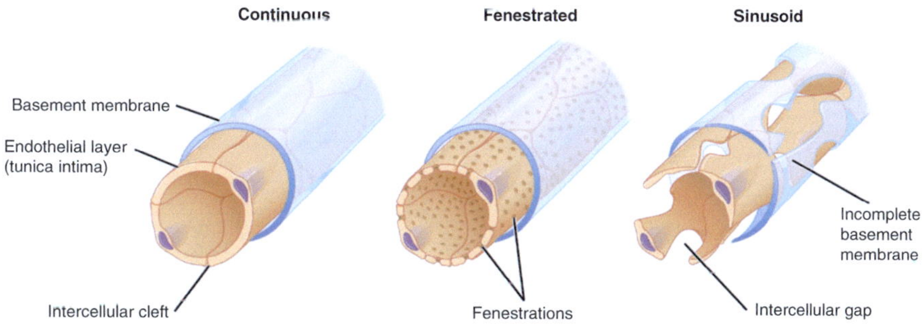

(Courtesy from Anatomy & Physiology by Lindsay M. Biga, Sierra Dawson,

Under normal conditions, the number of substances exchanged by diffusion is about 5000 times more than that exchanged by filtration and pinocytosis. Thus, diffusion can be regarded as the key mechanism in exchange of gases, solutes, and waste products between intravascular and interstitial compartments at the level of capillaries. Diffusion of a particular substance is seen to be more at the venular end of the capillaries than at the arteriolar end because of the increased number of pores in the venular side. Even though the capillary membrane is highly permeable, molecules larger than 60,000 MW units cannot penetrate the endothelium. The 0.5 μm thick glycocalyx lining the luminal side of the endothelium serves as a **molecular filter** in this regard. The extravasations of larger solute particles like proteins from intravascular to interstitial compartments in disease states like edema are either due to an increase in the size of pores or fenestrations or due to development of additional pathological pores due to disruption of endothelial cells [10, 11].

3.6 Diffusion Across Capillary Endothelium

Lipid-soluble substances can diffuse across the endothelial cell membrane with ease, while diffusion of lipid-insoluble substances is restricted to the regions of endothelial discontinuity. Smaller molecules like ions have lower **reflection coefficient** (property by which molecules are denied access through the capillary membrane), while albumin and other larger molecules have higher reflection coefficient. So, the rate of diffusion is inversely related to the molecular size [12].

Based on size, molecules can be divided into two categories: flow-limited and diffusion-limited substances (Fig. 3.4). Smaller molecules when passing through capillaries get easily diffused out under favorable conditions and as a result their concentration in the interstitial fluid compartment is high in the arteriolar side. It is hardly possible to detect these substances on the venular end unless the flow is increased. Such substances are called **flow-limited** substances. On the other hand, larger molecules cannot leave the intravascular compartment easlly so they can be detected at the venular end. These substances are called **diffusion-limited**

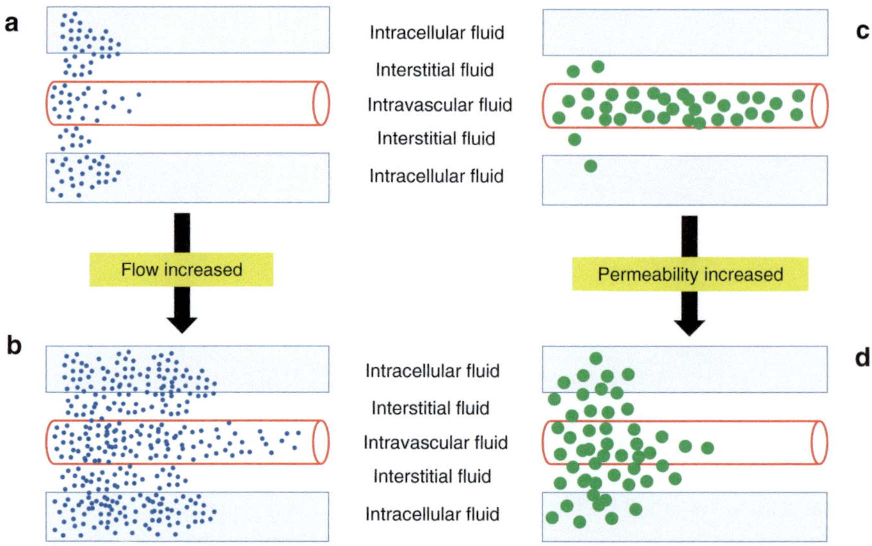

Fig. 3.4 (**a**) Flow-limited transport across capillary wall in which smaller solute particles (blue dots) reach negligible concentrations after passing only for a short distance down the capillary. If the blood flow is increased in the capillary as in (**b**), then the smaller solute particles can be detected for a longer distance along the capillary. (**c**) shows diffusion-limited transport in which larger solute particles (green dots) cannot cross the capillary membrane easily. So, they are detectable for longer distances along the length of capillary. But if the capillary permeability is increased as in (**d**) then the diffusion of larger solute particles is increased

substances. Diffusion of flow-limited substances from the intravascular compartment through the interstitial fluid to the adjacent intracellular compartments is also hampered if there is expansion of the interstitial compartment increasing the distance between the capillaries and the parenchymal cell wall as in edema [11, 13].

3.7 Capillary Filtration as Regulated by Pressure Gradients

Starling (1896) expounded that the magnitude and direction of water movement across the capillary membrane are determined by the algebraic sum of the hydrostatic and osmotic pressures that exist across the membrane [14]. The hydrostatic and osmotic pressures of the intravascular and interstitial compartments that determine the fluid dynamics are termed **Starling forces**. Filtration rate is proportional to the hydraulic drive across the capillary minus the osmotic suction. Hydraulic drive is the capillary filtration pressure minus the interstitial pressure. Osmotic suction is the plasma colloid osmotic pressure minus the interstitial colloid osmotic pressure. A rise in the **hydrostatic pressure** in the intravascular compartment pushes the fluid out while a fall in the same draws fluid into the particular compartment. The capillary hydrostatic pressure increases when the capillary blood flow increases. On the other hand, a rise in the **oncotic pressure** draws water into the intravascular compartment and a rise in the interstitial fluid osmotic pressure draws water out of the intravascular compartment. An increase in arteriolar resistance and a decrease in venular resistance decrease capillary hydrostatic pressure, while a decrease and increase in arteriolar and venular resistances, respectively, demonstrate an opposite effect. The oncotic pressure is mainly determined by the plasma proteins particularly albumin which on account of its larger molecular weight cannot leave the intravascular compartment to a larger extent under physiological conditions.

The net fluid movement across the capillary wall (capillary filtration coefficient) can be given by the formula, $\boldsymbol{Q_f = k\,[(P_c - P_i) - (\pi_c - \pi_i)]}$, where P_c is the capillary hydrostatic pressure, P_i is the interstitial fluid hydrostatic pressure, π_c is the capillary osmotic pressure, π_i is the interstitial osmotic pressure, an k is the filtration constant for the capillary membrane (Fig. 3.5). Conventional school of thought that filtration occurs at the arteriolar ends of the capillaries and absorption at their venular ends because of the hydrostatic pressure gradient along the capillaries has been replaced by direct observations which revealed that many capillaries show only filtration (e.g., renal glomerulus) and many show only absorption (e.g., intestinal mucosa) along their entire length.

The value of capillary filtration coefficient (Q_f) not only depends on the algebraic sum of the hydrostatic and osmotic forces (ΔP) but also on the capillary wall surface area available for filtration (A_m), the distance across the capillary wall (Δx), and the viscosity of the filtrate (η). So, the Starling equation can be rewritten using **Poiseuille law** for flow through tubes as $\boldsymbol{Q_f = kA_m\Delta P/\eta\Delta x}$, where the viscosity of filtrate and dimensions of the capillary wall are essentially constants for a particular tissue. In any given tissue, the filtration coefficient per unit area of the capillary surface is constant under physiological conditions, and thus, it can be used to estimate the relative number of open capillaries available for filtration or absorption in tissues. For example, increased metabolic activity in a muscle during exercise causes opening up of more capillaries (**capillary recruitment**) by relaxing precapillary vessels. This results in greater filtering surface area for capillary exchange to meet the increased metabolic demands. In resting tissues, most of the capillaries are collapsed (**inactive capillaries**) and blood bypasses them to flow through the thoroughfare meta-arterioles to the venules. In metabolically active tissues, the **precapillary sphincters** are dilated by local metabolic vasodilators and blood starts flowing through the capillaries (**active capillaries**). In all tissues, for most of the time the balance of pressures favors filtration of fluid across the capillary membrane into the interstitial fluid [12, 15, 16].

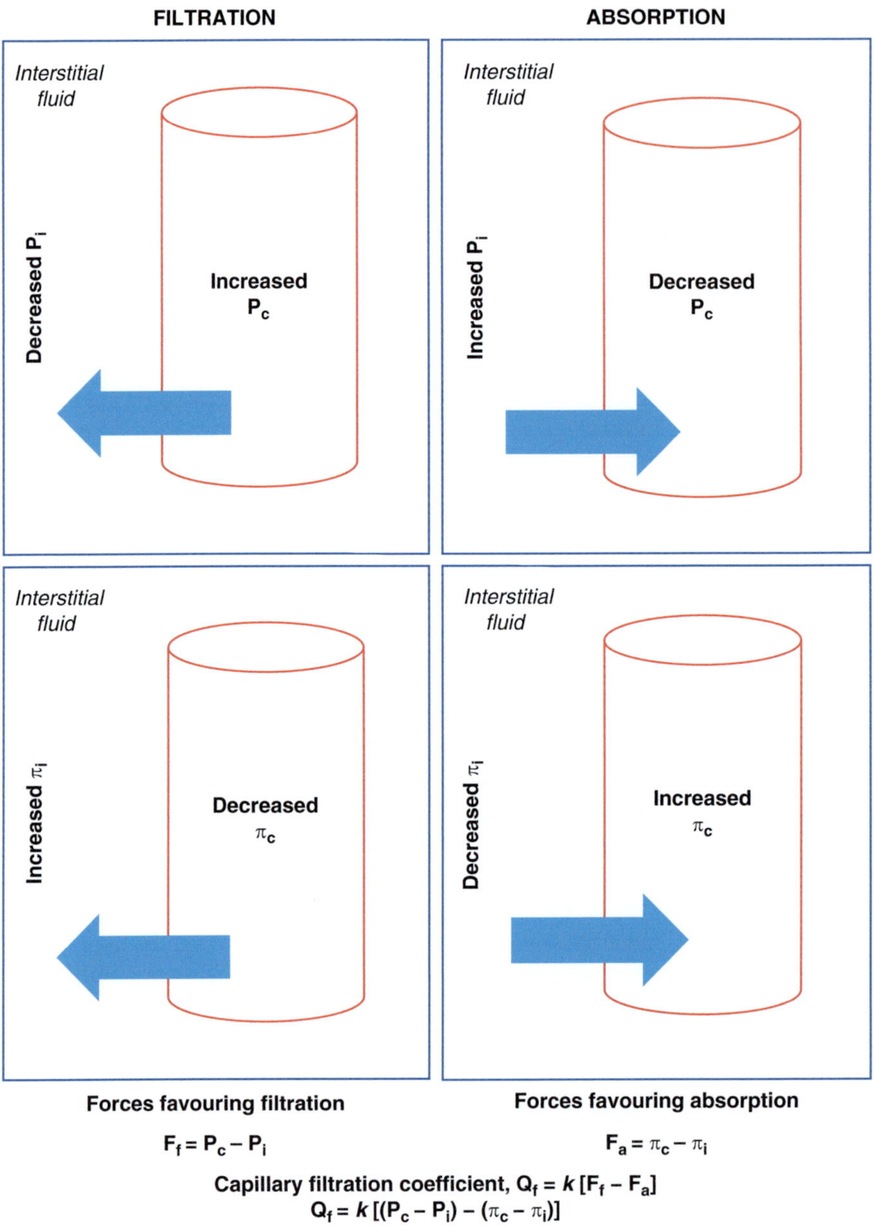

Fig. 3.5 Schematic representation of the Starling forces determining the fluid movement across capillary wall. P_c is the capillary hydrostatic pressure, P_i is the interstitial fluid hydrostatic pressure, π_c is the capillary osmotic pressure, π_i is the interstitial fluid osmotic pressure, and k is the filtration constant for the capillary membrane. Blue arrows denote the direction of fluid movement

3.8 Lymphatic Circulation

The excess fluid in the interstitial space after capillary filtration is called lymph. The composition of lymph is similar to the plasma except that its protein content is low due to the low permeability of the capillary endothelium to large molecular weight proteins. After capillary filtration, the excess fluid from the interstitium is removed by the lymphatic vessels. Lymphatic vessels are of two types: initial and collecting lymphatics (Fig. 3.6). **Initial lymphatics** as the name suggests are located at the beginning and they drain into the collecting lymphatics. Initial lymphatics lack valves and smooth muscles on their walls. In contrast to capillaries, they do not possess tight junctions or fenestrations. Their endothelial cells are held by loose junctions which allow small molecules to cross the lymphatic vessel wall.

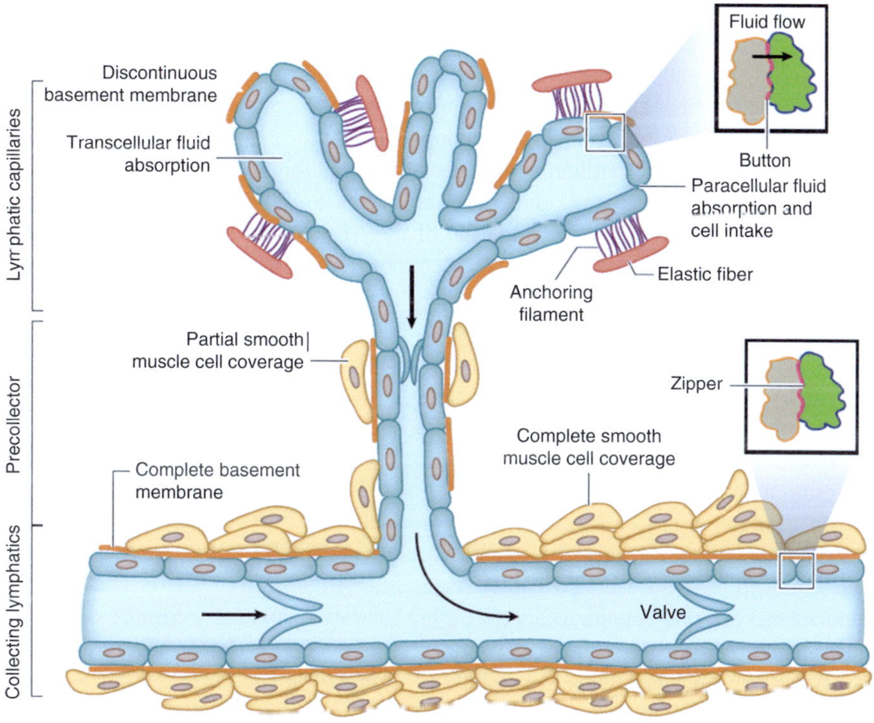

Fig. 3.6 Schematic diagram of the lymphatic vascular tree. The endothelium of initial lymphatic capillaries is only partially covered by basement membrane. Button structures located at the initial capillary walls facilitate interstitial fluid and cellular entry into the lymphatic capillaries through both paracellular and transcellular routes. Lymphatic capillaries converge into pre-collectors, which also have incomplete BM and partial smooth muscle cell coverage. Pre-collectors further converge into collecting lymphatics, which have complete basement membrane and smooth muscle cell layers. Lymphatic valves in collecting lymphatics allow only unidirectional lymph flow. Zippers located in the collecting lymphatic walls do not allow movement of fluids and solutes. (Courtesy from Annual Review of Physiology 2018. 80:49–70; Lymphatic Dysfunction, Leukotrienes, and Lymphedema; Xinguo Jiang, Mark R. Nicolls, Wen Tian and Stanley G. Rockson)

Initial lymphatics drain into the collecting lymphatics connected in a serial fashion. **Collecting lymphatics** as opposed to their initial counterpart possess valves and smooth muscles on their walls. Their main function is to push the lymph collected by the initial lymphatics into the thoracic large veins. The rhythmic contractions of the smooth muscle in their walls and the negative intra-thoracic pressure that develops during inspiration are the principal factors aiding this significant task of collecting lymphatics [17, 18].

3.9 Pathophysiology of Edema

Edema is an accumulation of excess fluid in the body. The excess fluid can be accrued outside (**interstitial edema**) or inside (**intracellular edema**) the cells. The term edema when not specifically designated simply and always implies the former, i.e., a large increase in the interstitial fluid volume. Peripheral edema is a nonspecific finding common to a wide range of medical conditions and can therefore pose a diagnostic challenge. The causes range from benign conditions that can be managed at the community level to even major organ failures requiring specialist referral or hospitalization. Peripheral edema is most commonly caused by extravasation of fluid from the vasculature into the interstitium as a result of altered vascular hemodynamics. Excessive accumulation of interstitial fluid is generally viewed as detrimental to tissue function because edema formation increases the diffusion distance for oxygen and other nutrients, which may compromise cellular metabolism in the swollen tissue. For the same reason, edema formation also limits the diffusional removal of potentially toxic by-products of cellular metabolism. These are especially important problems in the lungs, where pulmonary edema can significantly impair gas exchange [1].

The kidneys are enveloped by a tough fibrous capsule, the brain is surrounded by the cranial vault, and skeletal muscles in the volar and anterior tibial compartments are encased in tight fascial sheaths. As a consequence of the inability of these tissues to readily expand their interstitial volume, relatively small increments in transcapillary fluid filtration induce a large increase in interstitial fluid pressure. This, in turn, reduces the vascular transmural pressure gradient and physically compresses capillaries, thereby reducing nutritive tissue perfusion. In the intestine, unrestrained transcapillary filtration leads to exudation of interstitial fluid into the gut lumen, a phenomenon referred to as filtration secretion or secretory filtration. Filtration secretion may compromise the absorptive function of the delicate intestinal mucosa and appears to occur as a result of the formation of large channels between mucosal cells in the villous tips when interstitial fluid pressure increases by greater than 5 mm Hg. Ascites, or the pathologic accumulation of fluid in the peritoneal cavity, occurs in cirrhosis and is caused by fluid weeping from congested hepatic sinusoids secondary to elevated portal venous pressure. Ascites can predispose afflicted individuals to peritoneal infections, hepatic hydrothorax, and abdominal wall hernias [19]. Edema may occur due to the any of the following reasons: (1) increased capillary hydrostatic pressure, (2) reduced capillary oncotic pressure, (3) decreased interstitial hydrostatic pressure, (4) increased interstitial osmotic pressure, and (5) lymphatic flow defects. **Hydrostatic edema** refers to accumulation of excess interstitial fluid which results from elevated capillary hydrostatic pressure, while **permeability edema** results from disruption of the physical structure of the pores in the microvascular membrane such that the barrier is less able to restrict the movement of macromolecules from the blood to interstitium. **Lymphedema** represents a third form and may result from impaired lymph pump activity, an increase in lymphatic permeability favoring protein flux from lumen to interstitial fluid, lymphatic obstruction as in filariasis, or surgical removal of lymph nodes, as occurs in the treatment of breast cancer.

Increased capillary hydrostatic pressure is caused by local metabolites that cause dilation of the precapillary sphincter. This increases the capillary blood flow and thus the capillary hydrostatic pressure. The precapillary : postcapillary resistance ratio falls in the above case as precapillary resistance is decreased by sphincter relaxation. Sympathetic activation causes contraction of precapillary sphincter, thereby raising the above ratio. When a person continuously stands for prolonged period or if a person has cardiac failure or if the lower limb venous valves are incompetent or in cases of venous obstruction or hypervolemia, blood pools in the venous system of the dependent areas of the body. This increased venous pressure is transmitted back to the capillaries, resulting in elevated capillary hydrostatic pressure that pushes fluid out into the interstitial compartment (**transudation**).

Reduced oncotic pressure results from hypoproteinemia in liver diseases, nephrotic syndrome, malnutrition, starvation, and protein-losing enteropathy. **Increased interstitial osmotic pressure** occurs when osmotically active metabolites get accumulated in an exercising tissue at a rate faster than the lymphatics could remove them. When there is capillary endothelial damage due to cytokines and free radicals as in anaphylaxis, infections, transfusion reactions, etc., there is leakage of plasma proteins via pathological pores that develop on the capillary endothelial cells. This causes **exudation** of plasma proteins into the interstitial compartment and exerts osmotic effect drawing more fluid into it. **Increased capillary permeability** can also be produced by principal inflammatory mediators like histamine, kinins, substance P, etc. and capillary injury (toxins and burns) that causes significant plasma leak causing edema in anaphylaxis and other inflammatory pathologies. Drugs like benzopyrones (Coumarin) have been successful in treating high protein edema including lymphedema where there is high protein accumulation in the interstitium. **Benzopyrones** cause proteolysis and increase the protein phagocytosis by macrophages, thereby removing the osmotically active proteins from the interstitial compartment. This reduced the interstitial osmotic pressure, thus pushing the fluid back into the intravascular compartment. This class of drugs aids in decreasing edema and limb softening, thereby reducing complications like secondary infections. However, the hepatotoxicity reported with coumarin therapy is to be remembered.

Inadequate lymph flow is caused either by lymphatic obstruction or when the rate of filtration is so high as compared to the fluid removal capacity by the lymphatics. Common causes are filariasis and post-radical mastectomy (Table 3.1). In

Table 3.1 Classification of edema on the basis of pathophysiology

Hydrostatic Edema	Permeability Edema	Lymphedema
Increased capillary hydrostatic pressure (P_c)	Inflammation and anaphylaxis	Obstruction of existing lymphatics, e.g., filariasis
Decreased interstitial fluid hydrostatic pressure (P_i)	Toxins	Absent lymphatics, e.g., post-radical mastectomy
Decreased capillary oncotic pressure (π_c)	Burns	
Increased interstitial fluid oncotic pressure (π_i)		

radical mastectomy, the axillary lymph nodes are removed which reduces lymph drainage on the ipsilateral side. In **filariasis**, the microfilaria larva migrates to lymphatics and obstructs them either directly or by fibrosis caused by the provoked inflammatory reactions. Over a period of time, massive edema of the legs and scrotum (elephantiasis) results.

3.10 Thermodynamical Considerations in Edema Therapeutics

Colloidal proteins are in random motion in solution and exert a pressure (π) at any surface that reflects them. The asymmetry in pressure results in free water movement. A solute dissolving in a solvent causes disruption of order resulting in an increase in entropy (S), a decrease in free energy (G), and a decrease in activity coefficient (γ). The decrease in G results in less random thermal movement and collisions which results in relatively more movement of solute-free solvent across membranes until a new equilibrium of G and S is reached. The osmotic pressure of a solution contained in a beaker open to the atmosphere is not a pressure which it actually exerts; it is in fact to be regarded as one of the thermodynamic properties of this solution similar to, say, its freezing point. For example, when a solution is said to have an osmotic pressure of 20 atmospheres, this does not mean that the solution necessarily exerts this pressure, but only that the solution would be in equilibrium with pure solvent through a semi-permeable membrane, if an excess pressure of this amount was applied to the system. In his now classic observation, **van't Hoff** noted that osmotic pressure for an ideal solution acted like a gas according to the ideal gas law, **PV = nRT**. So, the question arises whether alterations can be made to the plasma to restore free entropy and avoid the need for diuretics or albumin infusions? Theoretically, some day we could treat edema of nephritic syndrome by restoring free entropy to the plasma rather than through the use of diuretic, avoiding their well-known complications.

3.11 Various Physiological Conditions Affecting Edema Formation

3.11.1 Effect of Gravity

Elevation of an extremity after musculoskeletal injury is a universal treatment aimed at decreasing effusion and edema formation. It is generally accepted that elevation affects edema formation by altering the influences of gravity. When the position of an extremity is along the gravity, the force of gravity increases hydrostatic pressure in the peripheral blood vessels while also increasing resistance to venous and lymphatic flow. This results in an increase in fluid movement into the tissues, thereby increasing extremity volume. By placing the injured extremity in an elevated position, the force of gravity assists the return of fluids back to the heart via the venous and lymphatic systems and decreases hydrostatic pressure by resisting flow into the elevated peripheral vessels [3, 20].

3.11.2 Effect of Diet and Nutrition

Marked reductions in the circulating levels of proteins, especially albumin, are another cause of edema relating to intravascular factors. Hypoproteinemia may result from rapid loss of proteins across a compromised glomerular barrier in diseased kidneys, impaired hepatic synthesis of plasma proteins in liver disease, severe malnutrition or protein-losing enteropathy (which limits the availability of substrate for protein synthesis), or from infusion of intravenous fluids lacking macromolecules. The ensuing reduction in the colloid osmotic pressure gradient ($\pi_c - \pi_t$), which favors reabsorption in the non-steady state and opposes the hydrostatic pressure gradient that favors filtration, induced by hypoproteinemia can result in a large transcapillary flux of protein-poor fluid into the interstitial spaces. Like capillary hypertension, this effect is opposed by elevations in tissue hydrostatic pressure, which increases lymph flow, both of which serve to limit the accumulation of tissue fluid. Edema is also seen commonly in overweight and obese individuals. The causes are not always clear and can be multifactorial. Chronic venous insufficiency, lymphatic system impairment, as well as defective cardiac, respiratory, or renal functions can be attributed to obesity-related oedema.

3.11.3 Effect of Physical Activity and Posture

Leg swelling is considered to be blocked by leg exercise, because muscle activity pumps lymph and maintains a high interstitial pressure, but the effect depends on the type of exercise. Intermittent heel-up and stepping exercises could not prevent leg swelling. Continuous pedaling reduced leg swelling according to the power required to pedal. Continuous walking at a speed of 1 m/s also reduced leg swelling remarkably. Moderate leg movement could not completely prevent leg swelling but could reduce the swelling to half compared with the conditions where leg movement was strictly inhibited. The limb edema caused in sitting position was greater than when standing. Though the hydrostatic pressure in the lower legs during standing is theoretically about 30 mmHg higher than that during sitting, as the vertical height of the heart from ground is higher than when sitting, there are other factors which increase leg swelling in the sitting posture. The leg muscle activity in the sitting posture is less than that in the standing posture because the muscles do not need to work to maintain the standing posture. This results in low muscle pump activity and low interstitial pressure, which may increase the leg swelling. It is also to be noted that the chair seat presses on the veins in the hip and thigh areas and obstructs blood circulation in the legs, which also promotes leg swelling. In supine and prone positions, edema fluid gets accumulated in the dependent areas of the body. In a bedridden patient placed in supine position, edema can be demonstrated in the buttocks and back (Fig. 3.7a) and in prone position in the chest wall. Edema in lower third of leg (Fig. 3.7b) is very obvious and demonstrated in sitting posture (**dependent edema**).

3.11.4 Edema in Pregnancy

During normal pregnancy total body water increases by 6 to 8 l, 4 to 6 l of which are extracellular, of which at least 2 to 3 l are interstitial. At some stage in pregnancy 8 out of 10 women have demonstrable clinical edema. There is also cumulative retention of about 950 mmol of sodium distributed between the maternal extracellular compartments and the product of conception. Thus, changes in factors governing renal sodium and water handling accompany alterations in local Starling forces

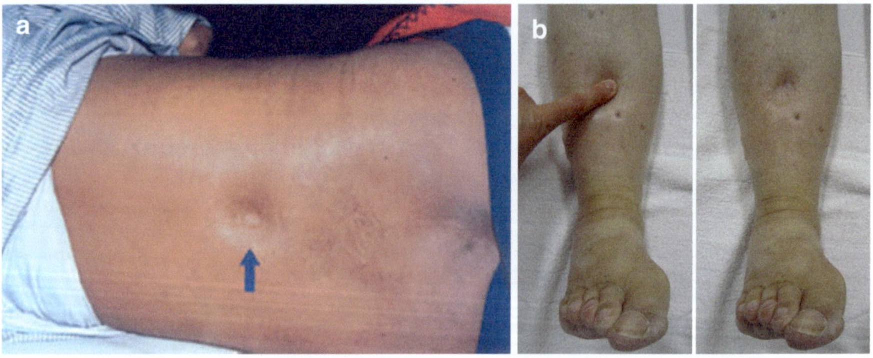

Fig. 3.7 Photographs showing the effect of gravity and posture on edema formation. (**a**) Arrow depicts the pitting edema formation in the dependent part on the back of a bedridden patient kept in supine position. (**b**) Godet sign is being elicited in a patient who has bilateral pedal edema probably due to prolonged standing. (Courtesy from Clinical Methods in Medicine: Clinical Skills and Practices; 2nd edition-2015; SN Chugh, Eshan Gupta)

whereby there is a moderate fall in interstitial fluid colloid osmotic pressure and a rise in capillary hydrostatic pressure, as well as changes in hydration of connective tissue ground substance. Salt and water are retained to increase plasma volume to meet the increased cardiac output required for the fetus and placenta. Inferior vena cava and iliac vein compression by the gravid uterus in the later stages of pregnancy can exacerbate edema formation.

3.11.5 Effect of Altitude Changes

Rapidly ascending to higher altitudes exposes individuals to hypoxic environments. The response of systemic vessels to hypoxia is vasodilation that increased the capillary hydrostatic pressure in the peripheral circulation leading to peripheral edema (**high-altitude peripheral edema—HAPE**). In contrast to this, lower limb edema can also occur at low altitudes (**low-altitude peripheral edema—LAPE**). Millions of permanent high-altitude residents, born at high altitude occasionally descend to sea level, for work or leisure. This is a change where the organism perfectly adapted to chronic hypoxia is suddenly exposed to a hypertoxic environment and needs to adapt to the new circumstance. One of the most striking symptoms that occur in these people is edema of lower limbs that can become more pronounced at 2 weeks of stay. A positive Godet sign develops in these individuals. The **Godet sign** is elicited by pressing for few seconds in front of the tibia bone. This displaces excessive fluid found in the interstitial subcutaneous spaces and gives rise to the formation of an evident concave impression. This sign is usually found in patients suffering from cardiac insufficiency, renal insufficiency, anasarca with low blood protein levels, or inflammation. Upon ascent to high altitude, there is central edema and that is why acute mountain sickness, high-altitude pulmonary edema, and high-altitude cerebral edema occur. Conversely, on descending to sea level, peripheral edema occurs. Going higher, oxygen needs to be transported preferably to the life-sustaining organs: brain, heart, and lungs, whereas going lower there is excessive amounts of oxygen and peripheral edema occurs possibly as a defense mechanism to reduce oxygen transport to the life-sustaining organs, as it is sensed toxic.

3.12 Pathological Conditions Presenting with Edema

3.12.1 Heart Failure

Heart failure (both left and right sided) is a common condition that presents with generalized peripheral edema. In heart failure, the inability of the heart to effectively circulate blood volume throughout the body leads to increased venous pressure that is transmitted to the capillaries. This causes extravasation of fluid into the interstitium, producing edema. A low-output state and hypoperfusion of vital organs lead to neurohormonal activation (stimulation of the sympathetic nervous system) which leads to peripheral vasoconstriction and increases cardiac rate and contractility, thereby increasing afterload and cardiac work. Though these events aim to restore circulatory homeostasis, they paradoxically worsen cardiac failure and exacerbate edema. Left heart failure (systolic or diastolic) causes pulmonary edema, as the increased central venous pressure is transmitted back to the pulmonary capillaries, giving rise to dyspnea. Right heart failure, on the other hand, causes peripheral edema, pleural effusions, and sometimes ascites which can be further exacerbated by severe tricuspid incompetence. The release of additional neurohormones of the renin–angiotensin–aldosterone system causes sodium and water retention, while arginine vasopressin (AVP) causes further water retention and peripheral vasoconstriction. The atrial (ANP) and B-type natriuretic peptides (BNP) are diagnostic markers of atrial and ventricular distension and are elevated in heart failure.

3.12.2 Hepatic Cirrhosis

Fulminant liver disease predominantly causes ascites, but patients also present with bilateral pedal edema. Severe hypo-albuminemia, salt and water retention, and formation of multiple arterio-venous fistulae are notable reasons of edema in liver failure. Ascites can be severe, and care is needed when performing paracentesis to prevent sudden fluid shifts out of the intravascular compartment. Plasma volume and oncotic pressure should be maintained by administering intravenous 20% concentrated albumin while performing slow and repeated paracentesis over a few days as per need. This helps to preserve the near-physiological functional fluid volume within the intravascular compartment.

3.12.3 Constrictive Pericarditis and Restrictive Cardiomyopathy

Constrictive pericarditis and restrictive cardiomyopathy are fewer common causes of peripheral edema. Patients with either of these conditions present with dyspnea, elevated jugular venous pressure, ascites, as well as peripheral edema. Left ventricular systolic functions are normal in echocardiography, but Doppler readings show pericardial constriction or restriction. Infiltrative diseases (amyloidosis), connective tissue diseases (scleroderma), and hypertrophic cardiomyopathy are notable causes of restrictive cardiomyopathy. Both constrictive pericarditis and restrictive cardiomyopathy require imaging and right heart catheterization for definitive diagnosis.

3.12.4 Renal Diseases

Nephrotic syndrome, acute renal failure, and fulminant renal failure can all give rise to peripheral edema. Nephrotic syndrome is characterized by proteinuria, low serum albumin levels, and high serum cholesterol levels. Diabetic nephropathy is another common cause of proteinuria in adults. Acute renal failure caused by severe renal insults and fulminant renal failure can be associated with oliguria or anuria accompanied by fluid retention, elevated central venous pressure, and generalized edema.

3.12.5 Medications

Calcium channel blockers (dihydropyridines)-induced peripheral edema is because of the unopposed precapillary arteriolar dilation which increases the fluid load on the cognate capillary network, thereby pushing fluid out into the interstitium. These effects may be minimized by administering calcium channel blockers at night and co-administering ACE inhibitors or angiotensin receptor antagonists. These agents act by causing post-capillary venular dilation, thereby reducing capillary hydrostatic pressure. Other drugs known to cause peripheral edema are NSAIDs, corticosteroids, antidepressants, estrogens, progesterones, thiazolidinediones, and vasodilators like minoxidil and hydralazine. Diuretics should not be used to treat peripheral edema caused by medications.

3.12.6 Thyroid Disease

Myxedema can occur in patients with severe hypothyroidism like Hashimoto thyroiditis. Myxedema is non-pitting and caused by dermatological changes, with deposition of glycosaminoglycans, rather than altered vascular hemodynamics. Pretibial myxedema can also occur in a minority of patients with Graves's disease and hyperthyroidism. Peripheral edema can be a feature of high-output cardiac failure in patients with severe hyperthyroidism.

3.12.7 Lymphatic Obstruction

Lymphedema is commonly caused by destruction of the local lymph nodes by surgery (e.g., mastectomy with axillary lymph node clearance) or radiotherapy. Another common tropical cause of lymphedema is filariasis. In lymphedema, the skin has a tethered to produce peau d'orange appearance and edema is mostly unilateral, occurring in the affected side.

3.12.8 Venous Incompetence or Deep Vein Thrombosis

Venous incompetence or a history of deep vein thrombosis can lead to impaired venous return. This may present with asymmetrical/bilateral peripheral edema but is often associated with unilateral swelling and pain with or without erythema. Varicose veins are a sign of venous incompetence which may or may not be associated with peripheral edema.

3.12.9 Dermatitis and Lipedema

Localized skin irritation can lead to an inflammatory infiltrate activated by cytokines, like tumor necrosis factor alpha and interleukin-8 and increased vascular permeability. This is usually associated with erythema and pruritus, but dermatitis or eczema occurring bilaterally in the lower extremities can mimic peripheral edema from other causes like cellulitis. Lipedema is caused by accumulation of fatty deposits, most commonly in the lower extremities. It can be bilateral and mistaken for lymphedema or venous incompetence but is differentiated from them by the absence of pitting and of involvement of the feet.

3.13 Conclusion

The causes of peripheral edema are varied, requiring a systematic approach to history taking and examination. Diagnosis is often a process of elimination of the common causes. Most patients who present early can be managed in the community. Patients with advanced cardiac, hepatic, or renal disease with gross peripheral edema warrant urgent specialist review or hospital admission. A high index of suspicion is required to detect rarer but potentially life-threatening causes of peripheral edema, such as constrictive pericarditis.

References

1. Berne RM, Bruce MK. Bruce AS Berne & levy physiology. 15th ed. Philadelphia, PA: Mosby/Elsevier; 2010.
2. Davies PF. Flow mediated endothelial mechano-transduction. Physiol Rev. 1995;75:519.
3. Auckland K. Why don't our feet swell in the upright position? News Physiol Sci. 1994;9:214.
4. Welsh DG, Segal SS. Endothelial and smooth muscle cell conduction in arterioles controlling blood flow. Am J Phys. 1998;274:H178.
5. Xia J, Duling BR. Patterns of excitation-contraction coupling in arterioles: dependence on time and concentration. Am J Phys. 1998;274:H323.
6. Bates DO, Lodwick D, Williams B. Vascular endothelial growth factor and microvascular permeability. Microcirculation. 1999;6:83.
7. Ganong (2012) Ganong's review of medical physiology. 7ed. New York: McGraw-Hill Medical.
8. Hall JE. Guyton and hall textbook of medical physiology. 13th ed. London, England: W B Saunders; 2015.
9. Michel CC, Neal CR. Openings through endothelial cells associated with increased microvascular permeability. Microcirculation. 1999;6:45.
10. Curry FE. Regulation of water and solute exchange in micro vessel endothelium: studies in single perfused capillaries. Microcirculation. 1994;1:11.
11. Rippe B, Haraldsson B. Transport of macromolecules across microvascular walls: the two pore theory. Physiol Rev. 1994;74:163.
12. Wright S, Cyril AK, Neil E. Applied physiology. 12th ed. London: Oxford University Press; 1971.
13. Vink H, Duling BR. The capillary endothelial surface layer selectively reduces plasma solute distribution volume. Am J Phys. 2000;278:H285.

14. Starling EH. On the absorption of fluids from the connective tissue spaces. J Physiol. 1896;19:312.
15. Widmaier EP, Vander AJ, Raff H, Strang KT. Vander's human physiology: the mechanisms of body function, 15th ed. New York, NY: McGraw-Hill Education. 2019.
16. Boron WF, Boulpaep EL. Medical physiology: a cellular and molecular approach. 2nd ed. Philadelphia, PA: Saunders/Elsevier; 2009.
17. Bijlani RL, Manjunatha S. Understanding medical physiology: a textbook for medical students. 4th ed. New Delhi: Jaypee Brothers Medical Publishers; 2011.
18. Best CH, Taylor NB, In Tandon OP, In Tripathi YB. Best and Taylor's physiological basis of medical practice. 13th ed. Wolters Kluwer (India); 2012.
19. Zucker IH, Gilmore JP. Reflex control of the circulation. 1st ed. Boca Raton, FL: CRC Press; 1991.
20. Auckland K, Reed RK. Interstitial-lymphatic mechanisms in the control of extracellular fluid volume. Physiol Rev. 1999;73:1.

Aetiopathogenesis in Lower Limb Oedema

4

Vaibhav Pandey and Mohammad Imran

4.1 Introduction

Edema of lower limb is a common clinical presentation of local and systemic disorders. The word "edema" is derived from the Greek word "*oidēma*," where *oidein* means "to swell." The swelling of the lower limbs may result from an increase in the amount of any of the tissue components, i.e., muscle, fat, blood, etc. From a clinical point of view, all the conditions which result in excessive accumulation of fluid in the lower limbs lead to edema. The etiology of edema of lower limb varies, and it is important to assess whether the swelling is congenital or acquired, acute or chronic, symmetric or asymmetric and is localized or part of generalized edema [1].

4.2 Pathogenesis

The body fluid is divided into different compartments, i.e., intracellular and extracellular, which are further divided into intravascular plasma volume (25%) and the extravascular interstitial space (75%). Maintaining a balance between these compartments is essential for maintaining homeostasis. Any disbalance between forces maintaining this balance will lead to abnormal accumulation of fluid and will lead to edema. Two forces in majority maintain this balance (Starling forces) [2].

1. Hydrostatic pressure: Hydrostatic pressure is defined as the physical force that fluids exerted against its enclosing barriers. So, blood/plasma within the vessels exerts a positive pressure on the vessel wall, with a tendency to move out.

V. Pandey (✉) · M. Imran
Department of Paediatric Surgery, Institute of Medical Sciences, Banaras Hindu University, Varanasi, India

S. K. Tiwary (ed.), *Approach to Lower Limb Oedema*,
https://doi.org/10.1007/978-981-16-6206-5_4

The interstitium has also a hydrostatic pressure which is usually negative, due to fluid pumping action of lymphatics.
2. Oncotic pressure refers to the osmotic pressure generated by the presence of solutes in plasma. The albumin is the most important factor for this osmolarity and because of its large size it does not cross the capillary barrier. The high concentration of proteins inside capillaries maintains a higher oncotic pressure within the intravascular compartment compared to the oncotic pressure within the interstitial fluid. This leads to an oncotic pressure gradient between these two compartments.

   The relation between these Starling forces determines the movement of fluids between the intravascular compartment and interstitial spaces. These forces drive the passive exchange of water between the capillary microcirculation and the interstitial fluid. These forces not only determine the directionality of net water movement between two different compartments but also determines the rate at which water exchange occurs.

These forces work in tandem with two other important factors, inherent to vessels for maintaining the homeostasis of fluid between the capillary microcirculation and the interstitium.

1. **Vessel wall permeability:** The permeability of the vessel wall to water varies a lot and is determined by the histological architecture of capillaries. This can vary by over two orders of magnitude in different capillary beds like glomerular capillaries. They have a fenestrated architecture and they display an extremely high permeability to water. The capillaries of brain have extremely tight architecture and thus the blood–brain barrier has extremely low water permeability. The damage to capillary with inflammation, toxin, drug, or temperature can result in change in permeability and thus can lead to edema (venous edema).
2. **Lymphatic system:** The lymphatic system is a one-way drainage system which, through lymphatic vessels and lymph nodes, returns fluid back into the vascular circulation. Chronic edema happens due to a failure to drain the interstitial tissues properly in the lymph drainage system. The persistent accumulation of protein in the interstitium leads to increased water retention and thus edema (lymphedema). Usually, the swelling is soft and shows "pitting" at the onset and often resolves on elevation (acute). But with time the tissues may become hard due to fibrosis and edema becomes non-resolving (sub-acute or chronic). The progression of chronic edema is variable. In some cases, the skin becomes dry and develops flakes. On the other hand, it can progressively become moist and fluid starts oozing from it and it becomes prone for recurrent infection. Chronic edema in the lower limb can develop as a result of a number of factors, including venous disease trauma, infection, arterial insufficiency, or following orthopedic surgery (detailed later).

The venous and lymphatic systems are intricately associated with each other. A progressive and prolonged venous hypertension leads to increased capillary permeability and thus increased fluid retention in the interstitium. The lymphatic system uniquely compensates and does not allow accumulation of fluid by over-draining. If this venous hypertension persists the lymphatic system compensation fails, resulting in edema. This is known aslympho-venous edema. If edema persists there is underlying interstitial fibrosis and it becomes chronic edema. In many cases, edema of the lower limb will therefore have both lymphatic and venous components.

The balance between these forces determines the net pressure which dictates the direction of fluid movement.

4.3 Starling Forces

- $\mathbf{J_v = K_f\,[(P_c - P_i)\text{-}(\Pi_c - \Pi_i)]}$
  - J_v = Net fluid movement (ml/min). A positive value indicates movement out of the circulation
  - K_f = Vascular permeability coefficient
  - P_c = Capillary hydrostatic pressure
  - P_i = Interstitial hydrostatic pressure
  - Π_c = Capillary oncotic pressure
  - Π_i = Interstitial oncotic pressure

4.4 Etiology

As the movement of fluid and in lower limbs is controlled by all the above forces, any factor causing change in these will disturb this homeostasis and cause lower limb edema. These factors can be local (affecting lower limb) or can be a part of systemic disorder. It is important to determine the location of swelling and its subsequent symptoms, including whether it is unilateral, bilateral equivalent, or bilateral but asymmetrical, along with any changes happening with the place and time of day with its intensity. Swelling may be asymptomatic, but signs such as pain, heaviness, symptomatic venous, or lymphatic skin changes or peri skin changes may be correlated with it. Common causes of leg swelling based on acuity and unilateral or bilateral symptoms are shown in Table 4.1. Unilateral swelling favors primary and secondary sources of venous or lymphatic compromise and bilateral or generalized swelling is rooted to systemic cause (Table 4.2).

Bilateral but asymmetric cases can have various etiologies or differing degrees of unilateral causes on each leg or a unilateral cause superimposed on a systemic disease context. Lymphedema and venous edema can both be bilateral differential and bilateral, but with venous etiologies below the IVC, bilateral equality is less common as the condition is often asymmetric at any point in time. As a precedent for both venous and lymphatic etiologies of edema, prior abdominal or pelvic operation, malignancy, or radiation background is also essential [3].

Systemic disease evaluation is important, particularly in elderly patients with multiple comorbid conditions that could lead primarily to their bilateral leg edema.

Table 4.1 Common causes of Leg Edema

<table>
<tr><th colspan="2">Unilateral</th><th colspan="2">Bilateral</th></tr>
<tr><th>Acute (<72 h)</th><th>Chronic</th><th>Acute (<72 h)</th><th>Chronic</th></tr>
<tr><td>Deep vein thrombosis</td><td>Venous insufficiency</td><td>Bilateral deep vein thrombosis</td><td rowspan="4">Common Causes
• Venous insufficiency
• Pulmonary hypertension
• Heart failure
• Idiopathic edema
• Lymphedema
• Drugs
Uncommon/Rare
• Premenstrual edema
• Pregnancy
• Obesity
• Renal disease (nephrotic syndrome, glomerulonephritis)
• Liver disease
• Secondary lymphedema (secondary to tumor, radiation, bacterial infection, filariasis)
• Pelvic tumor or lymphoma causing external pressure
• Dependent edema
• Diuretic-induced edema
• Dependent edema
• Preeclampsia
• Lipidema
• Anemia</td></tr>
<tr><td>Ruptured Baker's cyst</td><td>Secondary lymphedema (tumor, radiation, surgery, bacterial infection)</td><td>Acute worsening of systemic cause (heart failure, renal disease)</td></tr>
<tr><td>Ruptured medial head of gastrocnemius</td><td>Pelvic tumor or lymphoma causing external pressure on veins</td><td rowspan="2"></td></tr>
<tr><td>Compartment syndrome</td><td>Reflex sympathetic dystrophy</td></tr>
</table>

Table 4.2 Acute (<72 h) progressing to Chronic

Unilateral	Bilateral
• Primary lymphedema (congenital lymphedema, lymphedema praecox, lymphedema tarda) • Congenital venous malformations • May-Thurner syndrome (iliac-vein compression syndrome)51	• Primary lymphedema (congenital lymphedema, lymphedema praecox, lymphedema tarda) • Protein losing enteropathy, malnutrition, malabsorption • Restrictive pericarditis • Restrictive cardiomyopathy • BeriBeri • Myxedema

The development of edema and its type has a temporal association with factors. If the inciting cause is severe in intensity, it leads to acute edema. If the intensity is low and persists, it causes sub-acute or chronic edema. It is necessary to evaluate the length of symptoms, with acute swelling (<72 h) more typical of etiologies such as

DVT, illness, accident, deterioration of a medical condition such as congestive heart failure, or recent adjustments in medication. A sudden onset of limb swelling, a slow onset, or a more prolonged syndrome can be identified in patients. Venous insufficiency, lymphatic dysfunction, static foot conditions, or more long-standing pathological etiologies may be responsible for recurrent swelling. In comparison, swelling due to venous illness usually worsens throughout the day with dependency and improves with elevation. Also, venous edema is also a common phenomenon. Venous edema is also commonly associated with complaints of aching, heaviness, or fatigue of the limbs.

Pain is an important symptom to differentiate the etiology of lower limb edema. A musculoskeletal or joint condition might be indicated by focal pain. For a severely sore, regular swelling of limb, reflex sympathetic dystrophy (complex regional pain syndrome) must be considered. Lymphedema is typically painless and may display common symptoms of foot involvement and skin involvement [4, 5] Table 4.3.

Lipedema is a condition in which lower limbs are swollen due to deposits of fat beneath the skin. Usually, over time, it gets worse, there can be discomfort, and sufferers bruise quickly. Lipedema is nearly invariably bilateral, easily spares the feet, and has disproportionate pain, tenderness, and an abnormal tendency to bruise. It is necessary to note that the often-referenced clinical findings are not always the rule with these conditions.

Systemic disease evaluation is important, particularly in elderly patients with multiple comorbid conditions that could lead primarily to their bilateral leg edema. A cause may be new onset or exacerbations of heart, renal, hepatic, and endocrine problems. Malignant venous compression may indicate a history of unexplained weight loss or adenopathy. Any changes in regimens should be considered in relation to swelling onset.

Lower limb edema is one of common adverse drug reactions to multiple drugs. Like 50% of patients on amlodipine, a calcium channel blocker will develop pedal edema. The other common drugs are highlighted in Table 4.4 [4, 6].

Table 4.3 Causes of painful oedema of lower limb

• Painful swelling in lower limbs
• Deep vein thrombosis
• Cellulitis
• Superficial thrombophlebitis
• Joint effusion or hemarthrosis
• Hematoma
• Baker's cyst
• Torn gastrocnemius muscle
• Arthritis
• Fracture
• Acute arterial ischemia
• Dermatitis

Table 4.4 Common drugs causing lower limb oedema

• Antihypertensive drugs
• Calcium channel blockers
• Beta blockers
• Clonidine
• Hydralazine
• Minoxidil
• Methyldopa
• Hormones
• Corticosteroids
• Estrogen
• Progesterone
• Testosterone
• Other
➢ Nonsteroidal anti-inflammatory drugs
➢ Pioglitazone, rosiglitazone
➢ Monoamine oxidase inhibitors

It is very important to note that there are often several factors responsible for swelling in any given patient and it is incumbent on the physician to determine the relative contribution of each. This will allow a more complete diagnosis and help the physicians to prioritize management to address the most important or impactful etiologies.

Systemic Causes These lead to generalized edema or anasarca. All these disorders lead to intravascular volume contraction and thus excessive fluid retention. Due to dependent position of lower limbs, the edema appears first.

4.5 Heart Diseases

In heart diseases, edema happens as there is a rise in venous pressure, leading to an increase in hydrostatic pressure; this mechanism can be related to many heart diseases such as hypertensive cardiomyopathy, coronary artery disease, and others. Hypoperfusion causes an increase in sympathetic tone and the renin-angiotensin-aldosterone pathway, increasing hydro-saline retention, vascular tolerance, and cardiac inotropism with diminished left ventricular activity (forward hypothesis). The right-sided failure also leads to edema due to diastolic pressure transmission in a retrograde way (*backward hypothesis*) [7].

4.6 Liver Diseases

In liver cirrhosis, fluid accumulation is linked to portal hypertension (>12 mmHg) and elevated sinus pressure. Both portal vein obstruction and splanchnic vasodilation have been found to be involved in physiopathology. Indeed, hyperdynamic circulation, lowered vascular resistance and average blood pressure, and increased cardiac production describe liver cirrhosis. Even though intravascular hypovolemia is associated with interstitial fluid expansion, the reduction in blood pressure is experienced by baroceptors and causes a neurohormonal reaction with hydro-saline retention by RAAS activation and increased fluid retention [8].

4.7 Renal Diseases

Nephrotic syndrome is characterized by proteinuria. Several pathways, in particular the so-called underfilling and overload, are implicated in pathogenesis and are present to a certain degree in all patients and differ at various stages of the disease.

The *underfilling* is a chronic intravascular hypovolemia, due to oncotic capillary pressure reduction. The hydro-saline retention is responsible for vascular *overflow in patients with decreased renal function* [2].

4.8 Venous (or Lymphatic) Drainage Obstruction

Venous drainage obstruction results in increased hydrostatic pressure which in turn leads to increased fluid translocation to interstitial space and results in edema. Most common causes of venous drainage obstruction are thrombophlebitis and deep vein thrombosis.

4.9 Deep Vein Thrombosis

Deep vein thrombosis (DVT) is one of the most common cause of peripheral edema encountered in clinical practice. The classical description of swelling pain and raised temperature may be misleading. Although the swelling is an important feature and is seen in 90% of cases, raised temperature is usually absent. Increased temperature in the affected leg (>37.5 °C) has shown to be a negative predictor of DVT [9]. Usually it affects only one side, but rarely might be bilateral. D-dimer positivity increases the probability of DVT independently from the clinical risk group, but is not diagnostic [10].

4.10 Chronic Vein Insufficiency

Edema is one of the signs of venous insufficiency in the clinical presentation; other symptoms include discomfort, itching, feeling heavy in the legs, and cramps (especially during the night), while the most frequent signs are varicose veins, skin changes, and ulcers. The swelling is normally exacerbated by the standing posture (thus, at night, it is usually more severe). In 1994, the CEAP system was established, in order to stage the disease in relation to clinical presentations (C), etiology (E), anatomic distribution (A), and physiopathology (P) [11].

4.11 Reflex Sympathetic Dystrophy

When leg edema is associated with discomfort, reflex sympathetic dystrophy should be examined (RSD).RSD is a progressive neurological condition that affects the limbs and induces serious disabilities. It is typically preceded by trauma, upper or lower limb surgery, malignancy, and pregnancy. Typically, the symptoms are disproportionately severe to the swelling. The neurological symptoms associated are autonomic, vasomotor and sensory changes, elevated limb temperatures, hyperhidrosis, atrophy of the skin/muscle/bone, repetitive movements, tremors, and spasmodic muscles [12].

4.12 Lymphedema

It is a common cause of lower limb oedema. It typically develops due to reduced local lymphatic drainage with fluid overload and elevated interstitial lymphatic length; lymphedema is typically confined to the upper or lower extremities [13]. It is classified as *primary lymphedema,* caused by congenital abnormalities of lymphatic structures, and *secondary lymphedema,* due to many causes, such as malignancies, traumas, and infections.

4.13 Inflammatory Edema

Inflammatory reaction causes vast changes in the capillary endothelium. There is a massive increase in the permeability of plasma proteins. The increased interstitial protein draws and retains fluid with it, resulting in edema. The inflammatory process may be generalized or may be generalized or localized. The local inflammatory response may be due to infections, chemical substances, traumatic or mechanical agents, or immunological factors.

4.14 Summary and Conclusion

The etiology of lower limb edema is vast and ranges from simple local to complex systemic causes. A proper clinical history and thorough physical examination help a in excluding the different causes, but a systematic approach is mandatory in order to pinpoint the diagnosis from such a long list. The first and foremost approach is to identify whether the edema is unilateral or bilateral; then one should divide the causes on the basis of duration as acute and chronic. In a patient of pedal edema with acute onset (<72 h) of symptoms having either unilateral or bilateral involvement, a deep vein thrombosis should be ruled out using a Doppler examination in order to avoid life-threatening complications. If a systemic disorder has been ruled out or considered unlikely, the most common causes of bilateral leg edema are idiopathic edema (in young women) and chronic venous insufficiency (in older patients). The patients should be investigated for cardiac, renal, or hepatic causes in patients with chronic bilateral edema and systemic symptoms. This approach helps to utilize the patient's history and clinical examination, perform the required imaging to avoid over-testing, and follow a cost-effective approach.

Funding Nil.

References

1. Paramesparan K, Iqbal A, Shah A, Botchu R. Imaging of the unilateral swollen painful lower leg: deep vein thrombosis mimics. Indian J Musculoskelet Radiol. 2019;1(1):27–40.
2. Lent-Schochet D, Jialal I. Physiology, Edema. [Updated 2020 Jul 10]. In: StatPearls [Internet]. Treasure Island (FL): StatPearls Publishing; 2020 Jan-. Available from: https://www.ncbi.nlm.nih.gov/books/NBK537065/
3. Gasparis AP, Kim PS, Dean SM, Khilnani NM, Labropoulos N. Diagnostic approach to lower limb edema. Phlebology. 2020 Oct;35(9):650–5. https://doi.org/10.1177/0268355520938283. Epub 2020 Jul 6. PMID: 32631171; PMCID: PMC7536506.
4. Evans NS, Ratchford EV. The swollen leg. Vasc Med 2016;21(6):562–564. https://doi.org/10.1177/1358863X16672576. Epub 2016 Oct 12. PMID: 27738281.
5. Eldufani J, Elahmer N, Blaise G. A medical mystery of complex regional pain syndrome. Heliyon. 2020;6(2):e03329. https://doi.org/10.1016/j.heliyon.2020.e03329. PMID: 32149194; PMCID: PMC7033333.
6. Khadka S, Joshi R, Shrestha DB, Shah D, Bhandari N, Maharjan M, Sthapit S. Amlodipine-induced pedal Edema and its relation to other variables in patients at a tertiary level Hospital of Kathmandu, Nepal. J Pharm Technol. 2019;35(2):51–5.
7. Hartupee J, Mann DL. Neurohormonal activation in heart failure with reduced ejection fraction. Nat Rev Cardiol. 2017 Jan;14(1):30–8. https://doi.org/10.1038/nrcardio.2016.163. Epub 2016 Oct 6. PMID: 27708278; PMCID: PMC5286912.
8. Fountain JH, Lappin SL. Physiology, Renin Angiotensin System. [Updated 2020 Jul 27]. In: StatPearls [Internet]. Treasure Island (FL): StatPearls Publishing; 2020 Jan-. Available from: https://www.ncbi.nlm.nih.gov/books/NBK470410/
9. Tan KK, Koh WP, Chao AK. Risk factors and presentation of deep venous thrombosis among Asian patients: a hospital-based case-control study in Singapore. Ann Vasc Surg. 2007;21(4):490–5. https://doi.org/10.1016/j.avsg.2006.06.008. Epub 2007 Feb 26. PMID: 17628265.
10. Pulivarthi S, Gurram MK. Effectiveness of d-dimer as a screening test for venous thromboembolism: an update. N Am J Med Sci. 2014;6(10):491–9. https://doi.org/10.4103/1947-2714.143278. PMID: 25489560; PMCID: PMC4215485.
11. Zegarra TI, Tadi P. CEAP Classification of Venous Disorders. [Updated 2020 May 31]. In: StatPearls [Internet]. Treasure Island (FL): StatPearls Publishing; 2020 Jan-. Available from: https://www.ncbi.nlm.nih.gov/books/NBK557410/
12. Patel RH, Sheth R, Hus N. Complex regional pain syndrome caused by an axillary lipoma. Cureus. 2020;12(12):e12280. https://doi.org/10.7759/cureus.12280. PMID: 33510987; PMCID: PMC7828746.
13. Garza R 3rd, Skoracki R, Hock K, Povoski SP. A comprehensive overview on the surgical management of secondary lymphedema of the upper and lower extremities related to prior oncologic therapies. BMC Cancer. 2017;17(1):468. https://doi.org/10.1186/s12885-017-3444-9. PMID: 28679373; PMCID: PMC5497342.

Clinical Examination in Lower Limb Edema

5

E. Menegatti, M. Tessari, and S. Gianesini

5.1 Introduction

Edema is defined as an abnormal increase in the amount of liquid contained in the cells and/or in the intercellular spaces and tissues interstices.

The fluid between the interstitial and intravascular spaces is regulated by the capillary hydrostatic pressure gradient and the oncotic pressure gradient across the capillary. Differently from what believed years ago, the filtration process is far more complex than a simple balance between hydrostatic and oncotic pressure. Indeed, the filtration process is also mediated by a molecular sieve of various porosities determined by a matrix of glycoproteins and glycosaminoglycans present on the luminal surface of the endothelial cells [1].

The extraluminal fluid accumulation occurs when local and/or systemic conditions disrupt this equilibrium, leading to increased capillary hydrostatic pressure, increased plasma volume, decreased plasma oncotic pressure (hypoalbuminemia), increased capillary permeability, or lymphatic obstruction.

It can be a local condition that is, limited to a specific district of the body or a generalized condition, which is also accompanied by fluid pouring into the serous cavities (anasarca) [2, 3].

E. Menegatti · M. Tessari
Vascular Diseases Center, Department of Translational Medicine, University of Ferrara, Ferrara, Italy

S. Gianesini (✉)
Vascular Diseases Center, Department of Translational Medicine, University of Ferrara, Ferrara, Italy

Departement of Surgery, Uniformed Services University of the Health Sciences, Bethesda, MD, USA

S. K. Tiwary (ed.), *Approach to Lower Limb Oedema*,
https://doi.org/10.1007/978-981-16-6206-5_5

The major causes of edema include:

- Increase in intravascular pressure due to venous obstruction and/or reflux
- Increase in capillary vessel wall permeability
- Decrease in the intravascular osmotic pressure
- Excessive bodily fluids
- Lymphatic obstruction
- Local injury
- Infection
- Medication effect

The management of a patient with edema should start always with an accurate evaluation of the medical history and with a physical examination in order to clarify the etiology and the best instrumental diagnostic path aimed to design the proper therapeutic strategy [2].

5.2 Clinical History

An accurate history collection must include the description of:

- Sign and symptoms detailed report, including their timing
- Pain triggering factors
- Previous surgical, radiotherapy, or accidental trauma
- Pelvic venous disorders
- Abdominal conditions potentially altering the lymphatic drainage
- Comorbidities
- Medications, in particular the ones affecting the fluid homeostasis

The key element of the history should include the timing of the edema (acute if <72 h or chronic >72 h), specifying if it is unilateral or bilateral and whether it is posture dependent.

The most likely cause of bilateral chronic leg edema in women under 50 years old is idiopathic [4]. On the other end, the most common cause of lower limb edema in patients over 50 is chronic venous disease (CVD), which affects up to 30% of the population.

The most common cause of unilateral acute leg swelling is deep venous thrombosis (DVT), while less common causes can be popliteal cyst rupture, acute compartment syndrome, and gastrocnemius medial head traumatic rupture.

Chronic bilateral edema is due to the onset or exacerbation of chronic systemic conditions, such as heart failure, pulmonary hypertension, renal disease, hepatic disease, primary lymphedema, and medication.

Less common causes which can involve one or both limbs are secondary lymphedema (tumor, radiation, bacterial infection, or filariasis), pelvic masses causing external compression, May-Thurner syndrome, and congenital vascular malformation [2, 5].

The importance of the observation of edema variation following postural changes is another crucial point in clinical examination. The postural dependent edema caused by venous insufficiency is more likely to improve with elevation and worsen with prolonged orthostatic posture. This type of edema can improve overnight. To the contrary, the edema associated with decreased plasma oncotic pressure, such as malabsorption and liver and renal failure, does not significantly change with leg elevation [6].

Pain can play a crucial role in determining the cause of leg edema. This is particularly evident in a symptomatic venous thrombosis, for example.

Deep vein thrombosis and reflex sympathetic dystrophy are usually strongly painful and associated with redness and heat of the affected area. Chronic venous insufficiency and lymphedema are characterized by a low-grade aching often associated with heaviness, while edema of cardiac origin is usually painless.

Medication has to be considered when drawing the clinical history of the patient: antihypertensive drugs like calcium channel blockers, hormones such as steroids, and anti-inflammatory drugs can present edema as a side effect.

Finally, history of systemic disease involving the heart, kidney, liver, thyroid, tumor, pelvic obstruction, and radiation, has to be reported since they can be directly responsible for the onset of lower limb edema [2].

5.3 Physical Examination

In order to collect clinical information and formulate the differential diagnosis, an accurate physical examination is of primary importance.

Edema should be characterized for distribution, pitting sign, tenderness, skin changes, its association with varicose veins, and/or obesity.

5.3.1 Distribution

- Unilateral leg edema is generally due to a local cause such as deep vein thrombosis, venous insufficiency, or lymphedema.
- Bilateral edema can be due to a local cause or systemic disease, such as heart failure or kidney disease.
- Generalized edema is due to systemic disease.
- The dorsum of the foot is usually spared in lipedema, but prominently involved in lymphedema.

5.3.2 Tenderness

Tenderness to palpation over the edematous area is usually associated with deep vein thrombosis and lipedema, whereas lymphedema is usually non-tender. Variations can be observed in fluid vs sclerotic lymphedema.

5.3.3 Pitting

The edematous tissue appears swollen, pale, and, if incised, releasing abundant amounts of liquid. The presence of edema in the subcutaneous tissue is easily highlighted whenever a pressure is applied, resulting in a depressed area caused by the displacement of interstitial fluid. This is considered the main semeiotic sign of pitting edema [2, 7] (Fig. 5.1).

The assessment technique of the pitting edema consists in pressing firmly with the thumb for at least 2 s on each extremity [8]:

- Over the dorsum of the foot
- Bony portion of the tibia
- Lower calf above the medial malleolus

The grading of edema is determined by the pit depth (measured visually) and recovery time from grade 0 to 4. The scale is used to rate the severity and the scores are as follows:

- Grade 0: No clinical edema.
- Grade 1: Slight pitting (2 mm depth) with no visible distortion that rebounds immediately.
- Grade 2: Somewhat deeper pit (4 mm) with no readily detectable distortion that rebounds in fewer than 15 s.

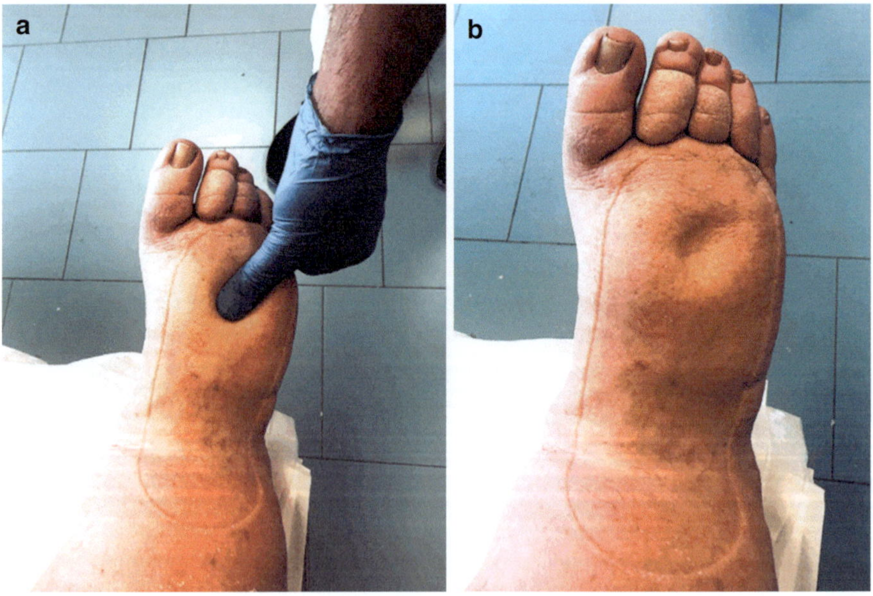

Fig. 5.1 Ptting edema represents a depressed area (**b**) that remains in the edematous tissue after pressure is applied (**a**)

- Grade 3: Noticeably deep pit (6 mm) with the dependent extremity full and swollen that takes up to 30 s to rebound.
- Grade 4: Very deep pit (8 mm) with the dependent extremity grossly distorted that takes more than 30 s to rebound.

Pitting edema occurs in deep vein thrombosis and venous insufficiency, but also in the early stages of lymphedema because of an influx of protein rich fluid into the interstitium, before fibrosis of the subcutaneous tissue. To the contrary, myxedema and the advanced fibrotic form of lymphedema typically do not pit.

5.3.4 Skin changes

Changes in skin temperature, color, and texture allow us to understand the cause of edema (Fig. 5.2): [9–11]

- Warty texture (hyperkeratosis) with papillomatosis and brawny induration are characteristic of chronic lymphedema.
- Acute DVT and cellulitis may produce increased warmth over the affected area.
- Brown hemosiderin deposits on the lower legs and ankles are consistent with venous insufficiency hypertension.
- Varicose veins, venous stasis, and dermatitis are often associated with edema and venous insufficiency.
- Lipodermatosclerosis of the pretibial and malleolar region is the result of venous insufficiency progression even leading to venous ulcer.

Examination of the feet is important in lower extremity edema. In patients with lymphedema, there is the impossibility to pinch a fold of skin on the dorsum of the foot at the base of the second toe (so-called Kaposi–Stemmer sign) [12, 13] (Fig. 5.3).

In patients with lipedema, which is an abnormal fat distribution and constitution resulting in disproportionate, painful limbs, the feet are generally spared, although the ankles often have prominent malleolar fat pads (cuff sign) [14, 15].

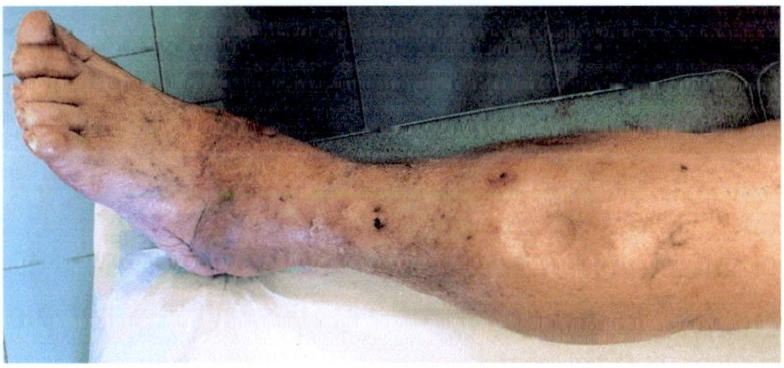

Fig. 5.2 Lipodermatosclerosis, dermatitis, and venous stasis from chronic venous insufficiency associated with edema

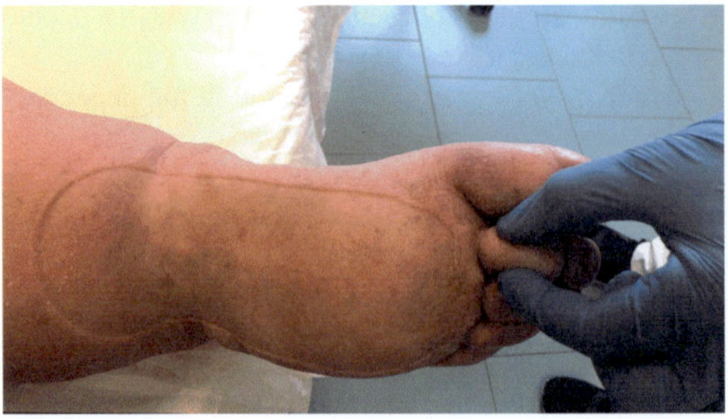

Fig. 5.3 Positive Kaposi–Stemmer sign

5.4 Diagnostic Studies

5.4.1 Laboratory Tests

Laboratory tests could be helpful to investigate systemic diseases, in particular if the etiology is still unclear. A list of laboratory tests will help to exclude systemic diseases: complete blood count, electrolytes, creatinine, urinalysis blood sugar, thyroid-stimulating hormone, and albumin [1].

5.4.2 Noninvasive Quantitative Methods to Assess Lower Limb Edema

A repeatable measurement that can size precisely the limb affected by edema or lymphedema is necessary, either to define the disease stage or to monitor its progression; furthermore, it is also useful to record the results induced by different medical therapies both conservative and surgical.

There are different noninvasive techniques described in the literature to assess peripheral edema. The limb volume can be measured by direct or indirect measurements [8].

5.4.3 Water Displacement (Volume Measurements) [16]

This method allows us to directly measure the limb volume using water immersion in a graduated displacement. The limb is immersed up to a specific level in a container previously filled with water. The volume that overflows in the adjacent container following the introduction of the leg represents an indicative parameter of limb volume.

The measurement of the leg should follow the correct standard reported in the literature: [15]

- Water level above the pretibial region
- Water temperature ranging from 28 °C to 32 °C;

– Subjects measured in sitting and resting position
– Volume assessment performed right before and right after the 5 exercise sessions
– Time of measurements between 9 and 12 a.m.

Despite it being a gold standard for measuring leg edema, this technique presents some defects: it requires considerable cooperation from the patient and a good joints mobility to place the limb inside the container; therefore, it cannot be used in case of important functional limitations. In case of skin lesions, it requires careful hygiene and accurate disinfection in the patient. It provides data regarding the immersed limb volume, but it does not give us indication regarding the edema distribution such as interstitial and intracellular components.

To the contrary, the method is suitable and useful for assessing the foot volume that could be difficult and unprecise using centimetric measurement.

5.4.4 Perometer [17]

This device evaluates the limb volume using infrared light sources stimulating specific sensors tracing the circular sections of the limb. This technique is precise and allows full leg evaluation. Its accuracy and repeatability are close to water plethysmography which remains up to now the gold standard.

5.4.5 Circumferential Method (with a Tape Measure) [18]

The limb volume can be calculated indirectly starting from a precise measurement of the limb circumferences at different levels using a flexible meter.

This measurement, compared to direct ones, presents the advantage of being rapid, inexpensive, and easily available in the clinical setting. It also provides the spatial distribution of edema, comparing the different limb segments giving the idea of the lower limb shape.

This technique shows an excellent inter-rater and test–retest reliability, but the obtained values are not comparable with the absolute volume measured with direct methods.

By assimilating the various limb segments to geometric solids, the volume is calculated applying mathematical formulas used for volume calculation. For this reason, the more the limb shape differs from theoretical solid on which the formula is based, the greater the error becomes.

The circumferences assessment can be taken at intervals of centimeters, or at predefined points by measuring the distance between these. The choice of smaller measurements ranges is based on the accuracy which also depends on the distance of the assessment points.

For consistent measurements, each upper or lower extremity is marked with a semi-permanent marker starting from bony prominences as reference. A critical point is the evaluation of the hand and the foot volume which has irregular shape, therefore hardly assimilating to geometric solids.

5.4.6 Bioimpedance (BIA)

BIA is a noninvasive technique able to measure the impedance of the human body, and it is founded on the ability of biological tissue to impede electric current, the so-called resistance. BIA is able to identify, even in a segmental way, the rate of extracellular water (ECW) out of total body water [19].

BIA use for lymphedema investigation was reported since the early 1990s, considering ECW evaluation as a fundamental parameter in the assessment of venous-lymphatic drainage alteration. Recently, it has been described for assessing the edema/lymphedema measurement during follow-up after rehabilitative interventions [20, 21].

In conclusion, after the preliminary evaluation, which can also be performed in a general medicine office, the patient should be addressed to a specialistic evaluation for detailed assessment and diagnostic integration by means for example of ultrasonography and eventually lymphoscintigraphy, which is the gold standard in lymphedema assessment. A detailed description on this diagnostic technique is reported in the related chapter of this textbook.

Maximum care must be dedicated to edema patients, particularly considering that a common condition like lymphedema is still considered a "hidden epidemic" because of its large epidemiology and is paradoxically often underdiagnosed and poorly managed condition.

References

1. Arokiasamy S, King R, Boulaghrasse H, Poston RN, Nourshargh S, Wang W, Voisin MB. Heparanase-dependent remodeling of initial lymphatic glycocalyx regulates tissue-fluid drainage during acute inflammation in vivo. Front Immunol. 2019;10:2316.
2. Trayes KP, Studdiford JS, Pickle S, Tully AS. Edema: diagnosis and management. Am Fam Phys. 2013;88:102–10.
3. Simon EB. Leg edema assessment and management. Medsurg Nurs. 2014;23:44–53.
4. Whayne TF Jr, Fisher MB. Idiopathic "Cyclic" edema: a frustrating and poorly understood clinical problem. Cardiovasc Hematol Agents Med Chem. 2018;16:88–93.
5. Ratchford EV, Evans NS. Approach to lower extremity edema. Curr Treat Opt Cardiovasc Med. 2017;19:16.
6. Topham EJ, Mortimer PS. Chronic lower limb oedema. Clin Med. 2002;2:28–31.
7. Bickley LS et al. Bates' guide to physical examination and history taking, 11th ed. Philadelphia, PA: Lippincott Williams & Wilkins. 2013. p. 505–6.
8. Brodovicz KG, McNaughton K, Uemura N, Meininger G, Girman CJ, Yale SH. Reliability and feasibility of methods to quantitatively assess peripheral edema. Clin Med Res. 2009;7:21–31.
9. Yale SH, Mazza JJ. Approach to diagnosing lower extremity edema. Compr Ther. 2001;27:242–52.
10. Ely JW, Osheroff JA, Chambliss ML, Ebell MH. Approach to leg edema of unclear etiology. J Am Board Fam Med. 2006;19:148–60.
11. Raffetto JD. Pathophysiology of chronic venous disease and venous ulcers. Surg Clin North Am. 2018;98:337–47.
12. Rockson SG. Current concepts and future directions in the diagnosis and management of lymphatic vascular disease. Vasc Med. 2010;15:223–31.

13. Jayaraj A, Raju S, May C, Pace N. The diagnostic unreliability of classic physical signs of lymphedema. J Vasc Surg Venous Lymphat Disord. 2019;7:890–7.
14. Kruppa P, Georgiou I, Biermann N, Prantl L, Klein-Weigel P, Ghods M. Lipedema-pathogenesis, diagnosis, and treatment options. Dtsch Arztebl Int. 2020;117:396–403.
15. Buso G, Depairon M, Tomson D, Raffoul W, Vettor R, Mazzolai L. Lipedema: a call to action! Obesity (Silver Spring). 2019;27:1567–76.
16. Rabe E, Stücker M, Ottillinger B. Water displacement leg volumetry in clinical studies–a discussion of error sources. BMC Med Res Methodol. 2010;13:10–5.
17. Reza C, Nørregaard S, Moffatt C, Karlsmark T. Inter-observer and intra-observer variability in volume measurements of the lower extremity using perometer. Lymphat Res Biol. 2020 Oct;18(5):416–21.
18. Kaulesar Sukul DM, den Hoed PT, Johannes EJ, van Dolder R, Benda E. Direct and indirect methods for the quantification of leg volume: comparison between water displacement volumetry, the disk model method and the frustum sign model method, using the correlation coefficient and the limits of agreement. J Biomed Eng. 1993;15:477–80.
19. Khalil SF, Mohktar MS, Ibrahim F. The theory and fundamentals of bioimpedance analysis in clinical status monitoring and diagnosis of diseases. Sensors (Basel). 2014;14:10895–928.
20. Cavezzi A, Urso SU, Paccasassi S, Mosti G, Campana F, Colucci R. Bioimpedance spectroscopy and volumetry in the immediate/short-term monitoring of intensive complex decongestive treatment of lymphedema. Phlebology. 2020 Jul 6:268355520938578.
21. Menegatti E, Pagani A, Avruscio G, Mucignat M, Gianesini S. The effects of thermal water physical exercise in patients with lower limb chronic venous insufficiency monitored by bioimpedance analysis. Diagnostics (Basel). 2020;10:889.

Investigations of Lower Limb Edema

6

Alberto Caggiati and Lorenza Caggiati

6.1 Introduction

The diagnosis of leg edema is currently based upon clinical history and laboratory investigations regarding systemic or local disorders (Table 6.1), followed by the local evaluation of objective signs.

In most cases, the local evaluation of limb edema is based upon the visual appearance of the leg, followed by skin palpation and, at the most, tape measurement of the ankle circumference.

Other techniques of edema quantification and characterization are poorly used in daily clinical practice, even be simple execution. Some of these techniques are

Table 6.1 Differential diagnosis of swollen legs

Causes of monolateral leg edema	
Local factors	Venous insufficiency, lymphatic disorders, skin diseases, inflammation or infections, trauma, previous surgery, osteoarticular, and/or neuromuscular disorders
Causes of bilateral symmetric leg edema	
Systemic diseases	Dyscrasia and dysproteinemia (renal and/or hepatic disorders), cardiac insufficiency, pulmonary disorders, malnutrition, hormonal disorders
Lifestyle	Obesity, sedentary
Drug therapies	Anti-inflammatory drugs, antihypertensive treatments, and others

A. Caggiati (✉)
Department of Anatomy, Sapienza University of Rome, Rome, Italy
e-mail: Alberto.Caggiati@uniroma1.it

L. Caggiati
Villa Margherita Hospital, Rome, Italy

S. K. Tiwary (ed.), *Approach to Lower Limb Oedema*,
https://doi.org/10.1007/978-981-16-6206-5_6

currently used only for research purposes. In turn, data obtained with these methods may help to refine the diagnosis as well as to furnish the information useful in decision-making regarding the therapy for each case.

In daily clinical practice, the more frequent cause of lower limbs edema is chronic venous disease (CVD). The presence of edema is currently considered an accurate index of CVD severity. In fact, grade 3 of the "C" score of the Clinical-Etiologic-Anatomic-Pathophysiologic classification (CEAP) consists of the presence of edema (C3) [1] Leg edema is also included in both the original and the modified versions of the Venous Clinical Severity Score (VCSS). The severity of edema is just classified as "absent" (grade 0), mild (grade 1, evening only), moderate (afternoon, grade 2), and severe (grade 3, morning) [2]. This grading is insufficient to quantify the severity of venous edema at all. In turn, a correct clinical categorization of venous edema needs a more detailed quantification of edema and characterization of tissue changes. Moreover, a correct quantification of edema is important for both the daily practice and research purposes. In addition, it seems appropriate to identify the pathogenesis of edema, necessary to plan the more appropriate treatment.

For all these reasons, even if patient history and visual inspection are enough to diagnose the presence of edema, more accurate tests are necessary for a correct overview of the clinical contest [3]. These can be shared in tests for the quantification of edema and tests for its characterization.

Quantification of edema can be performed by various methods, which can be summarized in the following three:

- Static leg circumference measurements
- Static leg volume measurements
- Dynamic leg volume measurements

Characterization of edema can be performed by radiologic (TC, MR), ultrasonographic, and physical techniques.

6.2 Static Leg Circumference Measurements

The simplest method consists of the direct measurement of the circumference of the leg at one or several points by a tape measure. Data obtained by these tests are compared with those from the contralateral leg (in the case of monolateral leg edema) or repeated to evaluate the efficacy of treatment.

More frequently, the leg circumference is evaluated 3–4 cm above the internal/medial malleolus or at the largest circumference of the calf. Accuracy of "hands-free" tape measurements can be improved using the "Leg-O-Meter" which allows for reproducible and consistent repeated evaluations because it takes into account the height at which the circumference has been measured. The Leg-O-Meter consists of a large tape measure fixed to a stand attached to a platform on which the

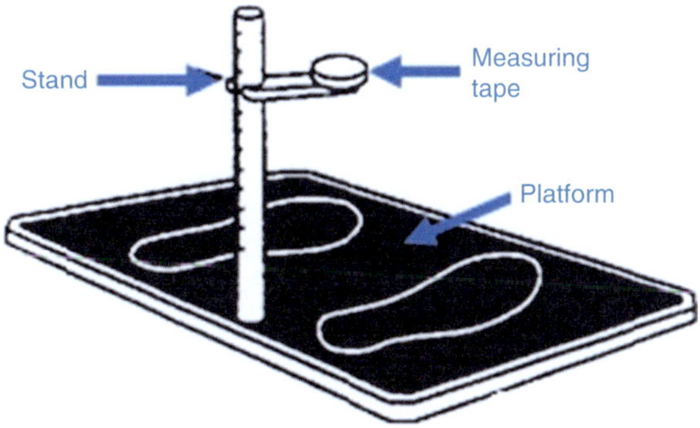

Fig. 6.1 The Leg-O-Meter

patient is in standing position. The tape measure is fixed at a fixed distance from the platform in order to obtain consistent standardized measurements by ensuring that repeated measurements are taken at the same point each time (Fig. 6.1) This is a simple and fast method and has been shown to be a reliable and standardized instrument to assess patients over time [4].

6.3 Static Leg Volume Measurements

The simplest method for leg volume measurements in static conditions is water displacement volumetry (WDV) and those based upon mathematical calculations on multiple measurements of limb circumference. Several other devices have been used to evaluate static leg volume: optoelectronic methods, computed tomography (CT), magnetic resonance (MR), and dual X-ray absorptiometry. The latter are expensive and not all of them have been validated. However, they seem to be the future investigations of choice because they allow us to discriminate the respective increase of volume of the superficial and deep compartments, as well as to furnish important information regarding the presence of muscular or osteoarticular lesions, possibly responsible for leg edema.

6.4 Water Displacement Volumetry (WDV)

WDV is generally regarded as the gold standard for measurement of lower limb volume and has become a routine screening test for assessment of leg edema (Fig. 6.2) [5]. It consists of a plexiglass box filled with water. When the leg is immersed, the displaced water spills out into a graduated receptacle. This is an inexpensive piece of equipment which allows us to measure the leg and foot volume in both the standing or sitting positions [6, 7].A variant water volumeter measures directly the level of the water in the container before and after the limb immersion. [6]

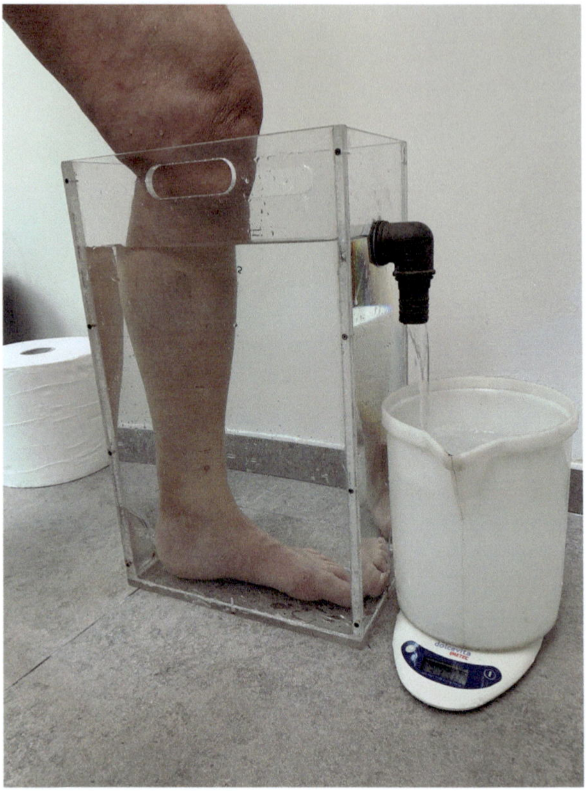

Fig. 6.2 The principle of WDV

6.5 The "Truncated Cone"

The "truncated cone" (Fig. 6.3) method is based upon the assumption that the leg approximates to the shape of one or more truncated cone(s) [8]. In its simplest version, this method is based upon the measurements of the leg circumference at the highest and lowest points of the leg segment under investigation, and on the distance between these two levels. A mathematical formula is then applied to these values to calculate the approximate volume of the leg segment between the two measurements. This technique does not include the volume of the foot.

An evolution of the truncated cone is based upon the application of the same Khunke's formula to multiple circumference measurements of the leg, with the volume measurement extending to the thigh by evaluating 11 perimeters which delimits 10 truncated cones [6, 9]. Limb volume is finally calculated as a summation of the multiple truncated cones. The perimeters are measured by weighted tapes attached every 4 cm to a semirigid stainless steel bar. The advantages of this simple device are the regular space, the horizontal position, and the reproducible traction on the tape. Both these techniques are currently used in scientific reports to evaluate the effects of pharmacologic, surgical, or physical treatments on the leg volume [5].

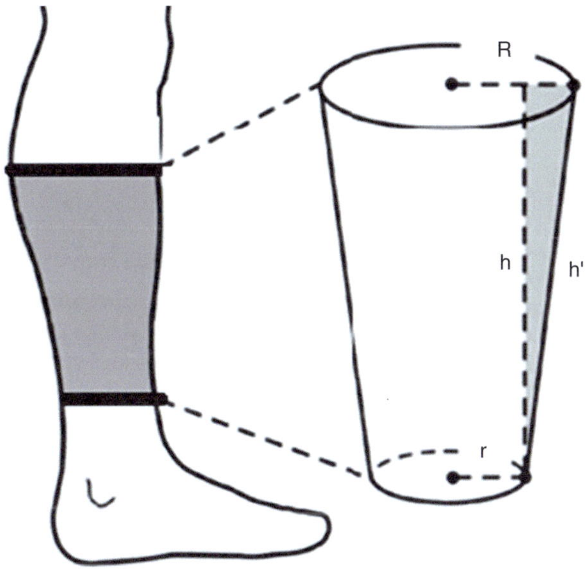

Fig. 6.3 The truncated cone

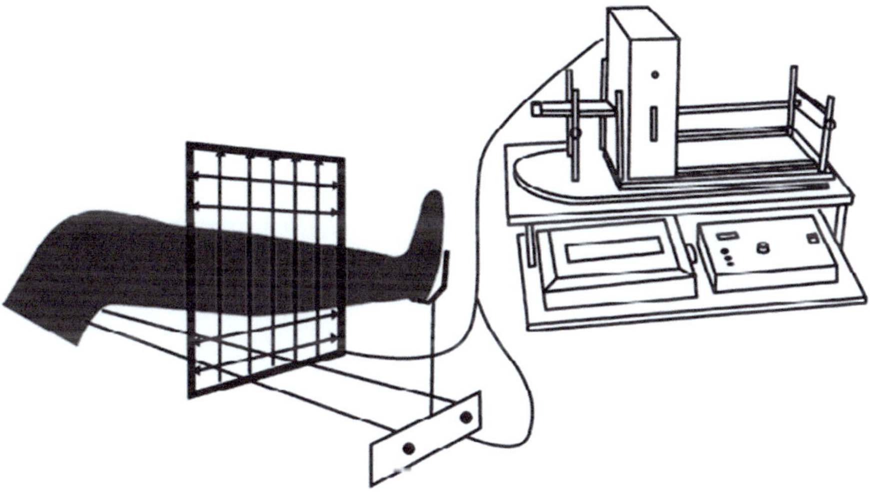

Fig. 6.4 Modified from Rabe et al., 2018

6.6 Optoelectronic Systems

Optoelectronic measurements of the leg volume are based upon infrared phototransistors which evaluate the circumference of the leg at multiple levels and calculate the volume electronically [10–13]. The leg passes through a four-sided sliding metal frame, which is equipped with infrared-detecting diodes. These emit an infrared beam that allows a three-dimensional image of the limb to be created indirectly. The volume of thin slices can then be calculated to provide an estimate of limb volume mainly in the supine position (Fig. 6.4).

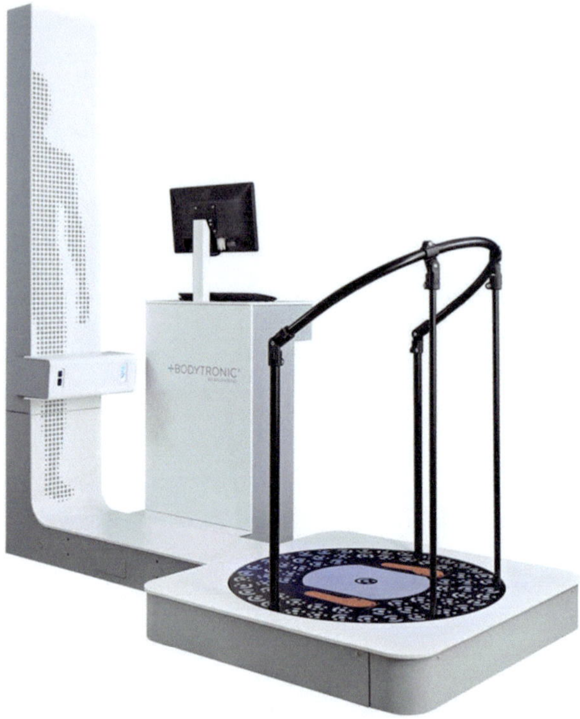

Fig. 6.5 The Bodytronic©

Recently, a novel optical three-dimensional (3D) volumetric measurement system (BODYTRONIC® 600) for the assessment of lower limb circumference and volume in standing position was introduced. Data obtained with Bodytronic was comparable to those furnished by CT [14] (Fig. 6.5).

6.7 Dynamic Volume Measurements

A few other techniques have been used to evaluate changes of leg volume provoked by special tests, i.e., postural, dynamic, or compressive maneuvers: strain gauge plethysmography and air plethysmography. These instruments evaluate changes of the calf circumference (strain gauge plethysmography) (Fig. 6.6) or of the calf volume (air plethysmography) (Fig. 6.7), for example during the elevation of the limb, during walking, during immersion, etc. [15, 16]. Accordingly, these methods are more an assessment of the venomuscular pump, vein competence, venous compliance, and/or venous outflow more than to quantify absolute volume variations [16].

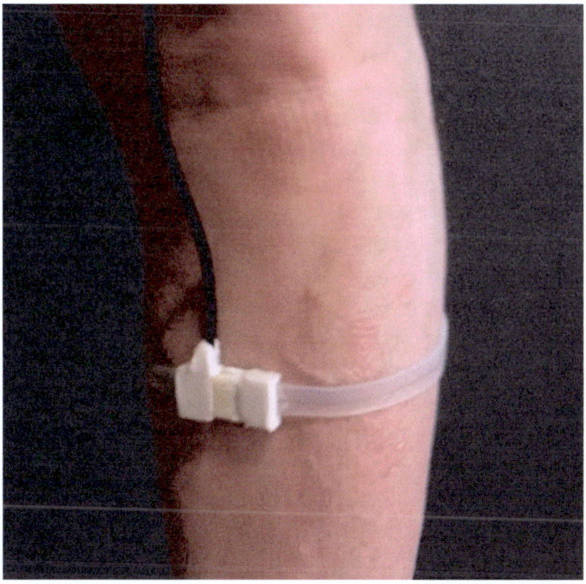

Fig. 6.6 Strain gauge plethysmography. By courtesy of Giorgio Bergamo, Microlabitalia, Padua (I)

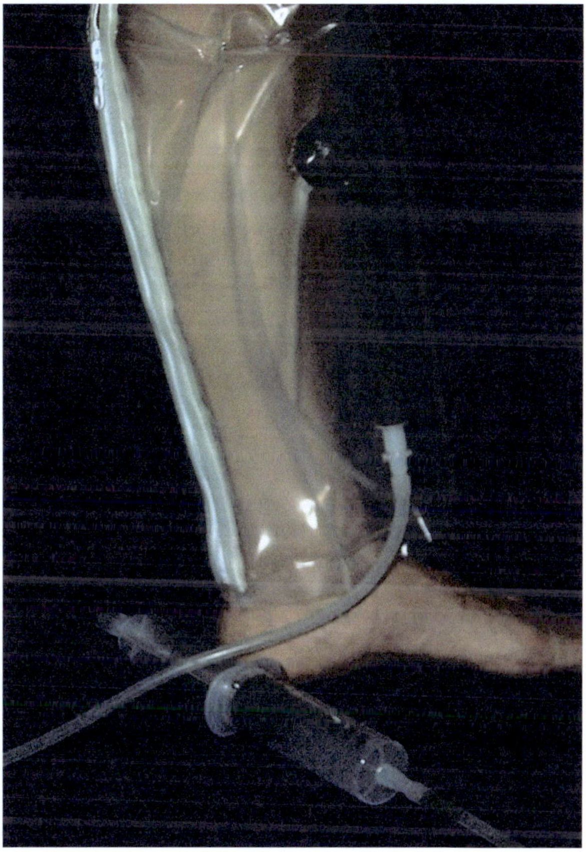

Fig. 6.7 Air plethysmography. By courtesy of Giorgio Bergamo, Microlabitalia, Padua (I)

6.8 Techniques for the Qualitative Evaluation of Leg Edema

In clinical practice, palpation is the most widely used technique to assess lower limb edema: the physician applies pressure with the index finger to a single point on the patient's ankle skin provoking or not a fovea (pitting or non-pitting edema). This maneuver allows us to evaluate the pit depth and the time necessary for the skin to return to its original appearance. The test is empirically graded with a score ranging from 0 to 4 (Table 6.2). While commonly used in clinical practice, this is an unvalidated, qualitative, and subjective measure of edema.

Pitting edema occurs in most diseases. Non-pitting edema occurs in thyroid disorders (myxedema), skin trauma, and infections. It is also reported to occur in lymphedema. However, in the first stages of lymphedema, skin edema may be compressible. Similarly, in the same conditions of venous disorders edema is not or poorly pitting. In these cases, pitting is painful and pain allows to exert only light and short compressions.

Recently, a new method was proposed to exactly measure the depth of the fovea, and a positive correlation between depth of the fovea and skin thickness was demonstrated [17].

Bioelectrical Impedance

Measurements of bioelectrical impedance are used to evaluate volume changes in human limbs [7, 18, 19]. A low intensity constant electrical current is applied to a subject's limb, and surface electrodes measure the resulting voltage. This technique is used to estimate relative changes in liquid distribution, also provoking a change in limb volume. A reduction of the leg bioimpedance with lower voltage with respect to the baseline corresponds to an increase of the fluid content of the limb and vice versa. Bioimpedance allows us to evaluate the extra- and intracellular water rates. In fact, due to the high impedance of the cell's membranes, using frequencies below 1 kHz, it is possible to evaluate the flow through extracellular fluid to quantify this parameter [20]. Bioimpedance can be performed without cloth removal and can be used in legs with dermatitis or ulcers (which cannot be tested by water immersion techniques). On the contrary, individuals with pacemakers and metal implants cannot be measured using this technique.

Table 6.2 Grading of skin pitting

Grade	Depth of the fovea	Definition
1	2 mm or less	Slight pitting, no visible distortion, disappears rapidly
2	2–4 mm	Somewhat deeper pit, no readably detectable distortion, disappears in 10–25 s
3	4–6 mm	Pit is noticeably deep. May last more than a minute. Dependent extremity looks swollen and fuller
4	6–8 mm	Pit is very deep. Lasts for 2–5 min. Dependent extremity is grossly distorted

6.9 Computed Tomography and Magnetic Resonance Leg Imaging

Computed tomography (CT) [21, 22] and magnetic resonance (MR) [23, 24] imaging may be used not only to measure the leg volumes but also to evaluate vascular, musculotendinous, or osteoarticular lesions in the deep or superficial compartments causing edema. CT and MRI can quantify edema in the different compartments of the limb. In particular, they are the only techniques allowing us to diagnose volume increase of the deep compartment. CT and MRI are also useful to possibly discriminate various causes of leg edema by differentiating lymphedema, lipedema, and venous edema.

In particular, MRI is even more used in the diagnosis and staging of limb lymphedema. Recent studies demonstrated the possible role of contrast less MRI in diagnosis of early-stage lymphedema in patients with borderline clinical measurements. MRI is particularly indicated in the long-term follow-up, especially if considering it is noninvasive and more readily accessible compared to lymphoscintigraphy or to lymphangiography.

6.10 Dual X-Ray Absorptiometry

Dual-energy X-ray absorptiometry (DXA) is capable of measuring regional body composition providing information about fat mass, lean mass, and bone mass for both total body and subregions. DXA was successful in the evaluation of limbs lymphedema and of lipedema of the leg [25–27].

6.11 Ultrasonography

High-frequency ultrasound allows us to visualize tissues of the superficial compartment. In swollen legs, US shows two patterns of subcutaneous thickening: (1) diffuse soaking with light increase of tissue echogenicity or (2) anechoic lacunae of variable size and extension. Moreover, US is the only technique allowing for an easy demonstration of dermal edema which can accompany or not subcutaneous edema.

Skin morphology is evaluated by the same probes used for Duplex evaluation of superficial veins. US allows us to exactly measure the thickness of the superficial compartment, its difference between the two limbs, and changes following treatment [28–30].

Besides skin thickness, US allows us to evaluate tissue echogenicity: the increase or reduction of tissue echogenicity corresponds respectively to increased cellularity (inflammation) or increase of water content. The latter can be diffused or concentrated in anechoic folds. Moreover, US allows us to identify the presence of dermal edema consisting of the increase of dermal thickness [29]. Edema of the dermis (alias: dermal edema, DE) may be present or not in legs with venous insufficiency.

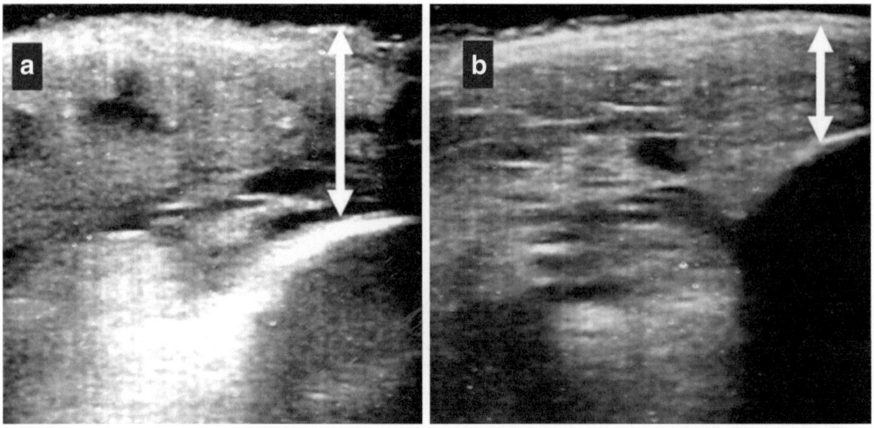

Fig. 6.8 Pitting test by US probe: (**a**) A positive squeezing test by US. (**b**) The thickness of the subcutaneous layer reduces significantly with disappearing of dermal edema

DE consists of an increase of water content of the dermis, with dermal thickening and hypoechogenicity. In most cases, edema is limited to the papillary dermis.

Tissue echogenicity is evaluated by the visual comparison of US findings from the swollen limb areas and the adjacent or contralateral homologous areas.

Finally, US allows us to better evaluate the pitting phenomena by compressing the skin with the probe instead of the finger. This maneuver allows us to quantify the compression-related reduction of skin thickness, the time of recovery of the initial conditions, and structural changes provoked by the pressure exerted on the skin. (Fig. 6.8). Skin squeezing by the US probe is negative in the presence of inflammatory processes and lipedema.

A positive squeezing test (Fig. 6.8) easily reveals those legs in which a mechanical treatment (manual or pneumatic lymphatic drainage, massotherapy, etc.) may effectively reduce the SCL or CL edema.

However, US does not allow for a differential diagnosis of the cause of leg edema. In fact, current knowledge is limited to the differential diagnosis between edema of the subcutaneous layer and increase in volume of the muscular compartment. With regard to subcutaneous edema, US allows us to discriminate between inflammatory and non-inflammatory causes.

Funding The author was kindly supported by Bauerfeind AG, Germany.

References

1. Vasquez MA, Rabe E, McLafferty CK, Shortell RB, Marston WA, Gillespie D, et al. Revision of the venous clinical severity score: venous outcomes consensus statement: special communication of the American venous forum ad hoc outcomes working group. J Vasc Surg. 2010;52:1387–96.

2. Wittens C, Davies AH, Baekgaerd N, Broholm R, Cavezzi A, Chastanet S, et al. Editor's choice. Management of chronic venous disease: clinical practice guidelines of the European Society for Vascular Surgery (ESVS). Eur J Vasc Endovasc Surg. 2015;49:678–737.
3. Rabe E, Carpentier P, Maggioli A. Understanding lower leg volume measurements used in clinical studies focused on venous leg edema. Int Angiol. 2018;37(6):437–43.
4. Berard A, Kurz X, Zuccarelli F, et al. And the VEINES group: reliability study of the leg-O-meter, an improved tape measure device, in patients with chronic venous insufficiency of the leg. Angiology. 1998;49:169–73.
5. Mosti G, Caggiati A. The effects of water immersion and walking on leg volume, ankle circumference and epifascial thickness in healthy subjects with occupational edema. Phlebology. 2021;36(6):473–80. https://doi.org/10.1177/0268355520984065. Epub 2021 Jan 6. PMID: 33407051
6. Rabe E, Stucker M, Ottilinger B. Water displacement leg volumetry in clinical studies. A discussion of error sources. BMC Med Res Methodol. 2010 Jan;13(10):5. https://doi.org/10.1186/1471-2288-10-5.
7. Wall R, Lips O, Seibt R, Rieger MA, Steinhilber B. Intra- and inter-rater reliability of lower leg water plethysmography, bioelectrical impedance and muscle twitch force for the use in standing work evaluation. Physiol Meas. 2017;38(5):701–14.
8. Devoogdt L, Van Nuland G, Christiaens C, Van Kampen M. A new device to measure upper limb circumferences: validity and reliability. Int Angiol. 2010,29(5):401–7.
9. Perrin M, Guex JJ. Edema and leg volume: methods of assessment. Angiology. 2000;51:9.12.
10. Blume J, Langenbahn H, Champvallins M. Quantification of edema using the volumeter technique: therapeutic application of Daflon 500 mg in chronic venous insufficiency. Phlebology. 1992;2(Suppl):37–40.
11. Tierney S, Aslam M, Rennie K, et al. Infrared optoelectronic volumetry, the ideal way to measure limb volume. Eur J Vasc Endovasc Surg. 1996;12:412–7.
12. Northfield JW, Holroyd B, et al. Validation of an optoelectronic limb volumeter (Perometer). Lymphology. 1997;30:77–97.
13. Veraart JCJM, Neumann HAM. Leg volume measurements with a modified optoelectronic measurement system. Phlebology. 1995;10:62–4.
14. Tischer T, Oye S, Wolf A, Feldhege F, Jacksteit R, Mittelmeier W, Bader R, Mau-Moeller A. Measuring lower limb circumference and volume - introduction of a novel optical 3D volumetric measurement system. Biomed Tech (Berl). 2020;65(2):237.
15. Mosti G, Bergamo G, Oberto S, Bissacco D, Chiodi L, Kontothanassis D, Caggiati A. The feasibility of underwater computerized strain gauge plethysmography and the effects of hydrostatic pressure on the leg venous Haemodynamics. EJVES Vasc Forum. 2020;47:60–2.
16. Rosfors S, Persson LM, Blomgren L. Computerized venous strain-gauge plethysmography is a reliable method for measuring venous function. Eur J Vasc Endovasc Surg. 2014;47(1):81–6.
17. Kogo H, Murata J, Murata S, Higashi T. Validity of a new quantitative evaluation method that uses the depth of the surface imprint as an indicator for pitting edema. PLoS One. 2017;12(1):e0170810.
18. Nishibe T, Nishibe M, Akiyama S, et al. Bioelectrical impedance analysis of leg edema and its association with venous functions in patients with saphenous varicose veins. Int Angiol. 2020;39:284–9.
19. Barnes MD, Mani R, Barrett DF, et al. How to measure changes in edema in patients with chronic venous ulcers? Phlebology. 1992;7:31–5.
20. Jaffrin MY, Morel H. Body fluid volumes measurements by impedance: a review of bioimpedance spectroscopy (BIS) and bioimpedance analysis (BIA) methods. Med Eng Phys. 2008 Dec;30(10):1257–69
21. Marotel M, Cluzan RV, Pascot M, et al. Tomodensitomtrie de 150 cas de lymphoedemes des membres inferieurs. J Radiol. 1998,79,1373–8.
22. Ling H, et al. Volumetric differences in the suprafascial and subfascial compartments of patients with secondary unilateral lower limb lymphedema. Plastic Reconstr Surg. 2020;145:1528–37.

23. Cluzan RV, Pereti IDDI, Alliot AF, et al. Cutaneous and subcutaneous changes in lymphedema analysed with high resolution MR imaging, indirect lymphography and lymphoscintigraphy. In: Whitte M, Whitte C, editors. Progress in lymphology XIV. Lymphology; 1994. p. 305–8.
24. Arrivé L, Derhy S, Dahan B, El Mouhadi S, Monnier-Cholley L, Menu Y, Becker C. Primary lower limb lymphoedema: classification with non-contrast MR lymphography. Eur Radiol. 2018 Jan;28(1):291–300.
25. Czerniec SA, Ward LC, Meerkin JD, Kilbreath SL. Assessment of segmental arm soft tissue composition in breast cancer-related lymphedema: a pilot study using dual energy X-ray absorptiometry and bioimpedance spectroscopy. Lymphat Res Biol. 2015 Mar;13(1):33–9.
26. Dietzel R, Reisshauer A, Jahr S, Calafiore D, Armbrecht G. Body composition in lipoedema of the legs using dual-energy X-ray absorptiometry: a case-control study. Br J Dermatol. 2015;173(2):594–6. https://doi.org/10.1111/bjd.13697. Epub 2015 Jul 2. PMID: 25641018
27. Hidding JT, Viehoff PB, Beurskens CH, van Laarhoven HW, Nijhuis-van der Sanden MW, van der Wees PJ. Measurement properties of instruments for measuring of lymphedema: systematic review. Phys Ther. 2016;96(12):1965–81.
28. Caggiati A. Utrasonography of skin changes in legs with chronic venous disease. Eur J Vasc Endovasc Surg. 2016 Oct;52(4):534–42.
29. Caggiati A, Caggiati L. Sonography of leg venous edema. Acta Phlebologica. 2018;19:59–62.
30. Caggiati A. Ultrasound of verrucous hyperplasia of the skin related to venous stasis and effects of compression treatment. J Vasc Surg Cases Innov Technol. 2019;5(3):225–7.

Differential Diagnosis of Lower Extremity Oedema

7

Sandeep Raj Pandey and Moorooteea Mehta Raaka Rai

7.1 Introduction

Lower extremity edema with a wide range of possible etiologies is a common problem in older patients. The diagnosis can be narrowed by categorizing the edema according to its duration, distribution, and accompanying symptoms. The differential diagnosis includes systemic illnesses such as heart failure, liver disease, malnutrition, and thyroid disorder; local conditions such as pelvic tumors, infection, trauma, venous thrombosis, chronic venous diseases, cellulitis, lymphoedema, and lipoedema; and various medications (antihypertensives, hormones, chemotherapy, NSAIDs, etc.) known to increase the risk of edema of the lower extremities. Patients with lower limb edema are frequently referred to vascular specialists for differential diagnosis evaluation and further management. Appropriate therapy is based on the presentation of edema and its identified etiology and differential diagnoses.

Detailed evaluation of lower extremity edema differential diagnoses mainly depends on:

History [1, 2]

1. **Duration** in acute is (<72 h) vs. chronic.
2. **Pain** is common in deep vein thrombosis, CRPS, less severe in venous insufficiency.

S. R. Pandey (✉)
Annapurna Hospital, Kathmandu, Nepal

M. M. R. Rai
Victoria Hospital, Quatre Bornes, Mauritius

S. K. Tiwary (ed.), *Approach to Lower Limb Oedema*,
https://doi.org/10.1007/978-981-16-6206-5_7

3. **If systemic disease:**

   Cardiac disease presents orthopnea and paroxysmal nocturnal dyspnea.
   Renal disease has proteinuria.
   Hepatic disease presents jaundice and ascites.

4. **Malignancy** condition presents lymphedema.
5. Ther's improvement with elevation/recumbency in venous insufficiency.
6. In OSA **there is** snoring and daytime somnolence.
7. **Medications:** B-blocker, calcium channel blockers, hormones, nonsteroidal anti-inflammatory drugs.

Physical Exam [1, 2]

1. **Distribution:** can be **unilateral, bilateral, or generalized**
2. **Quality:** can be pitting or non-pitting
3. **TTP:** DVT, cellulitis
4. **Varicose veins:** venous insufficiency
5. **Kaposi–Stemmer:** inability to pinch dorsum of foot at base of 2nd toe (lymphedema)

Lower extremity edema either unilateral or bilateral is acute or chronic:

Unilateral acute lower limb edema mainly occurs due to deep vein thrombosis, cellulitis, ruptured Baker's cyst, ruptured medial head of gastrocnemius, and compartment syndrome.

Unilateral chronic lower limb edema may occur due to venous insufficiency, lymphedema as a result of radiation, surgery, abdominal or pelvic malignancy, bacterial infection and complex regional pain syndrome, pelvic tumor or lymphoma causing external pressure on veins, congenital venous malformations, and May–Thurner syndrome (iliac-vein compression syndrome).

Bilateral acute lower limb edema mainly occurs due to drugs or bilateral deep vein thrombosis or acute worsening of systemic diseases (heart failure, renal disease).

Bilateral chronic lower limb edema occurs due to systemic disease mainly cardiac, renal (nephritic syndrome, glomerulonephritis), hepatic or pulmonary hypertension, venous insufficiency bilaterally, OSA, Lymphedema (secondary to tumor, radiation, bacterial infection, filariasis), lipedema, premenstrual edema, pelvic tumor or lymphoma causing external pressure, dependent edema, diuretic-indued edema, preeclampsia, anemia, protein losing enteropathy, malnutrition, malabsorption, restrictive pericarditis, restrictive cardiomyopathy, late pregnancy, and idiopathic edema.

7.2 Brief Details of Common Causes

7.2.1 DVT and Chronic Venous Disease

Deep vein thrombosis occurring mainly in the soleal plexus results in obstruction to venous flow. One of a swollen, warm, tender calf is the clinical picture of DVT. The resulting edema is pitting (Fig. 7.1) in nature and is usually much softer than in established lymphedema. Often, there are underlying risk factors, such as recent surgery or immobility, malignancy, a preceding long duration flight >6 h., or thrombophilia. The diagnosis is confirmed with duplex scanning or venography. Treatment is with anticoagulation [3].

One of the long-term sequelae of DVT is post-thrombotic syndrome (PTS). Here, there is reflux in the deep venous system, or deep venous insufficiency, resulting in chronic swelling of the limb, lipodermatosclerosis, and varicose veins, and in severe cases, venous ulceration (Figs. 7.2 and 7.3). On clinical grounds alone, this may be more difficult to differentiate from lymphedema, and further investigation, as outlined later in lymphedema details below in Sect. 2.3, may be required [3].

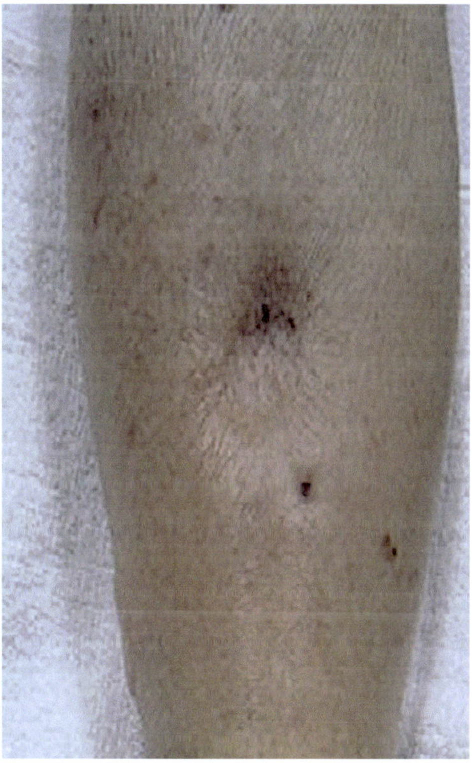

Fig. 7.1 DVT pitting edema

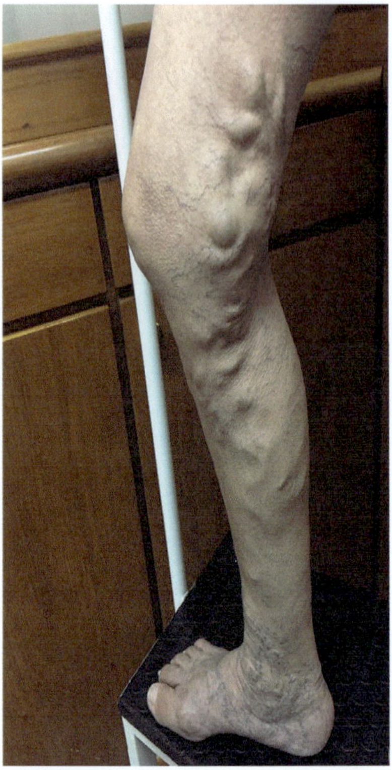

Fig. 7.2 Varicose veins

7.2.2 Cellulitis

Recurrent cellulitis can complicate venous disease (Fig. 7.4) of the lower limb, exacerbating swelling and venous hypertension and making venous ulcers harder to treat because lymph exudes through ulcers.

Key features which distinguish cellulitis are it is typically unilateral and acute and often presents with systemic symptoms (fever, leukocytosis).

Risk factors of cellulitis are immunosuppression, previous episodes, DM, PVD, etc.

7.2.3 Lymphedema

Lymphedema is found in both sexes, although women are investigated for this disease more often than men. It can be seen at any age as already noted, and two-thirds of cases are unilateral. The distal part of the leg is affected initially, with proximal extension occurring later. The feet are not spared. Patients with complete absence of lymphatics have a history of long-term swelling, while those with impaired lymphatics have a shorter history.

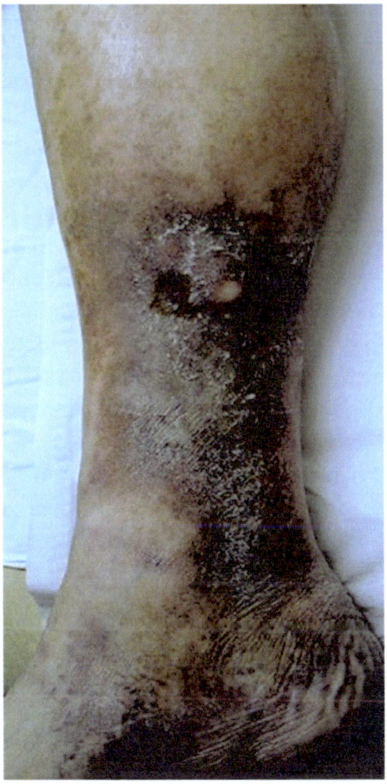

Fig. 7.3 PTS

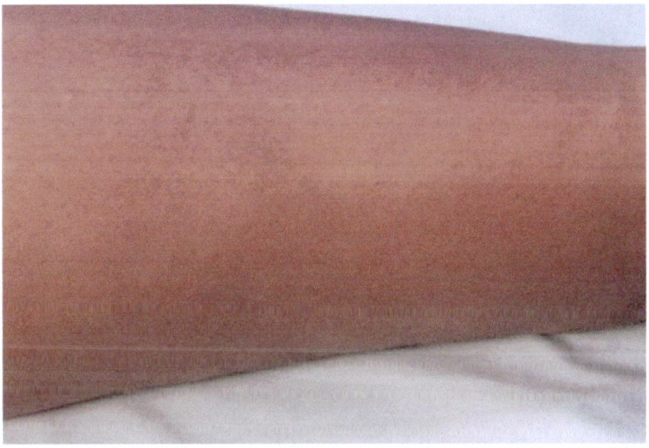

Fig. 7.4 Cellulitis edema

The initial symptom is usually painless swelling. The patient may also complain of a feeling of heaviness in the limb, especially at the end of the day and in hot weather. Symptoms may vary throughout the menstrual cycle [4].

On initial examination, the swelling is seen as pitting edema, but with time, fibrosis in the subcutaneous tissues causes the classical non-pitting signs [4]. The distribution is asymmetrical, and patients have a positive Stemmer sign (the inability to pinch the skin of the dorsum of the second toe between the thumb and forefinger) [5]. Early in the disease process, the edema can spread proximally (or distally), but this is uncommon after the first year. Radial enlargement, however, is usually progressive if treatment is not instituted. With time, skin changes are seen over the affected area; the skin becomes thicker (hyperkeratosis) and rougher (papillomatosis) and skin turgor is increased [4, 6]. In severe cases, the skin can break down, with lymph exuding through any skin breaks. This compromises healing and leads to an increased risk of infection. Recurrent infections, cellulitis, and lymphangitis are common. This unfortunately can lead to further deterioration in lymphatic drainage, ending in a vicious cycle of infection and worsening edema.

Lymphangiosarcoma is a rare late complication of lymphedema [4]. This was originally described in the lymphedematous arms of patients following radical mastectomy (Stewart Treves syndrome [7]) but has also been described in patients with Milroy disease [8]. It appears to be an earlier complication following radical mastectomy than in those with congenital lymphedema (average, 10 vs 38 years postdiagnosis) [9]. Treatment is primary radiotherapy, with surgery reserved for patients with discrete, nonmetastatic disease.

7.2.3.1 Primary Lymphedema

This is caused by a congenital abnormality or dysfunction in the lymphatic system and can be further classified according to age at initial examination (Fig. 7.5). The congenital form is detected at birth or in the first year of life and may either be sporadic or familial. The familial form is known as Milroy disease and is rare [10]. It is thought to result from an autosomal inheritance of a single gene [11]. The onset of lymphedema praecox is between the ages of 1 and 35 years [4]. The onset of lymphedema tarda occurs after 35 years of age [4].

The most common of these is the praecox variety. Primary lymphedema is more common in females, especially lymphedema praecox, where the onset is particularly common around menarche [5]. Symptoms may be linked to a minor trauma [12], suggesting that the abnormal lymphatics have coped under normal circumstances but are unable to cope with an increase in tissue fluid.

Alternatively, primary lymphedema can be classified according to the abnormality found in the lymphatics. Thus, it may be aplastic, hypoplastic, or hyperplastic. These terms suggest an abnormality in the development of the lymphatic system. While this is true for congenital lymphedema, cases of later-onset primary lymphedema might be due to an acquired abnormality. It is difficult to prove whether the abnormal lymphatics seen when these patients were investigated had existed in the same state since birth. Browse and Stewart have made a case for a new classification system that disposes of these terms [13].

Primary hypoplastic lymphedema can be further subdivided into proximal and distal hypoplasia. The most common form of primary lymphedema is distal hypoplasia. It is milder, often bilateral, and symptoms are confined to below the knee. Not surprisingly, proximal disease causes more severe symptoms, with whole-limb swelling. Patients with primary hyperplastic lymphedema have an increased

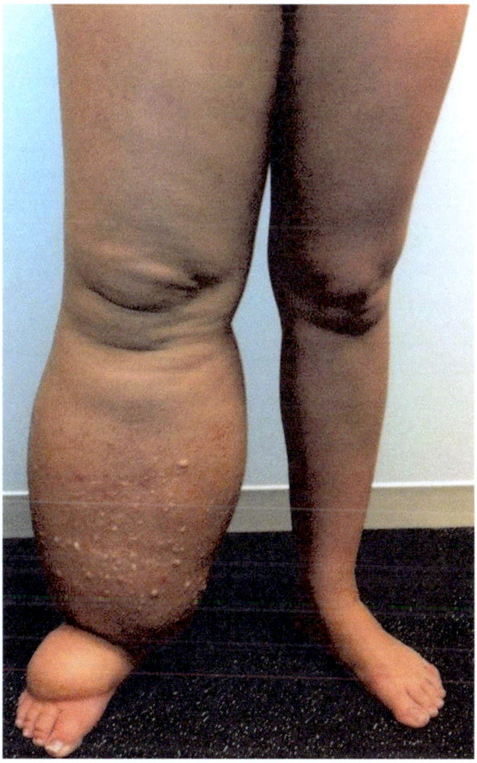

Fig. 7.5 Primary lymphedema

number and size of lymphatics. It is unusual in that it has a male preponderance and is more often familial [14]. An association with other congenital abnormalities is sometimes seen. The thoracic duct may be absent or abnormal in such patients.

7.2.3.2 Secondary Lymphedema

Secondary lymphedema is edema due to a reduction in lymph flow by an acquired cause. The causes of secondary lymphedema include trauma [15, 16], recurrent infection [17], and malignancy, including metastatic disease. In the developed world, the most common cause of secondary lymphedema is malignancy (including that resulting from cancer treatment). Lymphedema is common in the developing world secondary to infection with the parasitic nematode *Wuchereria bancrofti* (otherwise known as filariasis and in complicated stage elephantiasis), making this the most common cause of lymphedema worldwide (Fig. 7.6).

It is unusual for surgery alone to cause lymphedema, as lymphatics have excellent regenerative capabilities. Some series have shown significant lymphatic damage in more than 60% of patients undergoing varicose vein surgery [18]. Lymphedema is unusual after varicose vein surgery, but patients should be examined preoperatively, as vein stripping can significantly exacerbate mild lymphedema. Patients with venous disease have been shown to have impaired lymphatic drainage [18].

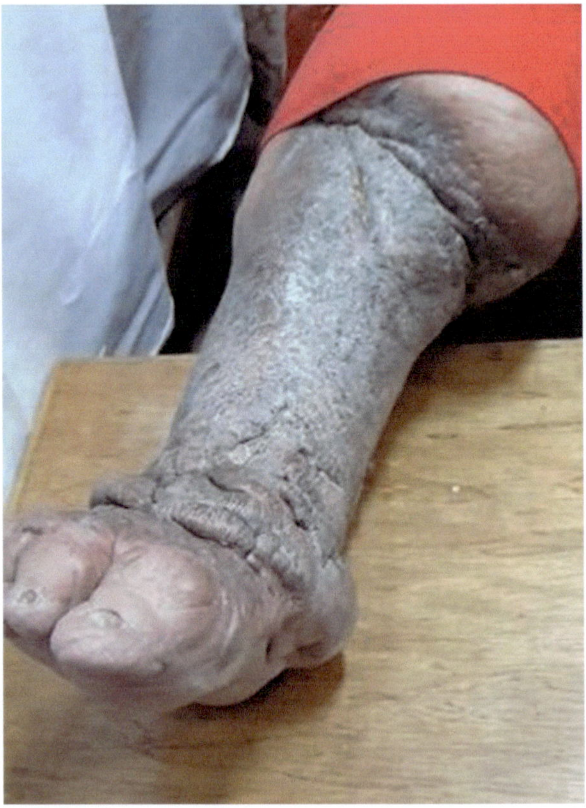

Fig. 7.6 Filariasis (elephantiasis)-secondary lymphedema

Even after radical lymph node excision for malignancy, lymphedema does not always ensue. When it does occur, it is often a late complication. The reasons for this late development are uncertain, but gradual failure of distal lymphatics, which have to "pump" lymph at a greater pressure through damaged proximal ducts, has been postulated. The transected lymphatics will regenerate after node clearance procedures. If combined with radiotherapy, however, the risk of lymphedema is higher, as fibrous scarring reduces regrowth of ducts [19].

7.2.4 Lipedema

Lipedema is also known as lipomatosis of the leg (Fig. 7.7). The clinical features of lipedema include early age of onset, female exclusivity, and positive family history in some patients [20, 21]. The clinical signs include elastic symmetrical enlargement of both legs with sparing of the feet. so-called riding breech thighs and stove pipe legs, [22] hypothermia of the skin, a negative Stemmer sign, and plantar positioning alterations. Weight loss does not affect leg appearance [21].

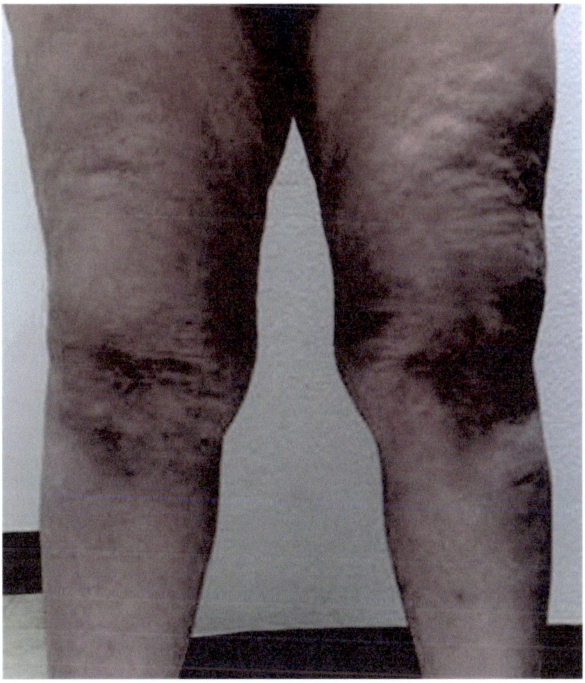

Fig. 7.7 Lipedema

7.2.5 Postoperative Swelling

Postoperative edema occurs predominantly after arterial reconstruction. The incidence of peripheral edema following arterial reconstruction is high, especially if the procedure is a femoropopliteal bypass [23]. If the swelling is significant (>4.5-cm increase in diameter), it is more likely to be due to thrombosis of the tibial or popliteal veins [24]. Following arterial reconstruction, there may be impairment of lymphatic drainage or lymphatic disruption secondary to the surgical dissection in the thigh and popliteal region. The swelling may persist for up to 3 months

7.2.6 Compartment Syndrome

Compartment syndrome occurs when excessive pressure builds up inside an enclosed muscle space in the body. Compartment syndrome usually results from bleeding or swelling after an injury.

Acute compartment syndrome usually develops over a few hours after a serious injury to an arm or leg. Some symptoms of acute compartment syndrome include:

- New and persistent deep ache in an arm or leg
- Pain that seems greater than expected for the severity of the injury
- Numbness, pins-and-needles, or electricity-like pain in the limb
- Swelling, tightness, and bruising

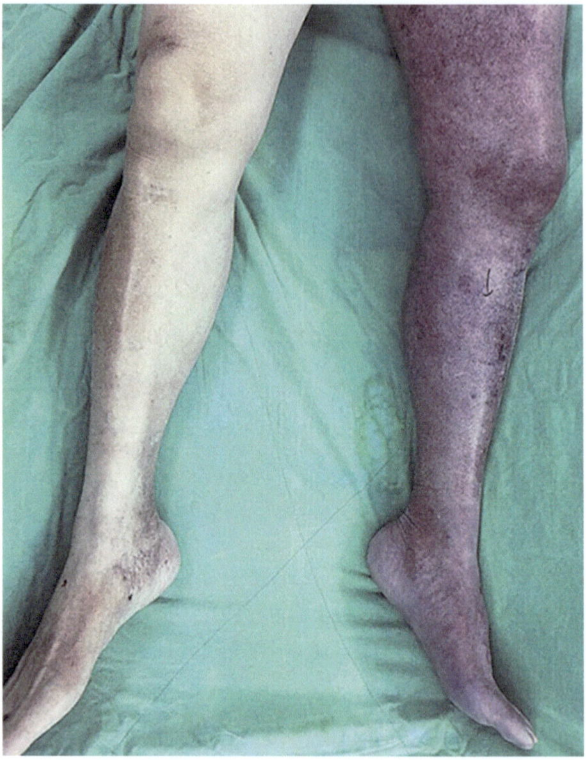

Fig. 7.8 Compartment syndrome

Emergency fasciotomy is needed to release edema.

Symptoms of chronic compartment syndrome (Fig. 7.8) (exertional compartment syndrome) include worsening of aching or cramping in the affected muscle (buttock, thigh, or lower leg) within a half-hour of starting exercise. Symptoms usually go away with rest, and muscle function remains normal. Exertional compartment syndrome can feel like shin splints and be confused with that condition.

7.2.7 Systemic Diseases

Lower extremity edema mainly seen in systemic diseases can be cardiac cause (Fig. 7.9) hepatic cause (Fig. 7.10), or renal cause. Cardiac also presents **JVD and crackles.** Hepatic presents **ascites, scleral icterus, and spider angiomas.** Renal presents oliguria or anuria.

7.2.8 Venous Malformation

Lower extremity edema also noted in congenital venous malformation such as KTS. (Fig. 7.11)

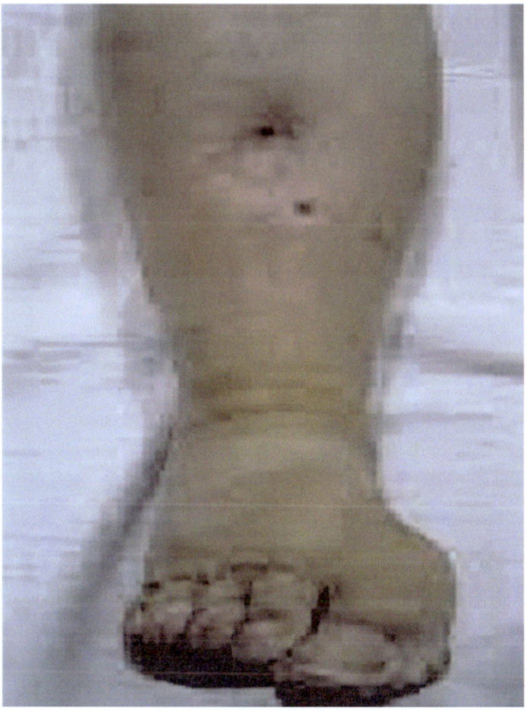

Fig. 7.9 Cardiac edema

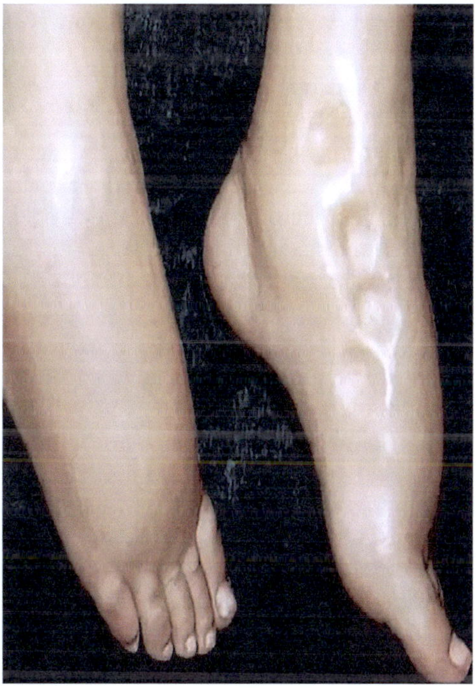

Fig. 7.10 Hepatic edema

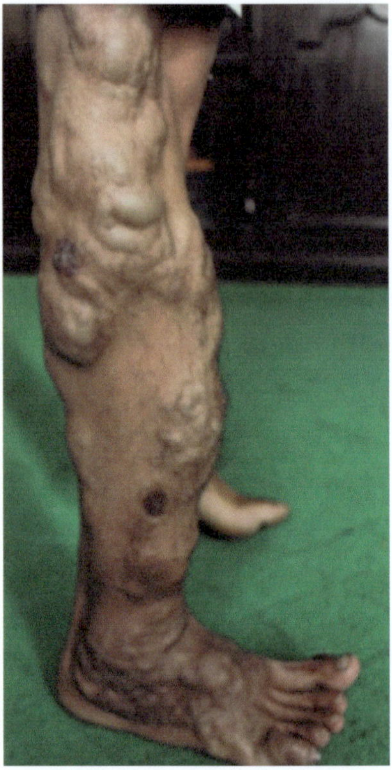

Fig. 7.11 Venous malformation in KTS

7.3 Summary

In approaching lower limb edema, a variety of etiologies and differential diagnoses must be considered to facilitate a systematic approach to patients presenting with either acute or chronic lower extremity edema in a unilateral or bilateral fashion.

Milestone-scientific literatures published globally during the last 10 years on differential diagnosis of lower extremity edema:

1. https://www.ncbi.nlm.nih.gov/pmc/articles/PMC7536506/
2. https://www.ncbi.nlm.nih.gov/pmc/articles/PMC5948740/
3. https://ddxof.com/lower-extremity-edema/
4. https://www.researchgate.net/publication/303916366_Management_of_Patients_With_Venous_Leg_Ulcers_Challenges_and_Current_Best_Practice
5. https://www.ncbi.nlm.nih.gov/pmc/articles/PMC6657795/
6. https://www.hindawi.com/journals/ulcers/2013/413604/
7. https://journals.sagepub.com/doi/10.1177/0268355519870690
8. https://www.msdmanuals.com/professional/gynecology-and-obstetrics/symptoms-during-pregnancy/lower-extremity-edema-during-late-pregnancy
9. https://pubmed.ncbi.nlm.nih.gov/7695655/

References

1. Trayes KP, Studdiford JS, Pickle S, Tully AS. Edema: diagnosis and management. Am Family Phys. 2013;88(2):102–10.
2. Ely JW, Osheroff JA, Chambliss ML, Ebell MH. Approach to leg edema of unclear etiology. J Am Board Family Med: JABFM. 2006;19(2):148–60.
3. Myint F, Platts A, Hamilton G. Thrombophilia. Peds. Vascular and Endovascular Surgery. WB Saunders Co Ltd 2001;415–50.
4. Schirger A. Lymphedema. Cardiovasc Clin. 1983;13:293–305.
5. Harwood CA, Bull RH, Evans J, Mortimer PS. Lymphatic and venous function in lipoedema. Br J Dermatol. 1996;13:41–6.
6. Lewis JM, Wald ER. Lymphedema praecox. J Pediatr. 1984;104:641–8.
7. Mortimer PS. Swollen lower limb-2: lymphoedema. BMJ. 2000;32:1527–9.
8. Stewart FW, Treves N. Lymphangiosarcoma in postmastectomy lymphedema: a report of six cases in elephantiasis chirurgica. Cancer. 1948;1:64–81.
9. Brostrom LA, Nilsonne U, Kronberg M, Soderberg G. Lymphangiosarcoma in chronic hereditary oedema (Milroy's disease). Ann Chir Gynaecol. 1989;78:320–3.
10. Chen KT, Gilbert EF. Angiosarcoma complicating generalized lymphangiectasia. Arch Pathol Lab Med. 1979;103:86–8.
11. Milroy WF. Chronic hereditary edema: Milroy's disease. JAMA. 1928;91:1172–5.
12. Salem AH, Mulhim AM, Grant C, Khwaja MS. Milroy's disease in a Saudi family. J R Coll Surg (Edin). 1986;31:143–6.
13. Allen EV. Lymphedema of the extremities. classification, etiology and differential diagnosis. Arch Int Med 1934;54606-624.
14. Wolfe JH, Kinmonth JB. The prognosis of primary lymphedema of the lower limbs. Arch Surg. 1981;116:1157–60.
15. Ter SE, Alavi A, Kim CK, Merli G. Lymphoscintigraphy: reliable test for the diagnosis of lymphedema. Clin Nucl Med. 1993;18:646–54.
16. Cambria RA, Gloviczki P, Naessens JM, Wahner HW. Noninvasive evaluation of the lymphatic system with lymphoscintigraphy: a prospective, semiquantitative analysis in 386 extremities. J Vasc Surg. 1993;18:773–82.
17. Richards TB, McBiles M, Collins PS. An easy method for diagnosis of lymphedema. Ann Vasc Surg. 1990;4:255–9.
18. Browse NL, Stewart G. Lymphoedema: pathophysiology and classification [review]. J Cardiovasc Surg. 1985;26:91–106.
19. Wright NB, Carty HM. The swollen leg and primary lymphoedema. Arch Dis Child. 1994;71:44–9.
20. Rudkin GH, Miller TA. Lipedema: a clinical entity distinct from lymphedema. Plast Reconstr Surg. 1994;94:841–7.
21. Harwood CA, Bull RH, Evans J, Mortimer PS. Lymphatic and venous function in lipoedema. Br J Dermatol. 1996;13:41–6.
22. Vrouenraets BC, Klaase JM, Bhyan K, Geel BN, Eggermont AM, Franklin HR. Long-term morbidity after regional isolated perfusion with melphalan for melanoma of the limbs: the influence of acute regional toxic reactions. Arch Surg. 1995;130:43–7.
23. Karakousis CP, Driscoll DL. Groin dissection in malignant melanoma. Br J Surg. 1994;81:1771–4.
24. Heyn R, Raney RB Jr, Hays DM, et al. Late effects of therapy in patients with paratesticular rhabdomyosarcoma: Intergroup Rhabdomyosarcoma Study Committee. J Clin Oncol. 1992;10:614–23.

Complications of Lower Limb Edema

8

Satendra Kumar

8.1 Introduction

Accumulation of excess fluid in interstitium which occurs as the capillary filtration exceeds the limits of lymphatic drainage, producing noticeable clinical signs and symptoms, is defined as edema. There are two fluid compartments in the human body, namely intracellular and extracellular spaces. Extracellular space contains one-third of total body water, which is further divided into intravascular plasma volume (25%) and the extravascular interstitial space (75%). Hydrostatic pressures and oncotic pressures maintain the fluid balance between these compartments. Apart from these, other two factors that play an important role in fluid balance are vessel wall permeability and lymphatic system. Any disturbance in this homeostasis leads to the accumulation of fluid in the interstitial space that is called edema [1].

There is renal retention of sodium and water to maintain intravascular volume and hemodynamic stability by diffusion of water and electrolytes into interstitial compartment. Mechanism of this cascade is via renal vasoconstriction reducing glomerular filtration, increases sodium reabsorption proximally mediated by angiotensin II and norepinephrine, and increases sodium and water reabsorption in the collecting tubules which is mediated by aldosterone and antidiuretic hormone. Endothelium-derived factors like nitric oxide and prostaglandins also limit sodium and water excretion, therefore promoting edema [2].

Albumin, one of the impermeable proteins, is a major contributor to maintaining intravascular oncotic pressure. A level below 2 g/dl of plasma often results in edema. Hypoproteinemia is seen in many conditions like nephrotic syndrome, severe nutritional deficiency, and severe liver disease in which hepatic synthetic function is impaired. Some drugs, like calcium channel blockers, especially dihydropyridines cause more selective arteriolar vasodilatation leading to peripheral edema. Apart

S. Kumar (✉)
Institute of Medical Sciences, Banaras Hindu University, Varanasi, India

S. K. Tiwary (ed.), *Approach to Lower Limb Oedema*,
https://doi.org/10.1007/978-981-16-6206-5_8

from these, other uncommon conditions are myxedema, lymphedema, and idiopathic edema. Impaired lymphatic transport leads to lymphedema causing accumulation of lymphatic fluid in the interstitium mostly in extremities [3].

8.2 Complications of Lower Limb Edema

8.2.1 Pain

Pain can present as a spectrum of discomfort ranging from fullness or heaviness, dragging, throbbing, and itching or aching to frank pain. It gets exacerbated by standing, progressive throughout the day. It is typically felt in the muscles in the calf or thigh which is relieved by rest and limb elevation.

Venous claudication leading to bursting pain is experienced during exercise, although rare. This is associated only with severe outflow obstruction. Night cramps may be occurring frequently, often after a long day of standing without exercise.

8.2.2 Superficial Thrombophlebitis

It is a common complication of varicose veins, probably due to over prominence of veins, which makes them more susceptible to local trauma. Spontaneous thrombophlebitis is rare and often associated with deep venous thrombosis. It may be caused by occult malignancy (Trousseau phenomenon). It is characterized by a tender, hot, thickened area along the course of a varicose vein, often extremely painful, which may be associated with fever and malaise. Long saphenous vein (60% to 80%) is most commonly affected followed by the small/short saphenous vein (10% to 20%) [4, 5]. If thrombophlebitis occurs in long saphenous vein, it has the potential to propagate beyond the sapheno-femoral junction into the common femoral vein, resulting in iliofemoral thrombosis which can result in pulmonary embolism (PE).

8.2.2.1 Investigations

Superficial thrombophlebitis used to be a clinical diagnosis traditionally. However, lately it has been realized that there is association of concomitant DVT or PE. Physical examination underestimates the severity of disease in up to 77% cases. Compressive ultrasonography can identify concomitant DVT, evaluate the extent of the thrombus, and confirm the diagnosis [6–8].

D-dimer testing has limited utility in diagnosing SVT. It is variably elevated in SVT and therefore cannot be used to distinguish isolated SVT from DVT [6].

8.2.2.2 Management

- In low-risk superficial thrombophlebitis management strategies are aimed to control symptoms and decrease the extension of thrombosis and risk for PE [6]. Low risk cases are defined as those not associated with the presence of or predisposition to other thromboembolic diseases. In these patients, nonsteroidal anti-inflammatory agents, heat, and anticoagulants can be used [9].

- High-risk cases are defined as those patients with an SVT of at least 5 cm in length in the lower extremity, SVT proximal to the knee, especially within 10 cm of the sapheno-femoral junction, the presence of severe symptoms, greater saphenous vein involvement, previous SVT/venous thromboembolic disease, active malignancy, or recent surgery [6]. These patients are a candidate to receive fondaparinux 2.5 mg/day subcutaneously for 45 days [10].
- Topical and surgical treatments were also evaluated in this Cochrane review. Rivaroxaban 10 mg daily for 45 days was found to be non-inferior to fondaparinux in the prevention of venous thromboembolic complications with a comparable safety profile in the SURPRISE trial [11]. Additionally, it recommended further study on the use of nonsteroidal anti-inflammatory agents and low-molecular-weight heparins [9].
- In case of Trousseau syndrome, the main objective is to eliminate the underlying malignancy. Heparin is the recommended treatment because multiple pathways contribute to the development of the thrombus. Fondaparinux has also been evaluated but found to be less efficacious than heparin [12].

8.2.2.3 Complications

Two significant complications of SVT are DVT and PE. It has been found in multiple studies that 6–36% of patients have concomitant DVT with SVT. These same studies clinically suspected concomitant PE in 2–13%, and regular performance of lung scans revealed that the rate of asymptomatic PE approached 33% [4]. Other retrospective studies from both primary and secondary/tertiary centers have reported coexisting DVT or symptomatic PE on initial presentation to be 25–30%. Symptomatic PE is present in about 5–7% of these patients [4, 5]. However, with the use of a more rigorous screening process in asymptomatic patients, the incidence of coexisting PE increased to 17%. 14–70% of patients with thrombus up to 3 cm from the sapheno-femoral junction progress to DVT, and they require prior treatment [8].

8.2.3 Dermatitis

The earliest cutaneous sequela of chronic venous insufficiency with venous hypertension is dermatitis which can lead to venous leg ulceration and lipodermatosclerosis. Chronic inflammatory changes lead to deposition of fibrin and hemosiderin with local edema, which can result in venous dermatitis or varicose eczema over time. It is seen in middle aged and elderly patients. It can also occur in young patients with acquired venous insufficiency due to surgery, trauma, or thrombosis. Retrograde flow related to incompetent venous valves, valve destruction, or obstruction of the venous system leads to venous hypertension causing dermatitis. It results in an inflammatory process that is mediated by metalloproteinases. Red blood cells extravasate in the interstitium and release ferric ions which upregulate these metalloproteinases [13].

There is a progressive loss of epithelium, which can result in spontaneous venous ulceration.

8.2.3.1 Investigations

Radiological examination—Venous Doppler studies may reveal deep venous thrombosis or severe valve damage due to past thrombosis.

8.2.3.2 Treatment

- Compression therapy—Compression therapy is done by specialized stockings that deliver a controlled pressure gradient (measured in mm Hg) to the affected leg. These are suitable for long-term management of edema but not for the healing of stasis ulcers. Compression stockings should be applied early in the morning before the patient rises from bed.
- High-level compression can be done by using elastic wraps compression (Unna) boots. Some more sophisticated devices such as end-diastolic compression boots can be used.
- Nonsteroidal calcineurin inhibitors like tacrolimus and pimecrolimus may be used in the management of stasis dermatitis [14].
- In patients with chronic quiescent stasis dermatitis can be managed with bland topical emollients to maximize epidermal moisture. Petroleum jelly is very effective and does not contain any contact sensitizers.

8.2.4 Lipodermatosclerosis

It forms a part of the pathological progression of venous disease that ultimately results in skin ulceration followed by progressive fibrosis. It is also known as sclerosing panniculitis as it is more encompassing nomenclature and more accurately reflecting the true nature of the process [15]. It is sometimes also called fat necrosis, folliculitis, or chronic cellulitis.

Acute lipodermatosclerosis was first described by Kirsner et al. in 1993 [16]. The area is red to violaceous, scaling, tender, and warm. The sharp demarcation of the induration noted in chronic LDS may be absent in acute stage. Well-demarcated, indurated, exquisitely tender "cellulitis" that involves the lower legs in patients should prompt the clinician to consider a diagnosis of LDS [17]. The chronic phase most often develops following the acute phase or may occur independently [18]. It is characterized by hyperpigmented thick, hard, tight, and contracted skin in the lower third of the patient's leg associated with pain mostly confined to the medial aspect. Skin tightening may eventually lead to constriction of the ankle region giving the leg the characteristic "inverted champagne bottle" appearance. Patients with classic chronic LDS may develop acute onset of pain and represent an "acute on chronic" form of LDS. The ulceration rate associated with LDS has been estimated to be around 13% in a recent retrospective analysis [15].

Risk factors for development of LDS [15, 17, 19]:

(1) Female gender
(2) High BMI
(3) Systemic hypertension
(4) History of venous abnormalities like chronic venous insufficiency

8.2.4.1 Investigations

- Doppler studies that assess the venous system, focusing on the sapheno-femoral junction in the popliteal fossa and the perforators between the knee and the ankle.
- Ultrasonography can be used for visualization of the water compartment of the dermis.
- Magnetic resonance imaging (MRI) can be a useful alternative to skin biopsy in cases where biopsy is contraindicated. Features of LDS on high-resolution MRI reveal thickening of the skin with typical distinct fibrous septa in the hypodermis with a "honeycomb" appearance [20].

8.2.4.2 Treatment

- Compression stockings are currently accepted as the most conventional treatment choice for LDS. Compression works by a variety of mechanisms from aiding venous returns to stimulating fibrinolysis [21].
- An anabolic steroid stanozolol, synthetic testosterone derivative, is approved for use in the treatment of hereditary angioedema. It has fibrinolytic properties that have also been used in the treatment of LDS, particularly its acute form [22].
- Danazol is another steroid derivative that is modified testosterone. Hafner et al. reported a case of a painful LDS successfully treated with danazol [23].
- Oxandrolone is another synthetic anabolic steroid, derived from dihydrotestosterone which can be used to treat LDS.

Less conventional treatment options include:

- Intralesional steroids: Intralesional triamcinolone at doses of either 5 or 10 mg/mL combined with compression results in alleviation of pain and prevents further progression of the disease [24].
- Pentoxifylline: Pentoxifylline may be effective in providing protection from endothelial damage via modulation of the effects of tumor necrosis factor-a (TNF-a) and via inhibition of the collagen metabolism [25].
- Surgical treatment: Excision of LDS skin area up to muscle fascia followed by split-thickness skin grafting can be done.
- Topical capsaicin: Topical creams with capsaicin are used in dermatology to treat pruritus, neuropathic sensations, and pain from a wide range of chronic conditions. Topical capsaicin reduces neurogenic inflammation by depleting substance P. Its fibrinolytic and antithrombotic effects are not well known [26].

8.2.5 Atrophic Blanche

It is a chronic condition. Symptoms are recurrent, painful ulcers of the lower leg, ankle, or dorsal foot, predominately occurring in young to middle-aged females with subsequent scar formation. On examination these present as a white atrophic stellate scar with peripheral telangiectasias. Coalescence of multiple areas may form a large scar, may break down spontaneously, or may following trauma form ulcers.

It occurs due to disturbances in fibrinolysis and/or coagulation leading to thrombo-occlusion of blood vessels in the superficial dermis [27]. Its correlation is seen with several prothrombotic factors including aPL antibodies, abnormalities in protein S and C, hyperhomocysteinemia, sticky platelet syndrome, antithrombin III deficiency, and factor V Leiden mutation.

8.2.5.1 Investigations

- Doppler studies and ankle-brachial index are aids to rule out venous stasis and arterial occlusion
- A skin biopsy to rule out cutaneous vasculitis.
- Screening coagulation studies to evaluate for antiphospholipid antibody syndrome.
- Lab work should include hemoglobin A1C.
- Complete blood count with differential.
- Basic metabolic panel.
- Antinuclear antibody (ANA).
- Rheumatoid factor and CRP to aid differentiation of diabetes mellitus, autoimmune syndromes, and malignancy.

8.2.5.2 Management

- In the absence of underlying disease, treatment of atrophie blanche includes antiplatelet, anticoagulation, and fibrinolytic therapies.
- Aspirin, dipyridamole, pentoxifylline, and heparin are used in treatment.
- Sulfasalazine, danazol, and stanozolol are also used as a single agent or in combination.
- Hyperbaric oxygen and PUVA have also shown good results.
- In refractory cases: rivaroxaban, oral steroids, prostanoids, and IVIG have been used with varying success.
- Patient education: smoking cessation, to avoid irritants and poorly fitting shoes.
- Basic wound care like leg elevation, compression therapy, and occlusive wound dressings [28–30].

8.2.6 Venous Ulcer

Venous ulcers are most common chronic wounds presenting on the lower extremities and feet. These are present in the skin over the ankles, either on the inner or outer aspect of the malleolus. On examination a venous ulcer is characterized by a shallow, exudative ulcer with granulating base and presence of fibrin, commonly located over bony prominences such as the gaiter area. Associated findings include edema, telangiectasias, corona phlebectatica, atrophie blanche, lipodermatosclerosis, and an inverted champagne bottle deformity of the lower leg.

8.2.6.1 Pathogenesis

Venous ulcers are formed because of dysfunctional micro- and macrocirculation. There is unrelieved or ambulatory hypertension within the veins of the calf often resulting from deep phlebothrombosis (DVT) that leads to destruction of venous valves resulting in their incompetence. This results in high venous pressures that are transmitted back to the capillaries and skin veins causing increased permeability, leakage, and deposition of hemosiderin within the skin changing its texture and elasticity. There are leucocyte trapping and subsequent microcirculatory impairment, pericapillary cuffs that trap nutrients and other substances, and tissue hypoxia leading to necrobiosis and ulceration, known as lipodermatosclerosis [31, 32].

8.2.6.2 Investigations

The diagnosis is based mainly on clinical examination. Arterial disease is excluded by ultrasound Doppler measurement of ankle-brachial systolic pressure index (ABI or ABPI). Ultrasound measurement of ABI or ABPI is recommended since palpation of the pedal pulses dorsalis is difficult in a swollen foot. Normal ranges of ABI or ABPI are as follows [33, 34].

0.9–1.2	Normal
≥ 0.5 to ≤0.9	Presence of peripheral arterial disease
≤ 0.5	Severe peripheral ischemia
≥ 1.2	Need to exclude aneurysmal changes or cardiovascular disease

Air plethysmography can be used for quantitative data on obstruction, calf muscle pumps ejection fraction, and reflux.

A tissue/wound swab can be taken when the ulcer shows clinical signs of infection.

Wound edge biopsy only if malignancy or other etiology is suspected.

8.2.6.3 Management

Venous ulcers are often treated with following modalities:

- Conservative management:

Compression therapy – it is standard treatment modality for initial and long-term treatment of venous ulcers in patients who do not have concomitant arterial disease. Compression therapy reduces edema and pain, improves venous reflux, and enhances healing. Multicomponent compression systems comprised of varied layers are more practical than single-component systems, and elastic systems are simpler than nonelastic systems [35].

Types of compression therapy:

Elastic: Elastic compression bandages conform to the size and shape of the leg and accommodate changes in leg circumference, thus providing sustained compression. It even has absorptive capacity and requires infrequent changing (about once a week). There is strong evidence for the use of multiple elastic layers vs. single layers to increase ulcer healing [36].

Inelastic: Inelastic compression wraps are impregnated with zinc oxide, e.g., Unna boots. They provide high compression only during ambulation and contraction. They are contraindicated in non-ambulatory patients or in those with arterial compromise. They have limited capacity for fluid absorption. They are best used for early, small, dry ulcers and for venous dermatitis because of the skin soothing effects of oxide [35].

Stockings: Compression stockings stimulate ulcer healing and forestall recurrence (recommended strength may be a minimum of 20 to 30 pressure unit but 30 to 40 mm Hg is preferred). It is knee-high, thigh-high, toes-in, or toes-out compression stockings according to patient preference. Once the ulcer has healed, continued use of compression stockings is recommended indefinitely [37].

Intermittent pneumatic compression: Intermittent pneumatic compression is taken under consideration when there is generalized refractory edema from venous insufficiency with lymphatic obstruction associated with significant ulceration of the lower extremity. Its effectiveness compared with other kinds of compression is unclear. Intermittent pneumatic compression improves ulcer healing when added to layered compression [38].

Debridement: Debridement is removal of necrotic tissue. It is used to expedite wound healing. Debridement is additionally sharp, enzymatic, mechanical, larval, or autolytic.

Enzymatic debridement using collagenase has been shown to effectively remove nonviable tissue.

Larval therapy using maggots could be a good method of debridement with added potential for disinfection, stimulation of healing, and biofilm inhibition and eradication.

Autolytic debridement uses moisture-retentive dressings and can be utilized additionally to other sorts of debridement.

Dressings are used to cover ulcers and promote moist wound healing. These are chosen according to wound location, size, depth, moisture balance, presence of infection, allergies, comfort, door management, ease and frequency of dressing changes, cost, and availability. Topical antiseptics like cadexomer iodine (Iodosorb), povidone-iodine (Betadine), peroxide-based preparations, honey-based preparations, and silver are also used to treat venous ulcers.

Medications:

- ***Pentoxifylline:*** It is a hemorheologic agent which improves microcirculation and oxygenation. It can be used effectively as monotherapy or with compression therapy for venous ulcers. Pentoxifylline plus compression improved healing of venous ulcers compared with placebo plus compression which was evident in seven randomized controlled trials [39].
- ***Aspirin:*** Aspirin can be used for treatment of venous ulcer, but there is inconsistent evidence concerning the benefits and harms of oral therapy [40].

- ***Statins:*** Statins have vasoactive and anti-inflammatory effects. In a small study, patients receiving simvastatin (Zocor), 40 mg once daily, had a higher rate of ulcer healing than matched patients given placebo [41].
- ***Phlebotonics:*** These are venoactive drugs; theoretically, these work by improving venous tone and decreasing capillary permeability. Drugs included in this group are saponins (e.g., horse chestnut seed extract), flavonoids (e.g., rutosides, diosmin, hesperidin), and micronized purified flavonoid fraction [42].
- ***Antibiotics:*** Venous ulcers can be colonized by bacteria. Colonization means presence of replicating bacteria without a host reaction or clinical signs of infection. Colonized venous ulcers need not be treated with antibiotics. Venous ulcers with obvious signs of infection should be treated with antibiotics. Oral antibiotics are preferred, and therapy should be limited to 2 weeks unless evidence of wound infection persists [43].

- Mechanical modalities:
  - Hyperbaric oxygen therapy: hyperbaric oxygen therapy in patients with chronic wounds found only one trial that addressed venous ulcers. Because of limited evidence and no long-term benefit, hyperbaric oxygen therapy is not recommended for treatment of venous ulcers [44].
  - Negative pressure wound therapy: Traditional negative pressure wound therapy systems are bulky and cannot be used with compression therapy. Negative pressure wound therapy is not recommended as a primary treatment of venous ulcers.
- Advanced wound therapy:
- If the venous ulcers that do not improve within 4 weeks of standard wound care, it should prompt consideration of adjunctive treatment options.
  - Cellular and tissue-based products: refractory venous ulcers can be treated with many cellular and tissue-based products which are approved for the treatment including allografts, animal-derived extracellular matrix products, human-derived cellular products, and human amniotic membrane-derived products. Compared with compression plus a simple dressing, one study showed that advanced therapies can shorten healing time and improve healing rates [45].
  - Skin grafting: In case of large ulcers (larger than 25 cm^2 [3.9 in^2]) in which healing is unlikely without grafting skin grafting should be considered. It can be used as secondary therapy for ulcers that do not heal with standard care [46].
- Surgical options:
- The goal of operative and endovascular management of venous ulcers is to improve healing and prevent ulcer recurrence. It is mainly of following types: Trendelenburg operation, endogenous ablation, ligation, subfascial endoscopic perforator surgery, and sclerotherapy. Recent trials show faster healing of venous ulcers when early endovenous ablation to correct superficial venous reflux is performed in conjunction with compression therapy compared with compression

alone or with delayed intervention if the ulcer did not heal after 6 months. The most common complications of endovenous ablation were pain and deep venous thrombosis [47, 48].

8.2.7 Cellulitis

Cellulitis is a non-necrotizing inflammation of the skin and subcutaneous tissues, caused due to acute infection which does not involve the fascia or muscles. It is characterized by localized pain, swelling, tenderness, erythema, and warmth. It is most commonly caused by streptococcal species. In cases of cellulitis due to carbuncle and furuncle Staph aureus is the causative organism.

8.2.7.1 Investigations

In case of mild, self-limiting cellulitis, no workup is needed as it resolves on its own but in case of moderate to severe cellulitis with systemic involvement, following laboratory investigations may be undertaken:

- Complete blood count: leukocytosis or leukopenia may be present.
- ESR/CRP: elevated in cases of severe cellulitis.
- Blood culture: may be needed in severe cellulitis.
- Renal function test: deranged renal profile in case of severe cellulitis with systemic involvement.
- Ultrasonography: for diagnosis of occult abscess and aspiration.
- CT/ MRI scan: In cases where necrotizing fasciitis is suspected.

8.2.7.2 Treatment

- Antibiotic treatment is effective in most cases with drainage of underlying abscess if present.
- In mild cases: Dicloxacillin, amoxicillin, or cephalexin orally on an outpatient basis.
- Clindamycin or a macrolide (clarithromycin or azithromycin): In patients who are allergic to penicillin.
- Severe cellulitis requires parenteral therapy with cefazolin, cefuroxime, ceftriaxone, nafcillin, or oxacillin for presumed streptococcal infection.

8.2.8 Lymphangiosarcoma

Lymphangiosarcoma is a rare complication of chronic lymphedema which is generally seen in patients with postmastectomy and radiation therapy for carcinoma breast in upper limbs. It can also occur in lower limb due to congenital, idiopathic, traumatic, filarial, or postsurgical causes of lymphedema [49].

8.2.8.1 Clinical Presentation

It is seen in chronic lymphedema after 10–15 years, characterized by skin changes in the form of purple colored raised cutaneous lesions which progress to ulceration. It has poor prognosis with 5 years survival rate of <5% with multimodality treatment [50].

8.2.8.2 Pathogenesis

In chronic lymphedema, there is accumulation of protein-rich interstitial fluid which alters the local immune response. This protein-rich fluid stimulates lymphangiogenesis for the development of collateral vessels. There is also compromised immune response leading to development of malignancy, specifically vascular tumors [51].

8.2.8.3 Investigations

1. Biopsy from the mass - To confirm the diagnosis. A lymphovascular invasive pattern may be seen. On immunohistochemistry markers, it may be positive for endothelial cell markers (CD31–CD36).
2. Antibody against factor VIII-related antigen: Markers for endothelial cells.
3. CD34 antigen - marker of vascular endothelial cells with no cross reactivity to the lymphatic endothelium.
4. Antikeratin antibodies - this finding confirms that the tumor cells are nonepithelial in origin.
5. Positive staining for laminin, CD31, collagen IV, and vimentin.
6. Metastatic workup - it includes chest x-ray to rule out lung metastasis. CECT thorax and USG abdomen to rule out any abdominal or lung secondaries.
7. Fluorodeoxyglucose (FDG) PET/CT scanning - delineate tumor spread, including metastases, and detect the possible malignant transformation.

8.2.8.4 Management

Chemotherapy and irradiation are used as adjuvants to surgery for the treatment of Stewart-Treves syndrome.

Multimodal therapy:

1. Hyperthermic isolated limb perfusion with tumor necrosis factor-alpha and melphalan.
2. Radical resection of the affected skin and subcutaneous tissue including the fascia.
3. Intra-arterial mitoxantrone/paclitaxel.
4. Immunotherapy may be beneficial as palliative treatment.
5. Expression of VEGF-C - good potential candidate for targeted antilymphangiogenic therapy.

Surgical therapy:

Amputation of the limb or forequarter is done rather than wide local surgical excision due to high rates of recurrence and metastasis. Metastatic disease should exclude surgical treatment unless surgery is useful for symptomatic improvement.

References

1. Little RC, Ginsburg JM. The physiologic basis for clinical edema. Arch Intern Med. 1984 Aug;144(8):1661–4.
2. Trayes KP, Studdiford JS, Pickle S, Tully AS. Edema: diagnosis and management. Am Fam Physician. 2013 Jul 15;88(2):102–10.
3. Ely JW, Osheroff JA, Chambliss ML, Ebell MH. Approach to leg edema of unclear etiology. J Am Board Fam Med. 2006 Mar-Apr;19(2):148–60.
4. Décousus H, Bertoletti L, Frappé P. Spontaneous acute superficial vein thrombosis of the legs: do we really need to treat? J Thromb Haemost. 2015 Jun;13(Suppl 1):S230–7.
5. Di Minno MN, Ambrosino P, Ambrosini F, Tremoli E, Di Minno G, Dentali F. Prevalence of deep vein thrombosis and pulmonary embolism in patients with superficial vein thrombosis: a systematic review and meta-analysis. J Thromb Haemost. 2016 May;14(5):964–72.
6. Scott G, Mahdi AJ, Alikhan R. Superficial vein thrombosis: a current approach to management. Br J Haematol. 2015 Mar;168(5):639–45.
7. Nasr H, Scriven JM. Superficial thrombophlebitis (superficial venous thrombosis). BMJ. 2015 Jun 22;350:2039.
8. Tait C, Baglin T, Watson H, Laffan M, Makris M, Perry D, Keeling D. British Committee for Standards in haematology. Guidelines on the investigation and management of venous thrombosis at unusual sites. Br J Haematol. 2012 Oct;159(1):28–38.
9. Maddox RP, Seupaul RA. What is the Most effective treatment of superficial thrombophlebitis? Ann Emerg Med. 2016 May;67(5):671–2.
10. Di Nisio M, Wichers IM, Middeldorp S. Treatment for superficial thrombophlebitis of the leg. Cochrane Database Syst Rev. 2018; Feb 25;2:CD004982.
11. Werth S, Bauersachs R, Gerlach H, Rabe E, Schellong S, Beyer-Westendorf J. Superficial vein thrombosis treated for 45 days with rivaroxaban versus fondaparinux: rationale and design of the SURPRISE trial. J Thromb Thrombolysis. 2016 Aug;42(2):197–204.
12. Varki A. Trousseau's syndrome: multiple definitions and multiple mechanisms. Blood. 2007 Sep 15;110(6):1723–9.
13. Sundaresan S, Migden MR, Silapunt S. Stasis dermatitis: pathophysiology, evaluation, and management. Am J Clin Dermatol. 2017;18(3):383–90. https://doi.org/10.1007/s40257-016-0250-0.
14. Maroo N, Choudhury S, Sen S, Chatterjee S. Oral doxycycline with topical tacrolimus for treatment of stasis dermatitis due to chronic venous insufficiency: a pilot study. Indian J Pharmacol. 2012;44(1):111–3. https://doi.org/10.4103/0253-7613.91878.
15. Jorizzo J, White WL, Zanolli MD, Greer KE, Solomon AR, Jetton RL. Sclerosing panniculitis: a clinicopathologic assessment. Arch Dermatol. 1991;127:554–8.
16. Kirsner R, Pardes JB, Eaglestein WH, Falanga V. The clinical spectrum of lipodermatosclerosis. J Am Acad Dermatol. 1993;28:623–7.
17. Bruce A, Bennett D, Lohse CM, Rooke TW, Davis MD. Lipodermatosclerosis: review of cases evaluated at Mayo Clinic. J Am Acad Dermatol. 2002;46:187–92.
18. Greenberg A, Hasan A, Montalvo BM, Falabella A, Falanga V. Acute lipodermatosclerosis is associated with venous insufficiency. J Am Acad Dermatol. 1996;35:566–8.
19. Herouy Y, May AE, Pornschlegel G, et al. Lipodermatosclerosis is characterized by elevated expression and activation on matrix metalloproteinases: implications for venous ulcer formation. J Invest Dermatol. 1998;111:822–7.
20. Chan C, Yang CY, Chu CY. Magnetic resonance imaging as a diagnostic tool for extensive lipodermatosclerosis. J Am Acad Dermatol. 2006;58(3):525–7.
21. Ahnlide I, Bjellerup M, Akesson H. Excision of lipodermatosclerotic tissue: an effective treatment for non-healing venous ulcers. Acta DermVenereol. 2000;80:28–30.
22. Helfman T, Falanga V. Stanozolol as a novel therapeutic agent in dermatology. J Am Acad Dermatol. 1995;33:254–8.

23. Hafner C, Wimmershoff M, Landthaler M, Vogt T. Lipodermatosclerosis: successful treatment with Danazol. Acta Derm Venereol. 2005;85:365–6.
24. Campbell L, Miller OF. Intralesional triamcinolone in the management of lipodermatosclerosis. J Am Acad Dermatol. 2006;55:166–8.
25. Goldman M. The use of pentoxifylline in the treatment of systemic sclerosis and lipodermatosclerosis. J Am Acad Dermatol. 1994;31:135–6.
26. Wang J, Hsu MF, Hsu TP, Teng CM. Antihemostatic and antithrombotic effects of capsaicin in comparison with aspirin and indomethacin. Thromb Res. 1985;37(6):669–79.
27. Mimouni D, Ng PP, Rencic A, Nikolskaia OV, Bernstein BD, Nousari HC. Cutaneous polyarteritis nodosa in patients presenting with atrophie blanche. Br J Dermatol. 2003 Apr;148(4):789–94.
28. Amato L, Chiarini C, Berti S, Massi D, Fabbri P. Idiopathic atrophie blanche. Skinmed. 2006 May-Jun;5(3):151–4.
29. Franco Marques G, Criado PR, Alves Batista Morita TC, Cajas García MS. The management of livedoid vasculopathy focused on direct oral anticoagulants (DOACs): four case reports successfully treated with rivaroxaban. Int J Dermatol. 2018 Jun;57(6):732–41.
30. Vasudevan B, Neema S, Verma R. Livedoid vasculopathy: a review of pathogenesis and principles of management. Indian J Dermatol Venereol Leprol. 2016 Sep-Oct;82(5):478–88.
31. Coleridge-Smith PJ, Thomas P, Scurr JH, Dormandy JA. Causes of venous ulceration: a new hypothesis. Br Med J (Clin Res Ed). 1988;296:1726–7.
32. Falanga V, Eaglestein WH. The trap hypothesis of venous ulceration. Lancet. 1993;17:1006–8.
33. Mani R, Margolis D, Shukla V, Akita S, Lazarides M, Piaggesi A, et al. Optimising technology use for chronic lower extremity wound healing: a consensus document. Int J Low Extrem Wounds. 2016;15(2):102–19.
34. Norgren L, Hiatt WR, Dormandy JA, Nehler MR, Harris KA, Fowkes FG, TASC II Working Group. Inter-society consensus for the management of peripheral arterial disease (TASC II). J Vasc Surg. 2007;45(Suppl S):S5–67.
35. Hettrick H. The science of compression therapy for chronic venous insufficiency edema. J Am Col Certif Wound Spec. 2009;1(1):20–4.
36. Dolibog P, Franek A, Taradaj J, et al. A comparative clinical study on five types of compression therapy in patients with venous leg ulcers. Int J Med Sci. 2013;11(1):34–43.
37. Nelson EA, Bell-Syer SE. Compression for preventing recurrence of venous ulcers. Cochrane Database Syst Rev. 2014;9:CD002303.
38. Nelson EA, Hillman A, Thomas K. Intermittent pneumatic compression for treating venous leg ulcers. Cochrane Database Syst Rev. 2014;5:CD001899.
39. Margolis DJ. Pentoxifylline in the treatment of venous leg ulcers. Arch Dermatol. 2000;136(9):1142–3.
40. Layton AM, Ibbotson SH, Davies JA, et al. Randomised trial of oral aspirin for chronic venous leg ulcers. Lancet. 1994;344(8916):164–5.
41. Evangelista MT, Casintahan MF, Villafuerte LL. Simvastatin as a novel therapeutic agent for venous ulcers: a randomized, double blind, placebo controlled trial. Br J Dermatol. 2014;170(5):1151–7.
42. Coleridge-Smith P, Lok C, Ramelet AA. Venous leg ulcer: a metaanalysis of adjunctive therapy with micronized purified flavonoid fraction. Eur J Vasc Endovasc Surg. 2005;30(2):198–208.
43. Bowler PG, Duerden BI, Armstrong DG. Wound microbiology and associated approaches to wound management. Clin Microbiol Rev. 2001;14(2):244–69.
44. Kranke P, Bennett MH, Martyn-St James M, et al. Hyperbaric oxygen therapy for chronic wounds. Cochrane Database Syst Rev. 2015;6:CD004123.
45. Falanga V, Sabolinski M. A bilayered living skin construct (APLIGRAF) accelerates complete closure of hard-to-heal venous ulcers. Wound Repair Regen. 1999;7(4):201–7.
46. Jankunas V, Bagdonas R, Samsanavicius D, et al. An analysis of the effectiveness of skin grafting to treat chronic venous leg ulcers. Wounds. 2007;19(5):128–37.

47. Gohel MS, Barwell JR, Taylor M, et al. Long term results of compression therapy alone vs compression plus surgery in chronic venous leg ulcers (ESCHAR): randomized controlled trial. BMJ. 2007;335(7610):83.
48. Gohel MS, Heatley F, Liu X, et al. EVRA trial investigators. A randomized trial of early endovenous ablation in venous ulceration. N Engl J Med. 2018;378(22):2105–14.
49. Durr HR, Pellengahr C, Nerlich A, et al. Stewart-Treves syndrome as a rare complication of a hereditary lymphedema. Vasa. 2004;33:42–5.
50. Danese CA, Grishman E, Dreiling DA. Malignant vascular tumors of the lymphedematous extremity. Ann Surg. 1967 Aug;166(2):245–53.
51. Ruocco V, Schwartz RA, Ruocco E. Lymphedema: an immunologically vulnerable site for development of neoplasms. J Am Acad Dermatol. 2002;47:124–7.

Chronic Lower Limb Edema

9

Ram Niwas Meena, Vipul Srivastava, Akanksha, and B. R. Akshay

9.1 Introduction

Although edema is the most prevalent cause of leg swelling, an increase in any region of the tissue can cause the limb to expand completely or partially [1]. An accurate diagnosis must be made, irrespective whether the swelling is acute or chronic, symmetrical or asymmetrical, localized or generalized, congenital or acquired. Asymmetrical lower limb swelling indicates a sign of chronic edema arising from venous or lymphatic disease, whereas symmetrical lower limb swelling implies a systemic or more central cause of edema, such as heart failure or nephrotic syndrome. Edema develops when the rate of capillary filtration (lymph generation) exceeds the rate of lymphatic drainage, either due to excessive transcapillary filtration, inadequate lymphatic flow, or both. The lymphatic system regulates the amount of extracellular fluid, which normally compensates for increased capillary filtration [2]. The lymph drainage system is overburdened by filtration, which causes most edemas. Increased capillary filtration can occur as a result of increasing venous pressure, hypoalbuminemia, or increased capillary permeability as a result of local inflammation [3].

An increase in fluid volume in the interstitial space causes edema, which is a perceptible swelling. In order to clarify the etiology and diagnosis, the care of a patient with edema should be based on epidemiology, previous medical history, and physical examination. In addition, recommendations and criteria for stratifying clinical risk and guiding hospitalization decisions should be proposed [4]. Chronic edema is defined as a persistent, abnormal swelling of the legs that does not go away overnight or with elevation and lasts more than 3 months [5].

R. N. Meena (✉) · V. Srivastava · Akanksha · B. R. Akshay
Department of General Surgery, Institute of Medical Sciences, Banaras Hindu University, Varanasi, India

S. K. Tiwary (ed.), *Approach to Lower Limb Oedema*,
https://doi.org/10.1007/978-981-16-6206-5_9

9.2 Pathophysiology

A capillary leak with fluid translocation to the interstitial space, renal water and sodium reabsorption might both be used to determine fluid retention, resulting in an endocrine salt retention mechanism. If the accumulation of hydro-saline is the major cause of edema, the fluid excess appears to be intravascular as well as extravascular (the so-called overfilling seen in primary nephropathies) [5].

9.3 Classification

There are two types of leg edema: venous edema and lymphedema . Due to enhanced capillary filtration, venous edema is a deposit of low viscosity, protein-poor interstitial fluid that cannot be accommodated by the regular lymphatic system. Lymphedema is characterized by an accumulation of protein-rich interstitial fluid in the skin and subcutaneous tissue as a result of lymphatic malfunction. Lipidemia, a third variety is more correctly described as a sort of fat maldistribution than real edema [6]. Various common and the less common cause of leg edema are shown in Table 9.1 and 9.2.

Table 9.1 Common causes of leg edema

Unilateral		Bilateral	
Acute (<72 h)	Chronic	Acute (<72 h)	Chronic
Deep vein thrombosis	Venous insufficiency		Venous insufficiency
			Pulmonary hypertension
			Heart failure
			Idiopathic edema
			Lymphedema
			Drugs
			Premenstrual edema
			Pregnancy
			Obesity

Table 9.2 Less common causes of leg edema

Unilateral		Bilateral	
Acute (<72 h)	Chronic	Acute (<72 h)	Chronic
Ruptured Baker's cyst	Secondary lymphedema (tumor, radiation, surgery, bacterial infection)	Bilateral deep vein thrombosis	Renal disease (nephrotic syndrome, glomerulonephritis)
Ruptured medial head of gastrocnemius	Pelvic tumor or lymphoma causing external pressure on veins	Acute worsening of systemic cause (heart failure, renal disease)	Liver disease

Table 9.2 (continued)

Unilateral		Bilateral	
Acute (<72 h)	Chronic	Acute (<72 h)	Chronic
Compartment syndrome	Reflex sympathetic dystrophy		Secondary lymphedema (secondary to tumor, radiation, bacterial infection, filariasis)
			Pelvic tumor or lymphoma causing external pressure
			Dependent edema
			Diuretic-induced edema
			Preeclampsia
			Lipidemia
			Anemia

9.4 Assessment of Edema

Edema is almost always diagnosed clinically. The commencement of swelling, the look of the limb, the existence of pain with pressure, and the impact of passive leg elevation on edema can all help you diagnose edema. A complete medical history and physical examination are required for evaluation.

The amount of the edema should be determined first in the initial assessment. Unilateral edema indicates a compression of the venous or lymphatic vessels caused by an intravascular or extrinsic process. Congestive heart failure, chronic liver failure, renal illness and hypoalbuminemia are all causes for generalized edema [Table 9.3]. Many different drugs have been linked to the development of edema [Table 9.4], and stopping these medications should be part of the first treatment regimen. Based on the history and physical examinations, laboratory and other diagnostic procedures should focus on the most likely causes.

9.4.1 Diagnostic Studies

The majority of individuals with leg edema over the age of 50 have venous insufficiency, but if the cause is unknown, a brief list of laboratory tests can help rule out systemic disease; complete blood count, urinalysis, electrolytes, creatinine, blood sugar, thyroid-stimulating hormone, and albumin.

In lymphedema, ultrasonography can accurately measure soft tissue changes in the superficial and deep layers, but it does not provide adequate information on anatomical structure [7]. For identifying the location and extent of venous reflux and deep venous thrombosis, duplex venous ultrasonography is regarded the most accurate noninvasive method. In assessing calf vein and iliac-vein thrombosis, this approach is less accurate. Ultrasound can be used to detect both popliteal aneurysms and cysts.

Table 9.3 Rare causes of leg edema

Unilateral		Bilateral	
Acute (<72 h)	Chronic	Acute (<72 h)	Chronic
	Primary lymphedema (congenital lymphedema, lymphedema praecox, lymphedema tarda)		Primary lymphedema (congenital lymphedema, lymphedema praecox, lymphedema tarda)
	Congenital venous malformations		Protein losing enteropathy, malnutrition, malabsorption
	May-Thurner syndrome (iliac-vein compression syndrome)		Restrictive pericarditis
			Restrictive cardiomyopathy
			Beri Beri
			Myxedema

Table 9.4 Medicines most commonly implicated in edema and their causative mechanisms

Drug class	Mechanism
Calcium channel blockers	Increased hydrostatic pressure resulting from an increase in capillary blood flow as a result of dilation of the small arteries
Corticosteroids	Increased hydrostatic pressure resulting from fluid retention
Nonsteroidal anti-inflammatory drugs	
Sex hormones and related compounds	

In the case of suspected DVT, venous ultrasonography is the imaging modality of choice. For proximal thrombosis, compression ultrasonography with or without Doppler waveform analysis has a high sensitivity (95%) and specificity (96%); however, the sensitivity is lower for calf veins (73%). The diagnosis of chronic venous insufficiency can also be confirmed with duplex ultrasonography.

Ultrasonography is unable to detect lymph flow. When a clinical diagnosis of lymphedema cannot be made, indirect radionuclide lymphoscintigraphy, which demonstrates absence or delayed filling of lymphatic channels, is the method of choice for evaluating lymphedema [8].

In cases of indeterminate lymphoscintigraphy interpretation or in individuals whom lymphedema is likely to be treated surgically, radio contrast lymphography is now reserved. This approach solely gives static anatomical data. It is invasive, is difficult to conduct, and has the potential to affect underlying lymphatic vessels, aggravating lymphedema [9].

CT scans can reveal structural changes in soft tissues as well as fluid volume alterations between compartments. On CT, lymphedema can be distinguished from venous edema by the appearance of edema restricted to the skin and subcutaneous tissue, with sparing of the underlying muscle.

If the clinical suspicion for DVT remains high, patients with unilateral lower extremity edema who do not show a proximal thrombus on duplex ultrasonography may require further imaging to diagnose the etiology of edema. To assess for intrinsic or extrinsic pelvic or thigh DVT, magnetic resonance angiography with venography of the lower extremities and pelvis might be employed [10]. The diagnosis of musculoskeletal etiologies such as a gastrocnemius rupture or a popliteal cyst may be aided by magnetic resonance imaging. When lymphedema is suspected, T1-weighted magnetic resonance lymphangiography can be performed for direct visualization of the lymphatic pathways [11].

Patients with obstructive sleep apnea and edema should get an echocardiogram to check their pulmonary arterial pressures. 93 percent of obstructive sleep apnea patients with edema reported higher right atrial pressures in one report [12]. Edema linked with obstructive sleep apnea has long been assumed to be caused by pulmonary hypertension [13].

9.5 Therapeutic Options

9.5.1 Conservative and Skin Care Treatment

Leg edema that is persistent and uncontrolled leads to induration of the subcutaneous tissues, exudation, and eventually ulceration. This procedure also promotes the spread of bacterial and fungal infections, which impair the limb's overall health in the long run [14]. Patients with this problem require a thorough explanation of the importance of lowering edema and subsequent prevention. Other factors that can help to prevent the long-term consequences of leg swelling include skin care and general hygiene, boosting mobility, discouraging unsupported limb reliance, and weight management [14]. Because many of these patients are physically unable to care for their own feet due to obesity, degenerative musculoskeletal problems, and concurrent systemic conditions, the podiatrist serves a vital role in ensuring sufficient foot care.

Some individuals' skin may be thick, causing dryness, hyperkeratosis, and even ulceration. To lubricate their skin, all patients will require effective washing, drying, and emollient therapy. Emollients calm, smooth, and lubricate the skin and are recommended when the skin is dry or has scaling/hyperkeratosis [15].

9.5.2 Compression Therapy

The term "passive vascular exercise" became popular in the early 1900s. Blood flow was thought to be improved by passive stretching of the muscular layers of blood vessels. Another notion considered was to use alternating cycles of suction and compression to increase pressure gradients in vessels. By expanding the walls during suction and entirely emptying the venous bed during compression, this also increases the capacity of the venous system. Local and systemic effects of compression therapy are thought to exist. It is more complicated than merely stretching the vessel wall's muscular layers. This explains why a variety of illnesses react to compression therapy, including occlusive arterial disease, venous ulcers, and lymphedema.

9.5.3 Types of Compression

9.5.3.1 Hosiery

Compression stockings are a practical way to treat individuals with swollen limbs. They are useful in avoiding venous stasis by increasing venous outflow and exerting sustained pressure [16]. Graduated compression stockings are available from a variety of manufacturers and are categorized as above or below the knee.

As a result, there is some evidence that employing progressive compression stocking therapy in the swollen limb has its downsides [17]. Another type of compression therapy, such as intermittent pneumatic compression, will be beneficial to a considerable proportion of patients. It is possible that if this type of compression is performed and overseen in patient or home-based treatment, compliance will improve. Finally, there are a variety of compression techniques to choose from, and therapy must be tailored to the patient's condition and circumstances.

9.5.3.2 Bandages

Bandages can be inelastic or elastic, and they can be single or multilayered. Venous ulcers have been proven to benefit from multilayer bandage treatments. The "four-layer" technique has long been considered the gold standard for venous leg ulcer healing; however, additional research suggests that "short stretch" bandages may be just as effective. The success of bandages is based on the experience of the nurse or caregiver using the bandage system. There are various bandaging systems with varied qualities and acting on different scientific concepts.

9.5.3.3 Intermittent Pneumatic Compression [IPC]

IPC is the use of compressed air generated by a specifically constructed pump to apply regulated pressure to the extremities via garments fitting the limb. These devices are made by a variety of companies and can be used on the entire limb, the calf and foot, the calf alone, or the foot alone [18]. The pressure, cycle time, inflation and deflation time, and hold time are among the settings that can be changed. The garments can be single or multicell, and the pressures created range from 20 to 140 mm Hg. The multicell garments, acts by a "milking action" from the distal to the proximal limb when applied.

9.5.4 Exercise and Positional Therapy

- During long flights and vehicle or train travel, the patient is encouraged to move his or her feet and walk occasionally.

- Walking and other forms of physical activity increases muscle pumping and develop leg muscles.
- The patient should alternate between standing on tiptoes and heels. The exercise is done 15 times in each cycle, a few times a day.
- The patient should lie down many times a day with legs elevated and knees gently bent.

9.6 Surgical Management of the Swollen Lower Limb

The cause of a unilaterally swollen limb determines whether surgery is required or not. In uncomplicated varicose veins with simple sapheno-femoral incompetence, significant limb swelling is uncommon. Minor edema can be easily alleviated by ligating the high saphenous vein and stripping the long saphenous vein. If there is substantial edema with varicose veins, it is likely that the deep system of veins has either perforator incompetence or valve incompetence. Importantly, individuals with recurrent varicose veins after varicose vein surgery, persistent or recurrent sapheno-femoral incompetence, or improperly performed surgery may experience leg edema, which can progress to CVI, and are therefore candidates for additional treatment. Deep venous disease that was previously undiagnosed could be present as a result of a previous venous ailment, such as deep venous thrombosis, which could have occurred as a result of trauma [19].

Patients with sapheno-femoral or sapheno-popliteal reflux disease who do not have deep venous disease should have surgery. In both primary and secondary lymphedema, there are insufficient lymphatic channels, causing lymphatic fluid to pool in the subcutaneous tissue. The procedure leaves you with a limb that is prone to recurrent infections and injuries, as well as a poor cosmetic result. There are a variety of surgical procedures for treating lymphedema, but they all require a high level of competence [20]. Due to lack of a clearly defined selection method to determine which patients may benefit from surgery, the majority of lymphedema patients are treated conservatively with combined approach of infection management, massage, elastic clothing, and elevation [21].

There are two types of surgical intervention:

1. Physiological: Efforts are made to restore function; those with obstructive primary lymphedema may benefit from this. Subcutaneous tunnels, buried dermal flaps, lympho-venous shunts and mental transposition have all been explored with varied degrees of success.
2. Excisional: Efforts are focused on minimizing the size of the limb to improve symptoms; this is ideal for those with obliterative lymphedema or secondary lymphedema. The majority of excisional procedures include the removal of subcutaneous tissue blocks, either with or without the overlying skin. Defects are either closed with split skin grafts, as described by Homans and Charles. Many procedures exist that are all weakly supported by data; this could be one of the reasons why surgery is only performed on a small percentage of patients.

9.7 Common Causes of Leg Edema

9.7.1 Lymphedema

Lymphedema affects the upper and lower extremities and is highly frequent following breast cancer surgery due to poor local lymphatic drainage, fluid overload, and increased interstitial lymphatic volume. Skin may also crack and lymph may leak, exposing the skin to bacterial infection and increasing lymphatic drainage, producing a vicious cycle [22].

The goal is to slow the disease progression, reduce the size of the affected extremities, alleviate symptoms, and lower the risk of infection. Patients with lymphedema should be treated conservatively at first, using various compression techniques, and subsequently, if issues persist, a new surgical modality should be considered.

9.7.2 Varicose Vein

Varicose veins can affect anywhere from 10 to 30% of people. Family history, age, and pregnancy are all risk factors for varicose veins, as is standing for lengthy periods of time. Varicose veins can cause a variety of symptoms, including discomfort, aching, soreness, itching or dermatitis, as well as deep vein thrombosis (DVT) [23]. Clinical manifestations and ultrasonography are used to diagnose varicose veins. The gold standard for diagnosing superficial venous incompetence is duplex ultrasonography.

9.7.3 CEAP Classification: C (Clinical Component)

C0	No visible or palpable signs of venous disease
C1	Telangiectases (dilated interdermal venules <1 mm) or reticular veins (nonpalpable subdermal veins 1–3 mm)
C2	Varicose veins (diameter of vein >3 mm)
C3	Edema
C4a	Pigmentation or eczema
C4b	Lipodermatosclerosis
C5	Healed venous ulcer
C6	Active venous ulcer

Conservative treatment with stockings and external compression is an acceptable option to surgery, but if cutaneous abnormalities or symptoms deteriorate despite these efforts, surgery is usually required. However, a patient's preference for surgery over conservative care or for cosmetic reasons alone are both legitimate relative justifications for surgery. Multimodality treatments for varicose veins are the most effective, incorporating modern minimally invasive to endovascular procedures, as well as compression. However, there is no single best accessible treatment option for varicose veins.

9.7.4 Deep Vein Thrombosis

A symptom of venous thromboembolism (VTE) is deep venous thrombosis (DVT). Although most DVT are asymptomatic and resolves without complications, DVT-related major pulmonary embolism (PE) is responsible for up to 300,000 deaths in the USA each year [24]. Anticoagulation, different thrombolysis drugs, and endovascular and surgical treatments such as thrombectomy and inferior vena cava filters to trap venous emboli while maintaining normal venous flow are among the alternatives for treating DVT.

9.8 Filariasis

Humans and animals are both affected by filariasis. Only eight kinds of filarial parasites have been identified, out of hundreds that have been described. Lymphatic filariasis causes lymphatic damage, chronic swelling, and elephantiasis of the legs, arms, scrotum, vulva, and breasts as a result of repeated bouts of inflammation and lymphedema [25].

9.8.1 Lymphatic Filariasis

All species that cause lymphatic filariasis are intermediate hosts and vectors of mosquitoes belonging to the genera Aedes, Anopheles, Culex, or Mansonia.

Nodes in the femoral and epitrochlear areas are the most typically affected. Abscesses can arise anywhere throughout the distal vessel, including the nodes. More abscesses appear to be caused by *B. timori* infection than by *B. malayi* or *W. bancrofti* infection [26]. Microfilariae can be seen in the blood, urine, skin biopsy, and slit lamp examination of the patient's eye. Diethylcarbamazine (DEC), ivermectin, suramin, mebendazole, flubendazole, albendazole, and doxycycline are antimicrobials used to treat filariasis.

9.8.2 Cellulitis

Acute inflammatory episodes, often known as "cellulitis," are common in persons with chronic edema and should be treated with antibiotics as soon as possible, especially if systemic symptoms are evident [30]. Lower limb cellulitis affects both men and women equally, although it becomes more common with advancing age; the aging population and obesity have both contributed to an increase in the frequency of lower limb cellulitis [27].

Bacteria infiltrating a damaged skin surface is a common cause of cellulitis. Breaks in the skin, such as cracks between toes or lower leg ulcers, are common entry points for germs. To rule out other potentially serious differential diagnoses, such as deep vein thrombosis, a prompt and accurate assessment with a diagnosis are essential. Septicemia and other problems can be avoided with early treatment.

Cellulitis should be treated with the aim of resolving symptoms, efficiently managing infection and avoiding hospitalization. Antibiotic treatment should be continued in lymphedema patients until all indications of acute inflammation have subsided, which normally takes at least 14 days after a definite clinical response has been detected. Cellulitis treatment in lymphedema patients is complicated, and help from lymphedema specialist services should be sought whenever feasible.

9.9 Summary and Recommendations

- When treating leg edema with an unknown cause, the physician should first rule out lipedema (fat maldistribution with sparing of the feet) and lymphedema (marked foot and toe involvement, verrucous thickened skin, non-pitting when chronic) because the evaluation and treatment for these disorders are different.
- Idiopathic edema (in young women) and chronic venous insufficiency (in older patients) are the most common causes of bilateral leg edema.
- In patients with persistent bilateral edema, the physician should assess the most frequent systemic causes (cardiac, renal, and hepatic) and determine which of them should be ruled out with additional testing based on the patient's history and physical examination. Pulmonary hypertension is a prevalent cause of sleep apnea and should be considered in patients who have a large neck circumference, loud snoring, or apnea observed by a sleep partner.
- A Doppler test should be used to rule out a deep vein thrombosis if the patient presents with sudden onset (<72 h) leg edema.

References

1. Gorman WP, Davis KR, Donnelly R. Swollen lower limb: general assessment and deep vein thrombosis. West J Med. 2001;174(2):132–6. PMCID: PMC1071280.
2. Scallan J, Huxley VH, Korthuis RJ. Capillary fluid exchange: regulation, functions, and pathology. San Rafael (CA): Morgan & Claypool Life Sciences; 2010. PMID: 21452435.
3. Lent-Schochet D, Jialal I. Physiology, Edema. [Updated 2021 May 9]. In: StatPearls [Internet]. Treasure Island (FL): StatPearls Publishing; 2021 Jan-. Available from: https://www.ncbi.nlm.nih.gov/books/NBK537065/
4. Ely JW, Osheroff JA, Chambliss ML, Ebell MH. Approach to leg edema of unclear etiology. J Am Board Fam Med. 2006 Mar-Apr;19(2):148–60. https://doi.org/10.3122/jabfm.19.2.148. Erratum in: J Am Board Fam Med. 2008 Jan-Feb;21(1):86. PMID: 16513903.
5. Williams A, Craig G. Chronic oedema: challenges for community nurses. J Commun Nurs. 2007;21(11):38–44.
6. O'Donnell TF Jr, Rasmussen JC, Sevick-Muraca EM. New diagnostic modalities in the evaluation of lymphedema. J Vasc Surg Venous Lymphat Disord. 2017 Mar;5(2):261–73. https://doi.org/10.1016/j.jvsv.2016.10.083. Epub 2017 Jan 16. PMID: 28214496; PMCID: PMC5325714.
7. Liang ZY, Long X, Yu NZ, Huang JZ. Diagnostic workup of lymphedema. Plast Aesthet Res. 2019;6:23. https://doi.org/10.20517/2347-9264.2019.33.

8. Tamura K, Nakahara H. MR venography for the assessment of deep vein thrombosis in lower extremities with varicose veins. Ann Vasc Dis. 2014;7(4):399–403. https://doi.org/10.3400/avd.oa.14-00068. Epub 2014 Dec 25. PMID: 25593625; PMCID: PMC4293190.
9. Kattula SRST, Avula A, Baradhi KM. Anasarca. [Updated 2021 Feb 16]. In: StatPearls [Internet]. Treasure Island (FL): StatPearls Publishing; 2021 Jan-. Available from: https://www.ncbi.nlm.nih.gov/books/NBK519013/
10. O'Hearn DJ, Gold AR, Gold MS, Diggs P, Scharf SM. Lower extremity edema and pulmonary hypertension in morbidly obese patients with obstructive sleep apnea. Sleep Breath. 2009;13(1):25–34. https://doi.org/10.1007/s11325-008-0200-z. Epub 2008 July 10. PMID: 18615260
11. Ely JW, Osheroff JA, Chambliss ML, Ebell MH. Approach to leg edema of unclear etiology. J Am Board Fam Med. 2006 Mar-Apr;19(2):148–60.
12. Easterbrook J, Walker MA. The unilateral swollen lower limb: etiology, investigation, and management. Int J Low Extrem Wounds. 2002;1(4):242–50.
13. Stephen-Haynes J. Skin and wound care in chronic oedema. In: Chronic Oedema Supplement. Wounds UK 2007;3(2):35–9.
14. Health Quality Ontario. Compression Stockings for the Prevention of Venous Leg Ulcer Recurrence: A Health Technology Assessment. Ont Health Technol Assess Ser. 2019 Feb 19;19(2):1–86. PMID: 30828407; PMCID: PMC6394515.
15. Lim CS, Davies AH. Graduated compression stockings. CMAJ. 2014 Jul 8;186(10): E391–8. https://doi.org/10.1503/cmaj.131281. Epub 2014 Mar 3. PMID: 24591279; PMCID: PMC4081237.
16. Delis KT, Azizi ZA, Stevens RJ, Wolfe JH, Nicolaides AN. Optimum intermittent pneumatic compression stimulus for lower-limb venous emptying. Eur J Vasc Endovasc Surg. 2000 Mar;19(3):261–9.
17. Campbell B. Varicose veins and their management. BMJ 2006;333(7562):287–292. https://doi.org/10.1136/bmj.333.7562.287. PMID: 16888305; PMCID: PMC1526945.
18. Ciudad P, Sabbagh MD, Agko M, Huang TCT, Manrique OJ, Carmen Román L, Reynaga C, Delgado R, Maruccia M, Chen HC. Surgical management of lower extremity lymphedema: a comprehensive review. Indian J Plast Surg. 2019 Jan; 52(1):81–92. https://doi.org/10.1055/s-0039-1688537. Epub 2019 May 14. PMID: 31456616; PMCID: PMC6664851.
19. Kareh AM, Xu KY. Surgical management of lymphedema. Mo Med. 2020 Mar-Apr; 117(2):143–8. PMID: 32308240; PMCID: PMC7144713.
20. Alguire PC, Mathes BM. Chronic venous insufficiency and venous ulceration. J Gen Intern Med. 1997;12:374–83.
21. Lin F, Zhang S, Sun Y, Ren S, Liu P. The management of varicose veins. Int Surg 2015 Jan; 100(1):185–189. https://doi.org/10.9738/INTSURG-D-14-00084.1. PMID: 25594661; PMCID: PMC4301287.
22. Fleck D, Albadawi H, Wallace A, Knuttinen G, Naidu S, Oklu R. Below-knee deep vein thrombosis (DVT): diagnostic and treatment patterns. Cardiovasc Diagn Ther. 2017;7(Suppl 3):S134–9. https://doi.org/10.21037/cdt.2017.11.03. PMID: 29399516; PMCID: PMC5778527
23. Syed A. A review of Filariasis. Int J Curr Res Med Sci. 2019;5(2):26–30.
24. Chandy A, Thakur AS, Singh MP, Manigauha A. A review of neglected tropical diseases: filariasis. Asian Pac J Trop Med. 2011 Jul;4(7):581–6.
25. Atkin L. Cellulitis of the lower limbs: diagnosis and management. Nurse Prescribing. 2017;15:588–92.
26. Ely JW, Osheroff JA, Lee Chambliss M, Ebell MH. Approach to leg edema of unclear etiology. J Am Board Family Med. 2006;19(2):148–60.
27. Dayna E., Gary Lymphedema diagnosis and management. Journal of the American Academy of Nurse Practitioners 2007;19(2):72–8. https://doi.org/10.1111/j.1745-7599.2006.00198.x.

DEEP Vein Thrombosis

10

Patrick Harnarayan, Dave Harnanan,
and Vijay Naraynsingh

10.1 Definition of Deep Vein Thrombosis

Deep vein thrombosis (DVT) occurs when thrombus forms in the deep veins of the limbs, and although many of these cases are asymptomatic, most (88%) typically involve the proximal veins, with 96% occurring in the pelvis and lower limb while 4% are found in the upper extremities [1]. Pulmonary embolism, the most feared complication, occurs when thrombus migrates into the lung accounting for the major cause of mortality [2].

10.2 History of Deep Vein Thrombosis

Thrombosis was known to ancient civilizations, appearing in Chinese writings in 2650 BC and was described as a pathological hemostasis [3]. The European entry to this landscape involves the Greek philosophers Plato (428–347 BC) who suggested that blood had "fibers" and Hippocrates, who observed that the blood of wounded soldiers on the battlefield "congealed" as it cooled (400 BC). The word "Thrombus" appears in the seventeenth-century texts, a transliteration of the Greek word Θρομβος which is "clot" designated in the 1850s by Virchow [4]. He demonstrated that a clot is formed when blood semi-solidifies ex vivo and a thrombus, in vivo.

Eventually, van Leeuwenhoek discovered the presence of red cells as a component of blood, previously thought to be fluid, and Marcello Malpighi (1628–1694) described the flow of blood in the capillaries of the lung (1661) and the effect of stagnation in these capillaries. John Hunter (1728–1793) noted the coagulated blood had a malevolent association with the veins which were afflicted with

P. Harnarayan · D. Harnanan · V. Naraynsingh (✉)
Department of Clinical Surgical Sciences, University of the West Indies, Trinidad and Tobago

S. K. Tiwary (ed.), *Approach to Lower Limb Oedema*,
https://doi.org/10.1007/978-981-16-6206-5_10

"inflammation of the internal walls." Baillie observed that obstruction of the inferior vena cava led to thrombosis and Cruveilhier correlated the changes in the lung, thought initially to be lobar pneumonia, noting clots in the pulmonary arteries. He astutely observed that when these lesions were found in the lung, "others could be found somewhere else within the venous system." Hunter concluded that DVT was a venous occlusion caused by clots [5] and performed venous ligations above the clots [6] to prevent fatal venous thromboembolism to the lungs [7].

Around 1846, Virchow indicated that pulmonary emboli arose from thrombi in the pelvic and femoral veins (quoted by Jorpes, 1946) and that these formed from eddies in pockets of larger valves of the veins [8]. By 1856, he had put forward the theory that there was a triad of interactions between decreased blood flow in the veins, vein wall injury, and abnormality in the blood and concluded that **thrombi** and **emboli** formed from moving, not static blood.

Unconfirmed reports are that the first clinical description of DVT came from the ancient Indian surgeon Sushruta [9] who was regarded as the "Father of Surgery" in India, and his influential treatise, the *Sushruta Samhita*, contains the first known description of basic surgical procedures. Phlegmasia alba dolens, seen historically during pregnancy and puerperium with extensive DVT compromising arterial flow, was described in 1784 and Phlegmasia cerulea dolens, the painful "blue" leg, due to obstruction in the deep as well as in the superficial venous system, in 1857. Homans sign, pain in the calf on dorsiflexion of the foot to clinically demonstrate DVT, was described in 1944 [10].

10.3 Epidemiology of Deep Vein Thrombosis

The reported incidence of DVT in the Western world is approximately 50–80/100,000 population with increases during winter and increasing age [11]. Studies in the USA and Sweden show that the weighted mean occurrence of a first-time DVT in the general population was 50.4/100,000 people with a 20–30/100,000 per year increase in the 30-49-year age group, up to 200/100,000 per year in the over 70 age group [12]. Women had a higher relative risk of DVT than men in the >65-year age group [13] and men a twofold increase above 75.5 years [14].

Ethnicity and variations by regions have a great influence on incidence. The incidence of DVT and venous thromboembolism (VTE) in the population of California, USA, considered variable in ethnicity was high among Caucasians (230 per 100,000) and African Americans (293 per 100,000) but had a low incidence in Latinos (139 per 100,000) and Asian-Pacific Islanders (60 per 100,000) [15]. In the Black Caribbean population, the overall annual incidence of DVT was 11.0 per 100,000 person years with a sharp rise with age (both genders), but rare in pregnancy [16].

Independent studies showed that people of European ancestry generally have a DVT rate of between 45 and 117 per 100,000 population [14, 17] with Britain, Denmark, Norway, and France showing varied incidences of 40, 65, 93, and 124 per 100,000 population [18–20].

The incidence in Asian Indian patients was thought to be lower than in the West, but one study found that Indian patients undergoing major lower limb surgery had a rate of 43.2%, comparable to Western figures [21], and in Southern India, researchers found 194.9 cases per 100,000 admissions over a 6-year period [22]. It is possible that VTE is quite similar in incidence to that in the West [9].

In other Asian populations, the incidence was also considered to be low, but in Singapore, the frequency of DVT at one hospital was found to be 158/100,000 admissions [23], while in Malaysia patients undergoing orthopedic procedures exhibited a high incidence (62.5%) of radiographically diagnosed DVT [24].

Japan showed an incidence of 19.2 per 100,000 population and a doubling of the incidence from 2006 [25]. This was explained by the change from a traditional Japanese to a more Westernized lifestyle, increased obesity, more diagnoses of malignancy, and liberal use of the oral contraceptive pill [26, 27].

10.4 Pathophysiology of Deep Vein Thrombosis: Mechanism and Pathology

Deep vein thrombosis (DVT) occurs because of the triad of venous stasis, vessel injury, and hypercoagulability [28] (Virchow 1856). Although venous stasis is considered to be the most prominent [29], by itself, it may not be capable of promoting thrombosis.

Thrombosis appears where there is altered blood flow in relation to the "pockets" next to the valves of the deep veins [30, 31]. It is thought that a drop in the velocity of blood causes stasis and hypoxia [32], and these two combine with existing inflammatory changes to initiate thrombosis [33, 34]. Many of the vessel-based anti-thrombotic agents like thrombomodulin [35] and endothelial protein C receptor (EPCR) are physically expressed on the valves [36].

It is also believed that hypoxia can lead to stimulation of procoagulant factors [32] which exist in the endothelium and promote cellular aggregation [34]. The presence of tissue factor (TF) lends to favorable conditions [37]since cellular elements containing TF are known to play a major role in thrombus formation [38]. Active malignancies appear to have fragment pieces (membrane particles) which have procoagulant activity [39, 40], one of which is TF [41]. In addition, some substrates possess sites for carbohydrate-binding adhesion molecules called Selectins, and one of these, P-Selectin, interacts with immunologic cells containing TF. P-Selectin has procoagulant properties and appears to be driven here by hypoxia [42], but it also binds to mucin cells produced by malignant tumors [43], and this interaction is thought to cause thrombosis in these patients.

This risk increases with age because the quantity of procoagulants increases with age, but this is not complemented by a corresponding increase in naturally occurring endothelial anticoagulants such as protein C [44]. This also decreases when there are extended periods of illness and immobilization [45].

10.5 Sites of Deep Vein Thrombosis

The most common site recorded in three large studies was the **femoral-popliteal** segment - 74% [46], 42% [47], 34% [48], followed by the **ilio-femoral segment** - 58% [46], 38% [48], 23% [49], and the **calf segment** - 69% [50], 40% [46], 32% [49].

Labrapoulos et al. [51] found that 40% of "normal" color-coded duplex scans had acute isolated calf DVT when the muscular veins were imaged. When the calf veins were independently assessed, the peroneal vein 81% [50], 41% [51], the posterior tibial vein 69% [50], 37% [51], and the soleal 39% and gastrocnemius 29% [51] were the most common non-muscular and muscular calf vein sites to demonstrate thromboses. Yoshimura et al. also found that muscular calf veins were the commonest site for DVT [52].

Unusual sites for DVT included the deep femoral vein (0.31%), the deep external pudendal vein (0.04%), and veins in Klippel-Trenaunay syndrome (0.12%): the muscular thigh branch, lateral thigh branch, and sciatic vein [53].

10.6 Pathology of the Edema of Deep Vein Thrombosis

Edema of the lower limb can be a significant finding in DVT. Its cross-sectional area, estimated by computerized tomography, is approximately 300 mls, 50% of which appears in the extracellular fluid [54]. In DVT, there is an increase of about 200 mls, most residing in this extracellular fluid [55].

The pathology of this edema appears to have its basis in the transcapillary forces at work in the limb. Under normal circumstances, these forces keep the fluid balance in dynamic equilibrium; however, this is disrupted in the presence of thrombosis [56].

Venous pressure at the foot in the upright patient exceeds 100 mmHg and at this pressure, transcapillary filtration is increased, which increases the fluid in the interstitium [57]. This increase in capillary filtration is thought to be the major cause of edema in DVT, but there is also a corresponding decrease in the resorption of fluid at the venous end of the capillaries [58]. The crucial factor usually preventing this is the calf muscle pump mechanism, which normally empties the sinusoids on contraction, e.g., during walking [59], and on relaxation the veins expand lowering the pressure significantly. However, this activity is severely impaired in DVT, since the deep venous pump system is not intact and may be paralyzed.

The lymphatic system also plays a role in edema of patients with DVT [60]. There is a reduction in the clearance of injected ^{131}I-labeled albumin from the subcutaneous tissue in patients with lymphedema, and there is an observed decrease in cutaneous lymphatic flow which is an important factor in the production of edema in DVT [61].

10.7 Risk Factors Associated with Deep Vein Thrombosis

Age and ethnicity are major risk factors, with DVT increasing with age for both male and females [62] with Afro-Americans and Caucasians having a greater risk of DVT than Hispanic and Asian-Pacific Islanders [15]. Surgery is an independent risk factor with the incidence of postoperative DVT increasing with patient age, duration of surgery [63], and type of surgery [64]. DVT also remains a life-threatening complication after major trauma [65], and at presentation, 25% of trauma patients show evidence of hypercoagulability [66]. Immobility brought about by prolonged bed rest, nursing home confinement [67], air travel [68], or hospitalization poses a greater than 100-fold risk of thrombotic events than in the community [69].

There is an increased risk of DVT in active malignancy [70] with first-time idiopathic DVT in normal individuals being a marker for malignant disease [71]. In the year which precedes this diagnosis, there is usually an unexplained rise in VTE associated with advanced disease [72] and also a sharp increase in the diagnosis of malignancy in the following years, persisting for up to 10 years after initial admission for DVT [73].

Medical disorders capable of inducing thromboses include chronic kidney disease, inflammatory bowel diseases (1.98-fold) [74], clinically proven HIV (2- to10-fold) [75], and heparin induced thrombocytopenia [76]. Diabetes mellitus (type 1 and 2), with diminished fibrinolysis, showed a tendency toward thrombosis twice that of the nondiabetic population [77]. Congestive cardiac failure patients are considered at risk of developing DVT, and the longer the hospital stay, the greater the risk [78]. Women have increased risks in pregnancy and the puerperium [79, 80], with the pill, hormonal treatment, and hormone replacement therapy [81, 82].

Hematological diseases such as polycythemia vera, leukemia, Hodgkin's and other lymphomas, myeloproliferative disorders [73, 83, 84], and relapsed and refractory multiple myeloma all have an increased risk of DVT [85, 86]. Anticoagulant factor deficiency in antithrombin III, proteins S and C [87], and the lesser known protein Z [88] also produce increased risks of DVT. The factor V Leiden thrombophilic gene mutation [89], prothrombin G2021OA gene mutation [90], and the novel prothrombin variant C20209T [91] are seen in patients with DVT and a strong family history of thrombophilia [92]. In addition, elevated levels of factor VIII carry a high risk of DVT [93] as seen in Afro-Caribbean populations where thrombin production is elevated [94].

The risk of incident DVT among varicose vein patients [95] appears due to increased inflammatory and hypercoagulation factor markers in their plasma [96]. Klippel-Trenaunay syndrome, due to venous stasis [97] and May Thurner syndrome by venous compression [98] also produce severe deep vein thromboses. Superficial venous thrombosis (SVT) considered a "benign" disease is now regarded as part of the paraneoplastic syndrome [99] since there is a clear association between migratory thrombophlebitis and malignancy [100], based on the observations of Trousseau [101]. SVT clearly is not always benign nor self-limiting as previously thought [102].

Table 10.1 Risk factors for deep vein thrombosis

High Risk
≫ Major surgery >3 h: Orthopedic, transplant, cardiovascular, trauma ≫ 75 yrs. old, current smoker, major trauma, # pelvis/femur/tibia ≫ Active malignancy +/− chemotherapy, oral contraceptive pill ≫ Acute spinal cord injury; neurological disease with leg paresis ≫ Stroke <1 month, BMI >50 kg/m^3
Medium Risk
≫ Major surgery (arthroscopic + laparoscopic surgery) >30 min ≫ 60–74 yrs old, confined to hospital bed >3 days with acute illness ≫ Recent VTE (DVT, PE), family history VTE, superficial venous thrombosis (SVT), varicose veins, venous malformations, venous compression ≫ Positive factor V Leiden and prothrombin 20210A, +ve lupus anticoagulant, elevated anticardiolipin antibodies, heparin-induced thrombocytopenia (HIT); other thrombophilia: proteins S, C, Z, and antithrombin III deficiencies. ≫ Central venous access, BMI ≥35 kg/m^3, non-contraceptive estrogen+progestins, immobilizing plaster cast, long-distance travel ≫ Inflammatory bowel disease, congestive cardiac failure, acute myocardial infarct <1 month, sepsis <1 month, pregnancy/ puerperium
Low Risk
Age >40 years, minor surgery, elective abdominal and thoracic surgery <30 min, no other risk factors
Age <40 years, minor surgery, uncomplicated abdominal or thoracic surgery, no other risk factors.

Caprini [103], Agarwal et al. [104],Grant et al. [105]

10.8 Diagnosis of Deep Vein Thrombosis

The diagnosis of a deep vein thrombosis (DVT) requires consideration of clinical findings, hematological investigations, and imaging. Additional consideration must be given to the level and extent of thrombus in the deep veins, whether the thrombus is completely or partially occlusive and if there are complications.

The diagnosis should be entertained in patients who present with acute unilateral leg swelling, erythema, warmth, tenderness, and engorged superficial veins [Fig. 10.1]. Since the clinical presentation of DVT is variable, scoring systems have been established to make a definitive diagnosis. The Wells score is a useful tool in evaluating and guiding management of DVT [Table 10.2]. The probability scores estimate the likelihood of DVT by incorporating signs, symptoms, and risk factors. According to the NICE guidelines, the sensitivity and specificity for DVT ranged from 77% to 98% and 37% to 58%, respectively [106].The Wells score clearly boasts of good sensitivity but lacks specificity and should not be used as a sole diagnostic modality.

10.9 D-Dimer

Following thrombus formation, the fibrinolytic response is activated resulting in the generation of plasmin and the release of fibrin degradation products including D-dimer. The D-dimer level is elevated in patients with acute DVT and can be

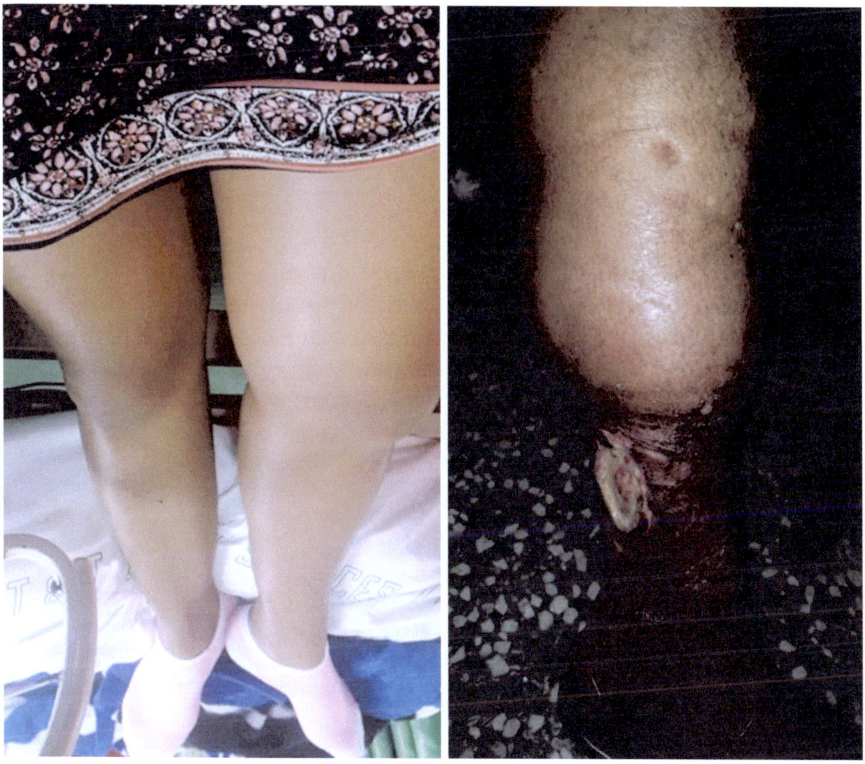

Fig. 10.1 Left: Acute unilateral limb edema with ilio-femoral DVT. Right: Post-thrombotic syndrome - lipodermatosclerosis with venous ulcer and proximal unilateral leg edema

Table 10.2 The Wells score [107]

Clinical Feature	Points
Active cancer (on treatment, treated in the last 6 months or palliative)	1
Paralysis, paresis, or plaster immobilization of the lower limb	1
Bedridden for 3 days or more, or major surgery in the past 12 weeks requiring general or regional anesthesia	1
Localized tenderness along the distribution of the deep venous system	1
Entire leg swollen	1
Calf Swelling 3 cm larger than the symptomatic side	1
Pitting edema confined to the symptomatic leg	1
Collateral superficial veins (non-varicose)	1
Previous DVT	1
Alternative diagnosis is at least as likely as DVT	−2
Clinical probability simplified score	Points
DVT likely	2 points or more
DVT unlikely	1 points or less

quantitatively assessed. It can also be elevated in conditions such liver disease, pregnancy, malignancy, and post-surgery. The sensitivity and specificity for D-dimer tests ranged from 75% to 100% and 26% to 83%, respectively, implying that this test is not suitable for confirming the presence of DVT, but can assist in eliminating it [106].

10.10 Ultrasound (US)

US is preferred as a first-line imaging modality for the diagnosis of DVT, and diagnostic criteria include non-compressibility, increased intraluminal echogenicity, absence of flow augmentation, and reduced or absent blood flow. US examination has high sensitivity and specificity for the diagnosis of symptomatic proximal lower extremity DVT when compared to conventional venography [Fig. 10.2]. The diagnostic performance is consistent in the femoral and popliteal veins, but less in the ilio-caval region and below the knee [108, 109]. It has improved diagnostic accuracy and reproducibility and is the preferred first-line diagnostic test for patients with suspected chronic DVT [110, 111].

10.11 CT Venography

Since ultrasonography may be influenced by body habitus and operator dependence, CT venography can be complementary in achieving diagnostic accuracy, proximal extent, and characterizing extrinsic compression in the case of pelvic masses and May-Thurner's syndrome [112–114]. CT venography can also be incorporated into an examination that includes pulmonary CT angiography for evaluation of both PE and proximal DVT [115]. In patients with suspected PE, a recent meta-analysis found that CT venography for the diagnosis of proximal DVT has a high sensitivity (95.9%) and specificity (95.2%) [Fig. 10.3] [116].

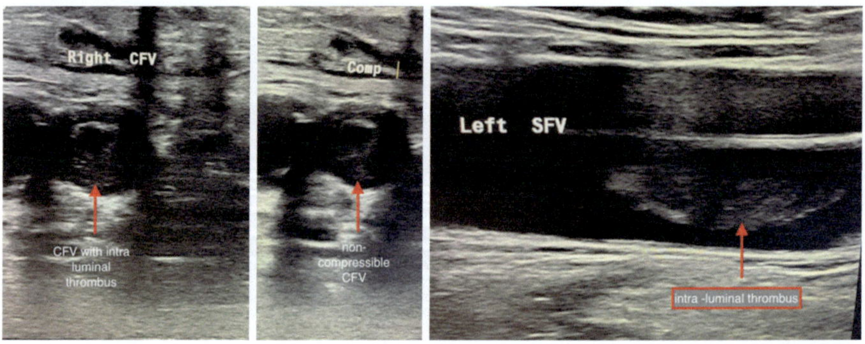

Fig. 10.2 (Right) Thrombus in common femoral vein will fail to compress on ultrasonography. (Left) Partially occlusive thrombus in superficial femoral vein

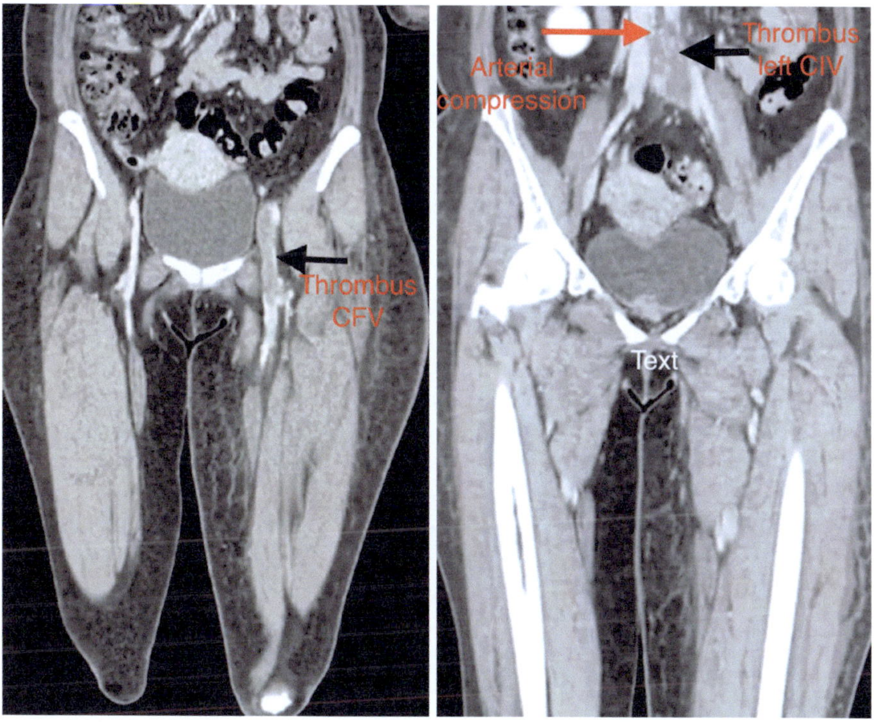

Fig. 10.3 (Right) CT venogram demonstrating thrombus in left CFV extending to the CIV. (Left) Diagnosis of May-Thurner's syndrome

10.12 Magnetic Resonance Venography

Magnetic resonance (MR) venography shares many of the clinical advantages of US, such as preventing exposure to ionizing radiation or iodinated contrast media. It also has the advantage of cross-sectional imaging for delineation of extravascular anatomy and identification of extrinsic venous compression, which may be an underlying cause of lower extremity DVT.

10.13 Venography

Ascending venography can accurately identify post-thrombotic changes in the deep venous system, the collateral patterns, and status of ilio-caval veins. It is useful for determining whether endovascular or surgical intervention is needed and which procedure is preferable. Descending venography can determine the extent of the reflux and may be useful for determining whether deep venous reconstructive surgery is needed and what type of surgery is feasible [117]. Imaging with intravascular ultrasound (IVUS) with cross-sectional views of the vein and adjacent structures has high diagnostic accuracy for ilio-caval thrombus burden or ilio-caval compression. This may influence the therapeutic options in terms of the accuracy and efficacy of endovascular venous techniques (Fig. 10.4) [118, 119].

10.14 Hematological Investigations

Thrombophilia is an acquired or inherited predisposition to venous thrombosis, and inherited thrombophilia includes deficiencies in one of the three natural anticoagulants—antithrombin III, protein C, and protein S, which have been linked with familial venous thrombosis.

According to the International Consensus Statement (2005), screening for thrombophilia should be performed in (1) all patients with a first episode of spontaneous VTE; (2) patients with VTE under the age of 50 years even with a transient predisposing factor; (3) patients with VTE whose only risk factor is oral contraceptive therapy, estrogen replacement therapy, or pregnancy; and (4) patients with recurrent VTE irrespective of the presence of risk factors. Genetic thrombophilia testing is not routinely recommended in all patients with DVT. [121]

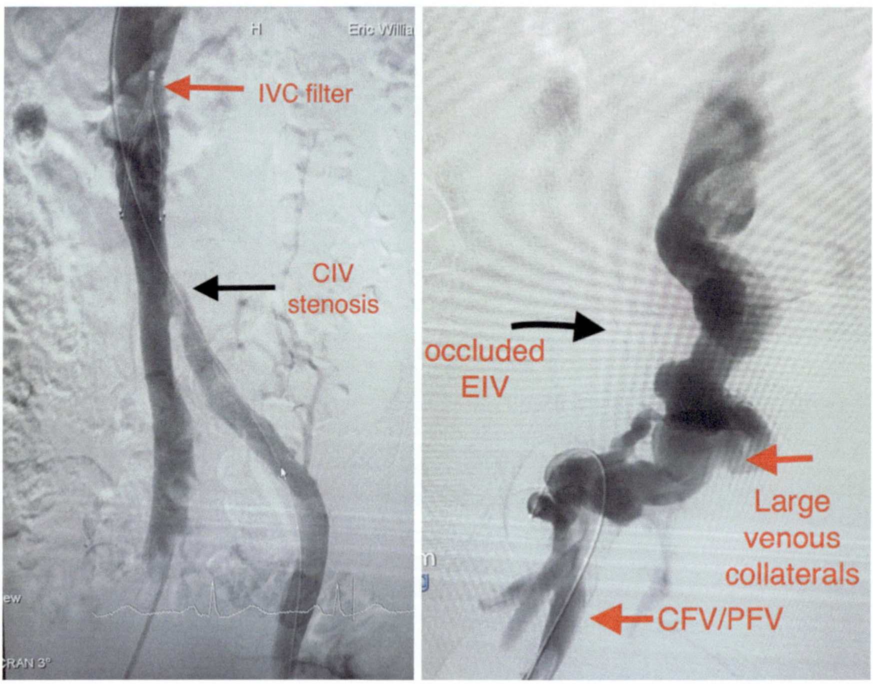

Fig. 10.4 (Right) Ascending venogram with IVC filter in situ filled with thrombus and left CIV stenosis. (Left) Chronically occluded external iliac vein with large collaterals

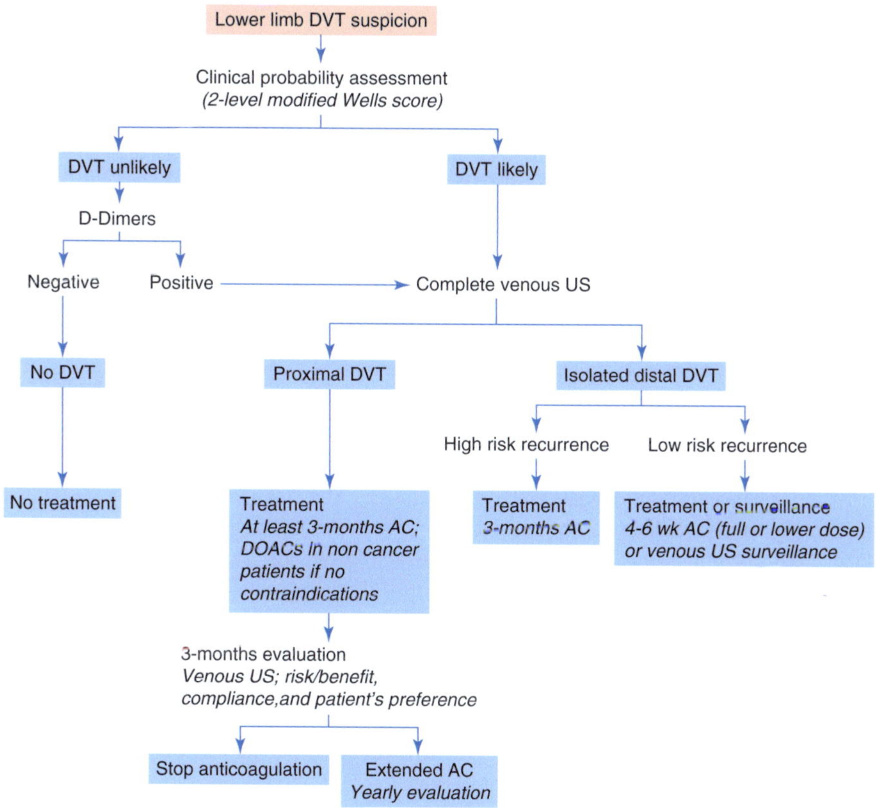

Fig. 10.5 Algorithm for the diagnosis of DVT. In patients with a low or unlikely clinical probability score, further diagnostic tests, such as the D-dimer test and duplex ultrasonography, can be performed to rule out DVT [120]

10.15 Treatment Strategies

Treatment of lower limb deep vein thrombosis can be considered and consists of three phases [122]:

- Initial treatment (5–21 days following diagnosis)
- Long-term treatment (first 3–6 months)
- Extended treatment (beyond 3–6 months)

10.16 Anticoagulation

In the initial phase of treatment, the patient receives parenteral therapy transitioning to vitamin K antagonists (VKA) or high-dose direct oral anticoagulants (DOAC). In patients with severe renal failure (creatinine clearance <30 mL/min), unstable renal function, or high bleeding risk, intravenous unfractionated heparin (UFH) may be preferable due to its short half-life and protamine sulfate reversibility. However, UFH is associated with dosing variability requiring laboratory monitoring and regular adjustments. Additionally, it is associated with high risk of heparin-induced thrombocytopenia [122]. For these reasons, low-molecular-weight heparin (LMWH) is the treatment of choice since they are as effective as UFH and probably safer [123]. Fondaparinux can also be used as parenteral agent [124].

Direct oral anticoagulants (DOACs) have emerged as valid options for long-term DVT treatment [122]. A meta-analysis (27,023 patients) showed similar VTE recurrence rates in patients receiving DOACs or conventional therapy (2.0% vs 2.2%, RR 0.90). Major bleeding (RR 0.61), fatal bleeding (RR 0.36), intracranial bleeding (RR 0.37), and clinically relevant non-major bleeding (RR 0.73) were significantly lower in DOAC-treated patients. DOACs as standalone therapy for DVT is gaining popularity [106, 125].

The risk of recurrence following discontinuation of anticoagulation after a first episode of DVT remains consistently around 30%. The risk is significantly increased in unprovoked DVTs (annual rate >7%) versus those with provoked DVT. Additionally, the risk of recurrence is higher for unprovoked DVTs than unprovoked PE [120].

For proximal DVT and/or PE, 3-months anticoagulation is the best option if transient and reversible risk factors were present. In all other patients, prolonging anticoagulation protects from recurrence (70–90%) but exposes to risk of unpredictable bleeding complications. Decision to discontinue anticoagulation should be individually tailored and balanced against bleeding risk, taking also into account patients' preferences and the associated cost.

10.17 Compression Therapy

PTS is a seriously burdensome complication of DVT that develops in 25–50% of patients [126, 127]. Its clinical features range from minor limb swelling and discomfort to severe leg pain, edema, skin changes, and even ulceration. Venous claudication and eventually lymphedema can severely affect quality of life of patients who develop PTS [128]. Compression therapy was thought to prevent PTS by reducing venous hypertension and reflux and can be used to treat leg complaints [129].

Kahn and colleagues reported the results of a multicenter randomized placebo-controlled trial of active treatment (knee-length stockings with 30–40 mmHg compression) versus placebo compression stocking (knee-length sham stockings without therapeutic compression) for 2 years in 806 patients to prevent PTS after a first proximal lower extremity DVT. The cumulative incidence of PTS was 14.2% for active compression stockings versus 12.7% for placebo compression stockings. These findings do not support routine wearing of compression stockings after DVT [130].

The efficacy of compression stockings in terms of reducing the incidence of PTS in patients with lower extremity DVT remains controversial; however, compression therapy associated with early mobilization and walking exercises has been effective in the relief of acute DVT symptoms and as such the decision for its early usage should be individualized. However, compression stockings may be required by patients to control their PTS symptoms beyond 2 years. This is more as a treatment for PTS rather than prevention of PTS.

10.18 Thrombolysis and Thrombectomy

Anticoagulation therapy is the main treatment option for acute femoropopliteal DVT, but anticoagulation in extensive ilio-femoral DVT is often not sufficient to prevent later development of chronic venous insufficiency and post-thrombotic syndrome [131–133].

Therefore, early thrombus removal is desirable. Surgical venous thrombectomy is recommended in selected patients who are candidates for anticoagulation but in whom thrombolytic therapy is contraindicated or not available [134]. In patients with limb-threatening venous ischemia, such as venous gangrene or phlegmasia cerulea dolens, aggressive thrombus removal should be considered if the patient's general condition is acceptable [135, 136]. Endovascular techniques for early thrombus removal for DVT consist of catheter-directed thrombolytic therapy (CDT) and/or percutaneous mechanical thrombectomy (PMT) [137]. Endovascular maneuvers at thrombus removal should be considered for patients with symptomatic ilio-femoral DVT who have symptoms of less than 14-days duration, good functional status, a life expectancy of 1 year or more, and a low risk of bleeding. When phlegmasia cerulea dolens or venous gangrene is present, aggressive endovascular thrombus removal should be performed on an emergency basis for limb salvage [132, 138, 139].

The threshold for thrombus removal strategies in acute femoropopliteal DVT should be higher than that for iliofemoral DVT. Multicenter registries have suggested a less favorable outcome for femoropopliteal than iliofemoral DVT treated with thrombolytic therapy [140].

CDT achieves early lysis of the blood clot, resulting in rapid relief of the symptoms and improved venous patency rates. The results of randomized trials and meta-analyses suggest that CDT improves quality of life without an unacceptable increase in bleeding [141–143]. Major bleeding complications have been reported at rates of 2–4% [144–146]. CDT is noted to preserve venous valvular function and decreased occurrence of PE and PTS [137].

Although CDT may be associated with asymptomatic radiographic evidence of PE, symptomatic PE appears to be a relatively rare complication of CDT. The incidence of clinical PE during CDT does not appear to exceed that in patients who receive anticoagulation therapy alone. According to the Prevention du Risque d'Embolie Pulmonaire par Interruption Cave (PREPIC) study, which was the first reported multicenter randomized controlled trial, the incidence of DVT at 2 years after inferior vena cava (IVC) filter placement was significantly higher than that in the no IVC filter group. In contrast, the overall survival rate was not significantly different between the two groups [147]. Therefore, routine placement of permanent IVC filters in patients undergoing CDT for DVT is not recommended in terms of short-term efficacy and long-term complications [138, 147, 148]. However, the introduction of retrievable filters has contributed to their increased overall usage. Filter Implantation to Lower Thromboembolic Risk in Percutaneous Endovenous Intervention (FILTER-PEVI) trial reported that IVC filter implantation during pharmaco-mechanical-thrombectomy (PMT) reduced the risk of iatrogenic PE eightfold (1.4% vs. 11.3%), without reducing mortality [149]. The use of periprocedural IVC filter may be considered in patients at high risk of PE, such as those with free-floating thrombus extending into the IVC, with marked limited cardiopulmonary reserve, or with mechanical thrombectomy alone [132, 149, 150].

Open surgical venous thrombectomy can be performed in selected patients when endovascular facilities are not available, such as those with a first episode of acute iliofemoral DVT, symptoms <14 days in duration, a low risk of bleeding, ambulatory with good functional capacity, and an acceptable life expectancy. In cases where these criteria are not met, conventional anticoagulation may be preferred over high-risk surgery (Fig. 10.6 [134]).

10.19 Surgical Treatment of Chronic Lower Extremity DVT

Despite therapeutic anticoagulation and elastic compression stocking therapy, a significant proportion of DVT patients may develop post-thrombotic sequelae. Because the iliac vein rarely recanalizes, patients with chronic iliofemoral DVT develop significant symptoms of PTS associated with valvular reflux and persistent venous obstruction [35, 46, 151]. Endovascular strategies at recanalization of the iliofemoral venous segments play an important role in improving presenting symptoms, reduction of venous disability, and/or healing of existing venous ulcers [138]. Recanalization was technically successful in 83% of occluded iliac veins with the 4-year primary and secondary patency rates approximately 35% and 72%, respectively [152, 153]. Although there are no high-level randomized controlled data, recanalization of chronic occlusive DVT can be performed safely and successfully and provide significant improvement in venous flow, ultimately leading to symptom relief and improvement in the quality of life.

Patients with chronic DVT who are not candidates for endovascular repair or those who failed attempts of endovascular revascularization can undergo open surgical reconstruction. Successful surgical bypass for iliofemoral venous occlusion refractory to endovascular therapy has been reported [154]. It has also been suggested that open procedures should be performed in cases of unsuccessful stenting attempts, stent failure, and long occlusions in which stenting may not be feasible [155].

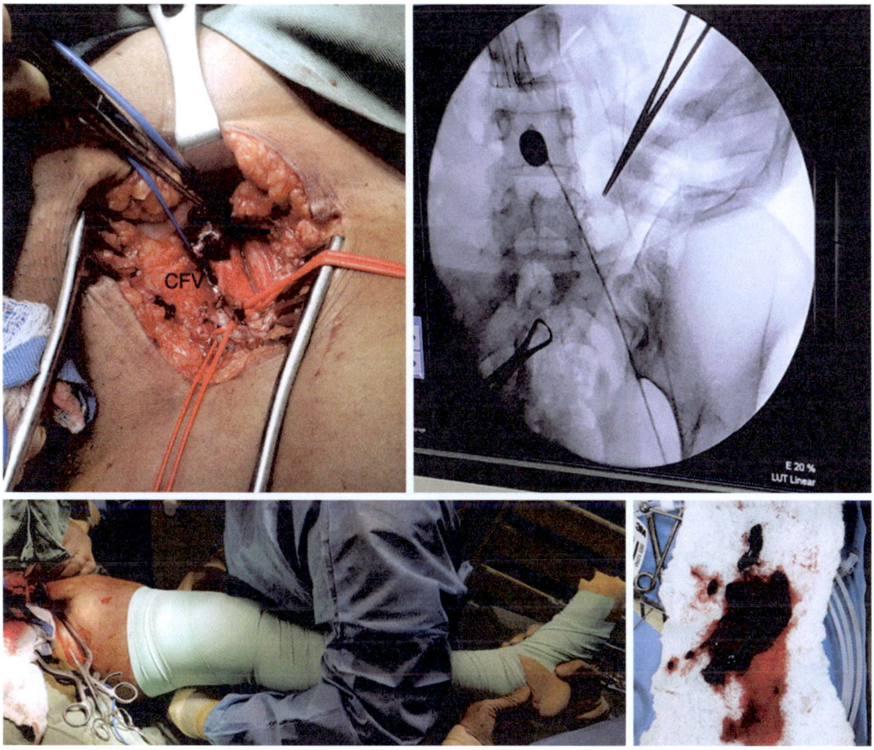

Fig. 10.6 Technique of open surgical venous thrombectomy - CFV exposure with proximal thrombus removal using embolectomy catheter/distal thrombus removal with the aid of an Esmarch bandage followed by completion venogram

Common open procedures for chronic DVT include a crossover bypass procedure (Palma-Dale procedure), in-line bypass surgery, and endo-phlebectomy. Endophlebectomy is an open surgical technique which demonstrated significant improvement in venous scores postoperatively. The venous clinical severity score was decreased from 17 to 9.8 after the operation and the Villalta scale was decreased from 13.6 to 6.0 postoperatively [156]. This technique can be combined with an endovascular recanalization of an occluded iliac venous segment as a hybrid technique with good long-term results [157, 158].

References

1. Muñoz FJ, Mismetti P, Poggio R, et al. Clinical outcome of patients with upper-extremity deep vein thrombosis: results from the RIETE registry. Chest. 2008;133(1):143–8. https://doi.org/10.1378/chest.07-1432.
2. Kearon C. Natural history of venous thromboembolism. Circulation. 2003;107:I22–30.

3. Dickinson B. Virchow's triad? South Med J. 2004;97:915–6.
4. Malone PC, Agutter PS. Springer. The aetiology of deep venous thrombosis: a critical, historical and epistemological survey. Springer Science & Business Media, 31 Dec 2007.
5. Mannucci PM. Venous thrombosis: the history of knowledge. Pathophysiol Haemost Thromb. 2002;32:2.
6. Wright IS. Thrombophlebitis. Bull N Y Acad Med 1941;17:348–7209–12. Medical – 318 pp.
7. Bagot CN, Ayra R. Virchow and his triad: a question of attribution. Br J Haematol. 2008;143:180–90.
8. McLachlin AD, McLachlin JA, Jory TA, Rawling EG. Venous stasis in the lower extremities. Ann Surg. 1960;152:678–83.
9. Stephen E, Samuel V, Agarwal S, Selvaraj D, Premkumar P. Deep vein thrombosis is not uncommon in India. Indian J Vasc Endovasc Surg. 2017;4:92–6.
10. Homans J. Diseases of the veins. N Engl J Med. 1944;231:51–60.
11. Bækgaard N. Incidence and location of deep vein thrombosis in the lower extremities: what do we know? Phlebolymphology. 2017;24(2):97.
12. Fowkes FJ, Price JF, Fowkes FG. Incidence of diagnosed deep vein thrombosis in the general population: systematic review. Eur J Vasc Endovasc Surg. 2003;25(1):1–5.
13. Kniffin WD Jr, Baron JA, Barrett J, et al. The epidemiology of diagnosed pulmonary embolism and deep venous thrombosis in the elderly. Arch Intern Med. 1994;154:861–6.
14. Cushman M, et al. Deep vein thrombosis and pulmonary embolism in two cohorts: the longitudinal investigation of thromboembolism etiology. Am J Med. 2004;117:19–25.
15. White RH, Zhou H, Romano PS. Incidence of idiopathic deep venous thrombosis and secondary thromboembolism among ethnic groups in California. Ann Intern Med. 1998;128:737–40.
16. Nossent JC, Egelie NC. Incidence and course of symptomatic deep venous thrombosis of the lower extremities in a black Caribbean population. Thromb Haemost. 1993;70(4):576–8.
17. Tagalakis V, Patenaude V, Kahn SR, Suissa S. Incidence of and mortality from venous thromboembolism in a real-world population: the Q-VTE study cohort. Am J Med. 2013;126:832.
18. Oger E. Incidence of venous thromboembolism: a community-based study in Western France. EPI-GETBP Study Group. Groupe d'Etude de la Thrombose de Bretagne Occidentale. Thromb Haemost 2000;83:657–60.
19. Huerta C, Johansson S, Wallander MA, Garcia Rodriguez LA. Risk factors and short-term mortality of venous thromboembolism diagnosed in the primary care setting in the United Kingdom. Arch Intern Med. 2007;167:935–43.
20. Severinsen MT, Johnsen SP, Tjonneland A, Overvad K, Dethlefsen C, Kristensen SR. Body height and sex-related differences in incidence of venous thromboembolism: a Danish follow-up study. Eur J Intern Med. 2010;21:268–72.
21. Agarwala S, Bhagwat AS, Modhe J. Deep vein thrombosis in Indian patients undergoing major lower limb surgery. Indian J Surg. 2003;65:159–62.
22. Pawar P, Ayyappan MK, Jagan J, Rajendra N, Mathur K, Raju R. Analysis of patients with venous thromboembolism in a multi-specialty tertiary hospital in South India. Indian J Vasc Endovasc Surg. 2020;7:29–33.
23. Lee LH, Gu KQ, Heng D. Deep vein thrombosis is not rare in Asia – the Singapore General Hospital experience. Ann Acad Med Singap. 2002;31:761–4.
24. Dhillon KS, Askander A, Doraismay S. Postoperative deep-vein thrombosis in Asian patients is not a rarity: a prospective study of 88 patients with no prophylaxis. J Bone Joint Surg Br. 1996;78:427–30.
25. Ota S, Matsuda A, Ogihara Y, Yamada N, Nakamura M, Mori T, Hamada M, Kobayashi T, Ito M. Incidence, characteristics and management of venous thromboembolism in Japan during. Pulmonary Circulat. 2018;82(2):555–60.
26. Helmerhorst FM, Bloemenkamp KW, Rosendaal FR, Vandenbroucke JP. Oral contraceptives and thrombotic disease: risk of venous thromboembolism. Thromb Haemost. 1997;78:327–33.
27. Tanaka H, Kokubo Y. Epidemiology of obesity. J Jpn Med Assoc. 2003;130:25–30. (in Japanese)

28. Virchow R, Beitr Z. Heparin in the treatment of Thrombosis. Exp Path. 2:227, 1846. Quoted by Jorpes JE. Oxford Medical Publications. 1946.
29. Wessler S, Reimer SM, Sheps MC. Biologic assay of a thrombosis-inducing activity in human serum. J Appl Physiol. 1959;14:943–6.
30. Paterson JC, McLachlin J. Precipitating factors in venous thrombosis. Surg Gynecol Obstet. 1954;98:96–102.
31. Gottlob M, May R. Part III. Pathologic venous valves. In: Gottlob R, May R, editors. Venous valves: morphology, function, radiology, surgery. New York, NY: Springer-Verlag; 1986. p. 82–92.
32. Hamer JD, Malone PC, Silver IA. The PO2 in venous valve pockets: its possible bearing on thrombogenesis. Br J Surg. 1981;68:166–70.
33. Lund FL, Diener L, Ericsson JLE. Post-mortem intraosseous phlebography as an aid in studies of venous thromboembolism: with application on a geriatric clientele. Angiology. 1969;20:155–76.
34. Myers DD, Hawley AE, Farris DM, et al. P-selectin and leukocyte micro particles are associated with venous thrombogenesis. J Vasc Surg. 2003;38:1075–89.
35. Sevitt S. The structure and growth of valve-pocket thrombi in femoral veins. J Clin Pathol. 1974;27:517–28.
36. Brooks EG, Trotman W, Wadsworth MP, et al. Valves of the deep venous system: an overlooked risk factor. Blood. 2009;114:1276–9.
37. Falati S, Liu Q, Gross P, et al. Accumulation of tissue factor into developing thrombi in vivo is dependent upon micro particle P-selectin glycoprotein 1 and platelet P-selectin. J Exp Med. 2003;197:1585–98.
38. Giesen PLA, Rauch U, Bohrmann B, et al. Blood-borne tissue factor: another view of thrombosis. Proc Natl Acad Sci USA. 1999;96(5):2311–5.
39. Dvorak HF, Quay SC, Orenstein NS, et al. Tumor shedding and coagulation. Science. 1981;212:923–4.
40. López JA, Kearon C, Lee AYY. Deep venous thrombosis. Hematol Am Soc Hematol Educ Program Book. 2004:439–56.
41. Rao LV. Tissue factor as a tumor procoagulant. Cancer Metastasis Rev. 1992;11:249–66.
42. Closse C, Seigneur M, Renard M, et al. Influence of hypoxia and hypoxia-reoxygenation on endothelial P-selectin expression. Thromb Res. 1997;85:159–64.
43. Kim YJ, Borsig L, Han HL, Varki NM, Varki A. Distinct selectin ligands on colon carcinoma mucins can mediate pathological interactions among platelets, leukocytes, and endothelium. Am J Pathol. 1999;155(2):461–72.
44. Lowe GDO, Rumley A, Woodward M, et al. Epidemiology of coagulation factors, inhibitors and activation markers: the third Glasgow MONICA survey I. illustrative reference ranges by age, sex and hormone use. Br J Haematol. 1997;97:775–84.
45. Silverstein RL, Bauer KA, Cushman M, Esmon CT, Ershler WB, Tracy RP. Venous thrombosis in the elderly: more questions than answers. Blood. 2007;110:3097–101.
46. Markel A, Manzo RA, Bergelin RO, Strandness DE Jr. Pattern and distribution of thrombi in acute venous thrombosis [published correction appears in Arch Surg 1992 Aug;127(8):923]. Arch Surg. 1992;127(3):303–309.
47. Cogo A, Lensing AW, Prandoni P, Hirsh J. Distribution of thrombosis in patients with symptomatic deep vein thrombosis. Implications for simplifying the diagnostic process with compression ultrasound. Arch Intern Med. 1993;153(24):2777–80.
48. De Maeseneer MG, Bochanen N, van Rooijen G, Neglén P. Analysis of 1,338 patients with acute lower limb deep venous thrombosis (DVT) supports the inadequacy of the term "proximal DVT". Eur J Vasc Endovasc Surg. 2016;51(3):415–20.
49. Messina LM, Sarpa MS, Smith MA, Greenfield LJ. Clinical significance of routine imaging of iliac and calf veins by color flow duplex scanning in patients suspected of having acute lower extremity deep venous thrombosis. Surgery. 1993;114(5):921–7.

50. Mattos MA, Melendres G, Sumner DS, et al. Prevalence and distribution of calf vein thrombosis in patients with symptomatic deep venous thrombosis: a color-flow duplex study. J Vasc Surg. 1996;24(5):738–44.
51. Labropoulos N, Webb KM, Kang SS, et al. Patterns and distribution of isolated calf deep vein thrombosis. J Vasc Surg. 1999;30(5):787–91.
52. Yoshimura N, Hori Y, Horii Y, et al. Where is the most common site of DVT? Evaluation by CT venography. Jpn J Radiol. 2012;30:393–7.
53. Labropoulos N, Bekelis K, Leon LR Jr. Thrombosis in unusual sites of the lower extremity veins. J Vasc Surg. 2008;47(5):1022–7.
54. Aukland K, Nicolaysen G. Interstitial fluid volume: local regulatory mechanisms. Physiol Rev. 1981;61:556–643.
55. Seem E, Stranden E. Transcapillary forces in subcutaneous tissue of lower limbs with deep venous thrombosis. Scand J Clin Lab Invest. 1986;46(5):417–22.
56. Starling EH. On the absorption of fluids from the connective tissue spaces. J Physiol. 1896;19(4):312–26.
57. Landis EM, Jonas L, Angevine M, Erb W. The passage of fluid and protein through the human capillary wall during venous congestion. J Clin Invest. 1932;11:717–34.
58. Wiederhielm CA. Dynamics of capillary fluid exchange: a non-linear computer simulation. Microvasc Res. 1979;18:48–82.
59. Kaza A, Cassada D, Fiser S, Long SM III, Tribble C. The cardiovascular system in the physiological basis of surgery. 3rd ed. Patrick O' Leary J, editor. Lippincott, Williams & Wilkins. Chapter 15, 2002. p. 389–417.
60. Fernandez MJ, Davies WT, Owne GM, Tyler A. Lymphatic flow in humans as indicated by the clearance of 125 I-labelled albumin from the sub-cutaneous tissue of the leg. J Surg Res. 1983;35:101–4.
61. Threefoot SA. The local spread of intradermally injected dye in edematous and non-edematous extremities. Clin Res. 1958;6:234.
62. Silverstein MD, Heit JA, Mohr DN, Petterson TM, O'Fallon WM, Melton LJ 3rd. Trends in the incidence of deep vein thrombosis and pulmonary embolism: a 25-year population-based study. Arch Intern Med. 1998;158(6):585–93.
63. Sweetland S, et al. Duration and magnitude of the postoperative risk of venous thromboembolism in middle aged women: prospective cohort study. BMJ. 2009;339:b4583.
64. White RH, Zhou H, Romano PS. Incidence of symptomatic venous thromboembolism after different elective or urgent surgical procedures. Thromb Haemost. 2003;90:446–55.
65. Toker S, Hak DJ, Morgan SJ. Deep vein thrombosis prophylaxis in trauma patients. Thrombosis. 2011;2011:505373.
66. Brohi K, Cohen MJ, Ganter MT, et al. Acute coagulopathy of trauma: hypoperfusion induces systemic anticoagulation and hyperfibrinolysis. J Trauma. 2008;64(5):1211–7.
67. Heit JA, et al. Risk factors for deep vein thrombosis and pulmonary embolism: a population-based case-control study. Arch Intern Med. 2000;160:809–15.
68. Dalen JE. Economy class syndrome: too much flying or too much sitting? Arch Intern Med. 2003;163:2674–6.
69. Heit JA, et al. Incidence of venous thromboembolism in hospitalized patients vs community residents. Mayo Clin Proc. 2001;76:1102–10.
70. Samama MM. An epidemiologic study of risk factors for deep vein thrombosis in medical outpatients: the Sirius study. Arch Intern Med. 2000;160(22):3415–20.
71. Prandoni P, Lensing AW, Büller HR, et al. Deep-vein thrombosis and the incidence of subsequent symptomatic cancer. N Engl J Med. 1992;327(16):1128–33.
72. White RH, Chew HK, Zhou H, et al. Incidence of venous thromboembolism in the year before the diagnosis of cancer in 528,693 adults. Arch Intern Med. 2005;165(15):1782–7.
73. Baron JA, Gridley G, Weiderpass E, Nyrén O, Linet M. Venous thromboembolism and cancer [published correction appears in Lancet 2000;355(9205):758]. Lancet. 1998;351(9109):1077–80.

74. Chung WS, Lin CL, Hsu WH, Kao CH. Inflammatory bowel disease increases the risks of deep vein thrombosis and pulmonary embolism in the hospitalized patients: a nationwide cohort study. Thromb Res. 2015;135(3):492–6.
75. Bibas M, Biava G, Antinori A. HIV-associated venous thromboembolism. Mediterr J Hematol Infect Dis. 2011;3(1):e2011030. https://doi.org/10.4084/MJHID.2011.030.
76. Shantsila E, Lip GYH, Chong BH, Heparin-induced thrombocytopenia. A contemporary clinical approach to diagnosis and management. Chest. 2009;135(6):1651–64.
77. Petrauskiene V, Falk M, Waernbaum I, Norberg M, Eriksson JW. The risk of venous thromboembolism is markedly elevated in patients with diabetes. Diabetologia. 2005;48(5):1017–21.
78. Bolorunduro O, Olatunde S, Singh A, Amer M, Akinboboye O, et al. Lower extremity deep vein thrombosis is associated with mortality among patients hospitalized with congestive heart failure: results from the Agency for Healthcare Research and Quality's Nationwide inpatient sample (1998-2007). J Vasc Med Surg. 2013;1:121.
79. Rosendaal FR. Risk factors for venous thrombotic disease. Thromb Haemost. 1999;82:610–9.
80. Heit JA, et al. Trends in the incidence of venous thromboembolism during pregnancy or postpartum: a 30-year population-based study. Ann Intern Med. 2005;143:697–706.
81. Chasan-Taber L, Stampfer MJ. Epidemiology of oral contraceptives and cardiovascular disease. Ann Intern Med. 1998;128:467–77.
82. Grady D, Hulley SB, Furberg C. Venous thromboembolic events associated with hormone replacement therapy. JAMA. 1997;278:477.
83. Gathof BS, Picker SM, Rojo J. Epidemiology, etiology and diagnosis of venous thrombosis. Eur J Med Res. 2004;9:95–103.
84. Tafur AJ, Kalsi H, Wysokinski WE, McBane RD, Ashrani AA, Marks RS, Crusan DJ, Petterson TM, Bailey KR, Heit JA. The association of active cancer with venous thromboembolism location: a population-based study. Mayo Clin Proc. 2011;86(1):25–30.
85. Zangari M, et al. Increased risk of deep-vein thrombosis in patients with multiple myeloma receiving thalidomide and chemotherapy. Blood. 2001;98:1614–5.
86. Knight R, DeLap RJ, Zeldis JB. Lenalidomide and venous thrombosis in multiple myeloma. N Engl J Med. 2006;354:2079–80.
87. Sanson BJ, et al. The incidence of venous thromboembolism in asymptomatic carriers of a deficiency of Antithrombin, protein C, or protein S: a prospective cohort study. Blood. 1999;94:3702–6.
88. Yin ZF, Huang ZF, Cui J, Fiehler R, Lasky N, Ginsburg D, Broze GJ Jr. Prothrombotic phenotype of protein Z deficiency. Proc Natl Acad Sci U S A. 2000;97(12):6734–8.
89. Folsom AR, Cushman M, Tsai MY, et al. A prospective study of venous thromboembolism in relation to factor V Leiden and related factors. Blood. 2002;99(8):2720–5.
90. Folsom AR, Cushman M, Tsai MY, Heckbert SR, Aleksic N. Prospective study of the G20210A polymorphism in the prothrombin gene, plasma prothrombin concentration, and incidence of venous thromboembolism. Am J Hematol. 2002;71:285–90.
91. Bani-Hani S, Siddiqui O, Patel A, Showkat A. C20209T prothrombin gene mutation associated deep venous thrombosis in a hemodialysis patient. Clin Nephrol Case Stud 2014;2:1–4. Published 2014 Jan 15.
92. Muñoz M, Vilos C, Cantín M. Prothrombin C20209T mutation in deep vein thrombosis: a case report. Int J Clin Exp Med. 2015;8(7):11225–9.
93. Wells PS, Langlois NJ, Webster MA, Jaffey J, Anderson JA. Elevated factor VIII is a risk factor for idiopathic venous thromboembolism in Canada—is it necessary to define a new upper reference range for factor VIII? Thromb Haemost. 2005;93:842–6.
94. Roberts LN, Patel RK, Chitongo P, Bonner L, Arya R. African-Caribbean ethnicity is associated with a hypercoagulable state as measured by thrombin generation. Blood Coagul Fibrinolysis. 2013;24(1):40–9.
95. Chang S, Huang Y, Lee M, et al. Association of Varicose Veins with incident venous thromboembolism and peripheral artery disease. JAMA. 2018;319(8):807–17.
96. Müller-Bühl U, Leutgeb R, Engeser P, Achankeng EN, Szecsenyi J, Laux G. Varicose veins are a risk factor for deep venous thrombosis in general practice patients. Vasa. 2012;41(5):360–5.

97. Nakano TA, Zeinati C. Venous thromboembolism in Pediatric vascular anomalies. Front Pediatr. 2017;5:158.
98. Peters M, Syed RK, Katz M, Moscona J, Press C, Nijjar V, Bisharat M, Baldwin D. May-Thurner syndrome: a not so uncommon cause of a common condition. Proc (Bayl Univ Med Cent). 2012;25(3):231–3.
99. Bergqvist D, Jaroszewski H. Deep vein thrombosis in patients with superficial thrombophlebitis of the leg. Br Med J (Clin Res Ed). 1986;292(6521):658–9.
100. Edwards E. Migrating thrombophlebitis associated with carcinoma. N Engl J Med. 1949;240:1031–5.
101. Trousseau A. Lectures on clinical medicine (delivered at the hotel-Dieu, Paris, France). London: The New Sydenham Society; 1872. p. 282–332.
102. Blumenberg RM, Barton E, Gelfand ML, Skudder P, Brennan J. Occult deep venous thrombosis complicating superficial thrombophlebitis. J Vasc Surg. 1998;27(2):338–43.
103. Caprini JA. Thrombosis risk assessment as a guide to quality patient care. Dis Mon. 2005;51(2-3):70–8.
104. Agarwal S, Lee AD, Raju RS, Stephen E. Venous thromboembolism: a problem in the Indian/Asian population? Indian J Urol. 2009;25(1):11–6.
105. Grant PJ, Greene MT, Chopra V, Bernstein SJ, Hofer TP, Flanders SA. Assessing the Caprini score for risk assessment of venous thromboembolism in hospitalized medical patients. Am J Med. 2016;129(5):528–35.
106. Schulman S, Konstantinides HY, Tang LV. Venous thromboembolic diseases: diagnosis, management and thrombophilia testing: observations on NICE guideline [NG158]. Thromb Haemost. 2020;120(8):1143–6.
107. Wells P, Anderson D, Rodger M, Forgie M, et al. Evaluation of the D-dimer in the diagnosis of suspected DVT. N Engl J Med. 2003;349:1227–35.
108. Ho VB, van Geertruyden PH, Yucel EK, Rybicki FJ, Baum RA, Desjardins B, et al. ACR appropriateness criteria(®) on suspected lower extremity deep vein thrombosis. J Am Coll Radiol. 2011;8:383–7.
109. Konstantinides SV, Torbicki A, Agnelli G, Danchin N, Fitzmaurice D, Galiè N, et al. 2014 ESC guidelines on the diagnosis and management of acute pulmonary embolism. Eur Heart J. 2014;35:3033–69.
110. Abai B, Labropoulos N. Duplex ultrasound scanning for chronic venous obstruction and valvular incompetence. In: Handbook of venous disorders: guidelines of the American venous forum. 3rd ed. Boka Raton, FL: CRC Press; 2008. p. 142.
111. O'Donnell TF Jr, Passman MA, Marston WA, Ennis WJ, Dalsing M, Kistner RL, et al. Management of venous leg ulcers: clinical practice guidelines of the Society for Vascular Surgery® and the American venous forum. J Vasc Surg. 2014;60(2 Suppl):3S–59S.
112. Begemann PG, Bonacker M, Kemper J, Guthoff AE, Hahn KE, Steiner P, et al. Evaluation of the deep venous system in patients with suspected pulmonary embolism with multidetector CT: a prospective study in comparison to Doppler sonography. J Comput Assist Tomogr. 2003;27:399–409.
113. Kanne JP, Lalani TA. Role of computed tomography and magnetic resonance imaging for deep venous thrombosis and pulmonary embolism. Circulation. 2004;109(12 Suppl 1):I15–21.
114. Zierler BK. Ultrasonography and diagnosis of venous thromboembolism. Circulation. 2004;109(12 Suppl 1):I9–I14.
115. Loud PA, Katz DS, Klippenstein DL, Shah RD, Grossman ZD. Combined CT venography and pulmonary angiography in suspected thromboembolic disease: diagnostic accuracy for deep venous evaluation. AJR Am J Roentgenol. 2000;174:61–5.
116. Thomas SM, Goodacre SW, Sampson FC, van Beek EJ. Diagnostic value of CT for deep vein thrombosis: results of a systematic review and meta-analysis. Clin Radiol. 2008;63:299–304.
117. Wahlgren CM, Wahlberg E, Olofsson P. Endovascular treatment in postthrombotic syndrome. Vasc Endovasc Surg. 2010;44:356–60.
118. Neglén P, Raju S. Intravascular ultrasound scan evaluation of the obstructed vein. J Vasc Surg. 2002;35:694–700.

119. Forauer AR, Gemmete JJ, Dasika NL, Cho KJ, Williams DM. Intravascular ultrasound in the diagnosis and treatment of iliac vein compression (May-Thurner) syndrome. J Vasc Interv Radiol. 2002;13:523–7.
120. Mazzolai L, Aboyans V, Ageno W, et al. Diagnosis and management of acute deep vein thrombosis: a joint consensus document from the European Society of Cardiology working groups of aorta and peripheral vascular diseases and pulmonary circulation and right ventricular function. Eur Heart J. 2018;39(47):4208–18.
121. Nicolaides AN, Breddin HK, Carpenter P, Coccheri S, Conard J, De Stefano V, et al. European Genetics Foundation; Cardiovascular Disease Educational and Research Trust; International Union of Angiology; Mediterranean League on thromboembolism. Thrombophilia and venous thromboembolism. International consensus statement. Guidelines according to scientific evidence. Int Angiol. 2005;24:1–26.
122. Becattini C, Agnelli G. Treatment of venous thromboembolism with new anticoagulant agents. J Am Coll Cardiol. 2016;67:1941–55.
123. Erkens PM, Prins MH. Fixed dose subcutaneous low molecular weight heparins versus adjusted dose unfractionated heparin for venous thromboembolism. Cochrane Database Syst Rev 2010;9:Cd001100.
124. Buller HR, Davidson BL, Decousus H, Gallus GM, Piovella F, et al. Subcutaneous fondaparinux versus intravenous unfractionated heparin in the initial treatment of pulmonary embolism. N Engl J Med. 2003;349:1695–702.
125. Van Es N, Coppens M, Schulman S, Middeldorp S, Buller HR. Direct oral anticoagulants compared with vitamin K antagonists for acute venous thromboembolism: evidence from phase 3 trials. Blood. 2014;124:1968–75.
126. Prandoni P, Lensing AW, Prins MH, Frulla M, Marchiori A, Bernardi E, et al. Below-knee elastic compression stockings to prevent the postthrombotic syndrome: a randomized, controlled trial. Ann Intern Med. 2004;141:249–56.
127. Kahn SR, Shrier I, Julian JA, Ducruet T, Arsenault L, Miron MJ, et al. Determinants and time course of the postthrombotic syndrome after acute deep venous thrombosis. Ann Intern Med. 2008;149:698–707.
128. Kahn SR. How I treat postthrombotic syndrome. Blood. 2009;114:4624–31.
129. Henke PK, Comerota AJ. An update on etiology, prevention, and therapy of postthrombotic syndrome. J Vasc Surg. 2011;53:500–9.
130. Kahn SR, Shapiro S, Wells PS, Rodger MA, Kovacs MJ, Anderson DR, et al. Compression stockings to prevent post-thrombotic syndrome: a randomised placebo-controlled trial. Lancet. 2014;383:880–8.
131. Bauersachs R, Berkowitz SD, Brenner B, Buller HR, Decousus H, et al. EINSTEIN investigators. Oral rivaroxaban for symptomatic venous thromboembolism. N Engl J Med. 2010;363:2499–510.
132. Meissner MH, Gloviczki P, Comerota AJ, Dalsing MC, Eklof BG, Gillespie DL, et al. Early thrombus removal strategies for acute deep venous thrombosis: clinical practice guidelines of the Society for Vascular Surgery and the American venous forum. J Vasc Surg. 2012;55:1449–62.
133. Nicolaides AN, Fareed J, Kakkar AK, Comerota AJ, Goldhaber SZ, Hull R, et al. Prevention and treatment of venous thromboembolism-- international consensus statement. Int Angiol. 2013;32:111–260.
134. Comerota AJ, Paolini D. Treatment of acute iliofemoral deep venous thrombosis: a strategy of thrombus removal. Eur J Vasc Endovasc Surg. 2007;33:351–60.
135. Juhan C, Alimi Y, Di Mauro P, Hartung O. Surgical venous thrombectomy. Cardiovasc Surg. 1999;7:586–90.
136. Weaver FA, Meacham PW, Adkins RB, Dean RH. Phlegmasia cerulea dolens: therapeutic considerations. South Med J. 1988;81:306–12.
137. Watson L, Broderick C, Armon MP. Thrombolysis for acute deep vein thrombosis. Cochrane Database Syst Rev. 2014;1:CD002783.

138. Vedantham S, Thorpe PE, Cardella JF, Grassi CJ, Patel NH, Ferral H, et al. Quality improvement guidelines for the treatment of lower extremity deep vein thrombosis with use of endovascular thrombus removal. J Vasc Interv Radiol. 2006;17:435–47; quiz 448
139. Kearon C, Akl EA, Ornelas J, Blaivas A, Jimenez D, Bounameaux H, Huisman M. Antithrombotic therapy for VTE disease. CHEST guideline and expert panel report. Chest. 2016;149:315–52.
140. Mewissen MW, Seabrook GR, Meissner MH, Cynamon J, Labropoulos N, Haughton SH. Catheter-directed thrombolysis of the lower extremity DVT: report of a national multicenter registry. Radiology. 1999;211:39–49.
141. Elsharawy M, Elzayat E. Early results of thrombolysis vs anticoagulation in iliofemoral venous thrombosis. A randomised clinical trial. Eur J Vasc Endovasc Surg. 2002;24:209–14.
142. Enden T, Kløw NE, Sandvik L, Slagsvold CE, Ghanima W, Hafsahl G, et al. Catheter-directed thrombolysis vs. anticoagulant therapy alone in deep vein thrombosis: results of an open randomized, controlled trial reporting on short-term patency. J Thromb Haemost. 2009;7:1268–75.
143. Enden T, Haig Y, Kløw NE, Slagsvold CE, Sandvik L, Ghanima W, et al. Long-term outcome after additional catheter-directed thrombolysis versus standard treatment for acute iliofemoral deep vein thrombosis (the CaVenT study): a randomised controlled trial. Lancet. 2012;379:31–8.
144. Grunwald MR, Hofmann LV. Comparison of urokinase, alteplase, and reteplase for catheter-directed thrombolysis of deep venous thrombosis. J Vasc Interv Radiol. 2004;15:347–52.
145. Sugimoto K, Hofmann LV, Razavi MK, Kee ST, Sze DY, Dake MD, et al. The safety, efficacy, and pharmacoeconomics of low-dose alteplase compared with urokinase for catheter-directed thrombolysis of arterial and venous occlusions. J Vasc Surg. 2003;37:512–7.
146. Shortell CK, Queiroz R, Johansson M, Waldman D, Illig KA, Ouriel K, et al. Safety and efficacy of limited dose tissue plasminogen activator in acute vascular occlusion. J Vasc Surg. 2001;34:854–9.
147. Decousus H, Leizorovicz A, Parent F, Page Y, Tardy B, Girard P, et al. A clinical trial of vena caval filters in the prevention of pulmonary embolism in patients with proximal deep-vein thrombosis. N Engl J Med. 1998;338:409–15.
148. Protack CD, Bakken AM, Patel N, Saad WE, Waldman DL, Davies MG. Long-term outcomes of catheter directed thrombolysis for lower extremity deep venous thrombosis without prophylactic inferior vena cava filter placement. J Vasc Surg. 2007;45:992–7.
149. Sharifi M, Bay C, Skrocki L, Lawson D, Mazdeh S. Role of IVC filters in endovenous therapy for deep venous thrombosis: the FILTERPEVI (filter implantation to lower thromboembolic risk in percutaneous endovenous intervention) trial. Cardiovasc Intervent Radiol. 2012;35:1408–13.
150. Sharifi M, Mehdipour M, Bay C, Smith G, Sharifi J. Endovenous therapy for deep venous thrombosis: the TORPEDO trial. Catheter Cardiovasc Interv. 2010;76:316–25.
151. Sevitt S. Organization of valve pocket thrombi and the anomalies of double thrombi and valve cusp involvement. Br J Surg. 1974;61:641–9.
152. Raju S, Neglén P. Percutaneous recanalization of total occlusions of the iliac vein. J Vasc Surg. 2009;50:360–8.
153. Neglén P, Oglesbee M, Olivier J, Raju S. Stenting of chronically obstructed inferior vena cava filters. J Vasc Surg. 2011;54:153–61.
154. Adams MK, Anaya-Ayala JE, Ismail N, Peden EK. Surgical femorocaval bypass for recalcitrant iliofemoral venous occlusion to endovascular treatment. Vasc Endovasc Surg. 2012;46:578–81.
155. Khanna AK, Singh S. Postthrombotic syndrome: surgical possibilities. Thrombosis. 2012; https://doi.org/10.1155/2012/520604.
156. Vogel D, Comerota AJ, Al-Jabouri M, Assi ZI. Common femoral endovenectomy with iliocaval endoluminal recanalization improves symptoms and quality of life in patients with postthrombotic iliofemoral obstruction. J Vasc Surg. 2012;55:129–35.

157. Garg N, Gloviczki P, Karimi KM, Duncan AA, Bjarnason H, Kalra M, et al. Factors affecting outcome of open and hybrid reconstructions for nonmalignant obstruction of iliofemoral veins and inferior vena cava. J Vasc Surg. 2011;53:383–93.
158. Verma H, Tripathi RK. Common femoral endovenectomy in conjunction with iliac vein stenting to improve venous inflow in severe post-thrombotic obstruction. J Vasc Surg Venous Lymphat Disord. 2017;1:138–42.

Chronic Venous Insufficiency

11

Varun N. Kumar and Ramesh K. Tripathi

11.1 Introduction and Epidemiology

The prevalence of leg edema (Fig. 11.1) as a manifestation of chronic venous insufficiency has been reported between 7.4 and 17.1% in men and 4.9–20.3% in women. Furthermore, the prevalence of CVI has been estimated from between <1 and 17% in men and between <1 and 40% in women [1]. Some of the variance in these values is due to differing criteria for what constitutes chronic venous insufficiency and sampling bias in the epidemiological studies. However, it is also known that different populations with exposure to different genetic and environmental factors show significant differences in the incidence of chronic venous insufficiency [2]. Regardless of the exact percentages, venous insufficiency is a common cause of both unilateral and bilateral leg edema. Its peak incidence is in the 5th decade of life, and it is approximately twice as common in females compared to males.

11.2 Anatomy and Physiology

Approximately 90% of blood from the lower limb is drained directly by deep veins, which follow the arteries supplying the lower limb. 10% is drained by superficial veins, which run above the deep fascia for most of their course [3] The physiological ejection fraction of the calf muscle pump is 65% and 15% for the thigh muscle pump [3–5]. When calf muscle dysfunction occurs, it impacts on the valve function too. One must keep in mind that treating valve function without addressing calf pump may lead to treatment failure.

V. N. Kumar · R. K. Tripathi (✉)
Faculty of Medicine, School of Biomedical Sciences, University of Queensland, Brisbane, QLD, Australia
e-mail: ramesh.tripathi@vascularsurgeon.org

S. K. Tiwary (ed.), *Approach to Lower Limb Oedema*,
https://doi.org/10.1007/978-981-16-6206-5_11

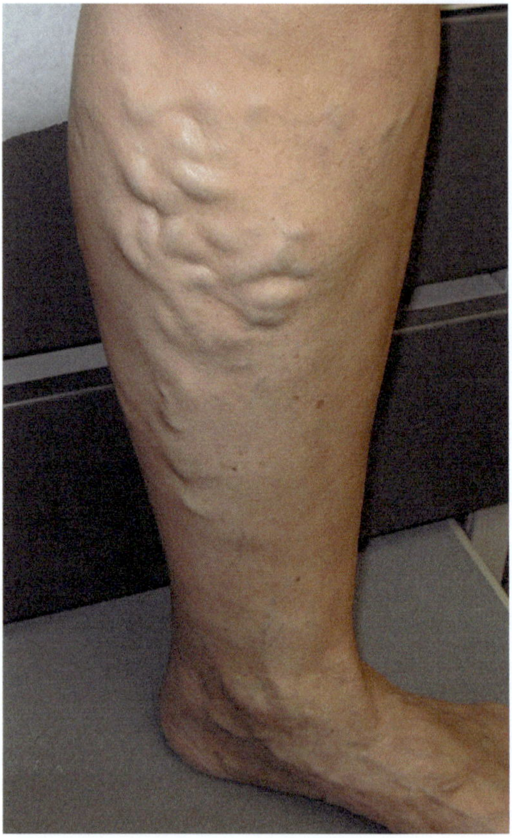

Fig. 11.1 CEAP C3 varicose veins with edema

The superficial venous system is responsible for temperature regulation, as a reservoir of blood and to deliver blood to the deep venous system. Medially, the great saphenous vein (GSV) originates from the dorsal venous arch at the ankle and runs to the pelvis, emptying into the femoral vein at the sapheno-femoral junction (SFJ). Its notable tributaries include the anterior accessory saphenous vein and the lateral accessory saphenous vein [3, 6]. The small saphenous vein (SSV) arises just underneath the lateral malleolus and travels up the leg posteriorly to join the popliteal vein at the sapheno-popliteal junction (SPJ). There are a multitude of perforators through which blood flows from superficial to deep vessels in physiological conditions [3] (Fig. 11.2a and b).

The common pathway of drainage of all the blood of the lower limb is through the femoral vein, up the external followed by the common iliac, into the inferior vena cava. In the case of IVC obstruction blood can drain through the ascending lumbar veins to the azygous and hemiazygos veins, as well as up the epigastric veins to the superior vena cava [7, 8].

Obstruction of the main pathways of venous return and the use of these small diameter collaterals results in a higher pressure distal to the pathology. More blood is pushed into the superficial venous system, which is more capable of distention as it is not constricted within muscle and dense fascia. However, in a system that only handles 10% of the lower limb blood flow, the introduction of more blood volume can lead to the maladaptive changes characteristic of chronic venous insufficiency.

11.3 Etiopathophysiology of Lower Leg Edema in CVI

The mechanism behind chronic venous insufficiency (CVI) is fundamentally an inflammatory state induced by the stress that venous hypertension places on cells of the vessel wall. As with injury in regions elsewhere in the body, vasoactive substances are released from the endothelium, adhesion molecules, chemokines, matrix metalloproteinases, and inflammatory mediators are expressed to create a local inflammatory response. Adhesion factors such as ICAM-1 have been associated

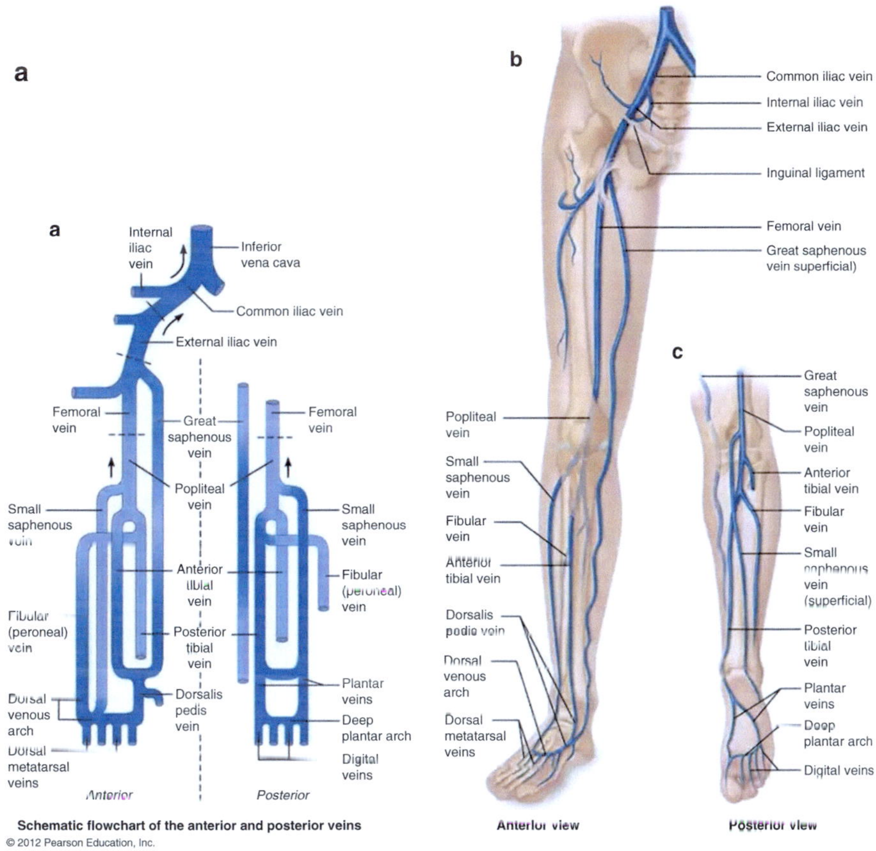

Fig. 11.2 (**a**) Anatomy of venous system of lower limbs; (**b**) Varicose veins and vein valve function

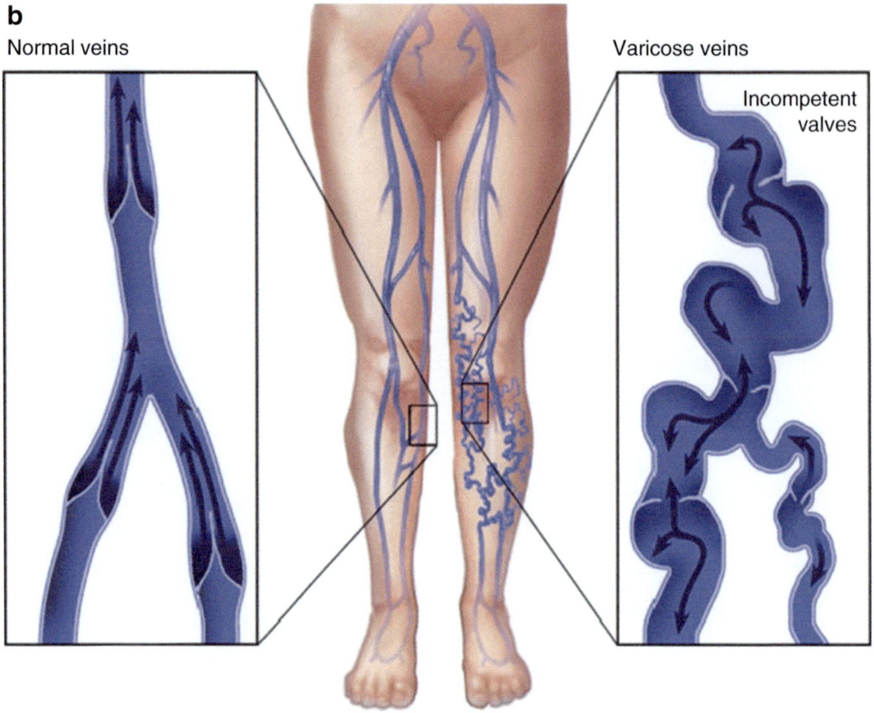

Fig. 11.2 (continued)

with the invasion of venous vales and vessel walls by monocytes and macrophages [9]. The overall result is disruption and disorganization of vessel walls with fibrosis, all of which leads to decreased vein compliance and further damage [5, 9]. Furthermore, stretching of the vessel wall may lead to a vicious cycle of further valvular incompetence causing more hypertension, dilation, and fluid leakage setting up a negative cycle in which the condition chronically progresses (Fig. 11.3).

Following from the pathophysiology, anything that increases lower limb venous pressure may contribute to the development of chronic venous insufficiency. These may include prolonged standing, musculo-venous pump failure, thoraco-abdominal pump failure, heart failure, decreased sympathetic tone, and obesity (increased intra-abdominal pressure) [2, 10].

An important cause of increased capillary hydrostatic pressure is estrogen. Estrogen inhibits vascular smooth muscle tone and proliferation, resulting in a greater diameter of vessels. The result is more fluid and hence more capillary hydrostatic pressure. This is why chronic venous insufficiency has a much greater prevalence in the female population [11]. During pregnancy, levels of estrogen are further elevated, and the developing fetus obstructs the inferior vena cava resulting in an increased risk of developing symptoms of chronic venous insufficiency.

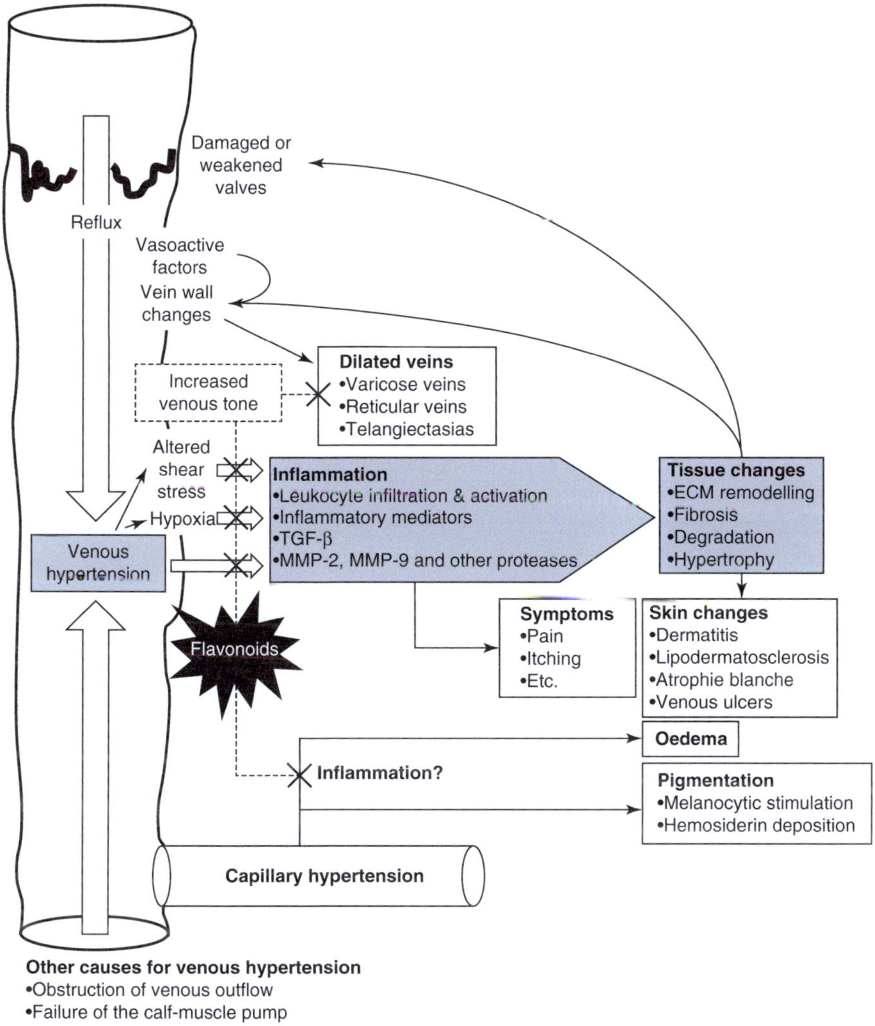

Fig. 11.3 Pathophysiological mechanisms in venous hypertension

While these underlying conditions may certainly contribute to chronic venous insufficiency, the most common cause of venous hypertension is deep venous obstruction (DVO). The etiology of DVO is broadly classified into deep vein thrombosis or scarring after DVT, or non-thrombotic iliac vein lesions (NIVL) [2].

A common cause of NIVL is May-Thurner syndrome. Also known as Cockett syndrome or Iliac vein compression syndrome, it occurs when the right common iliac artery compresses the left common iliac vein against the sacral promontory. This can lead to endothelial irritation and the formation of intraluminal "spurs" or "bands" which further affect blood flow [12]. It has been implicated in the etiology of leg edema and refractory leg ulcers and has been associated with varicose veins of the pelvic organs [12, 13]. It is present in 22–32% of the general asymptomatic population and 18–49% of patients with left lower limb DVT [14].

Other risk factors that make veins more vulnerable or weak to changes in venous pressure can also contribute to chronic venous insufficiency: advancing age, smoking, previous lower extremity trauma, and genetic disorders resulting in abnormal vein or connective tissue characteristics like Ehlers-Danlos type IV syndrome, Klippel-Trenaunay syndrome, hyperhomocysteinemia, and FOXC2 mutations (venous valve failure ➔ varicose veins) [15]. Additionally, a number of multifactorial genetic or epigenetic changes may predispose one to CVI through deformed, shrunken, or generally abnormal valves in the venous system of their lower limb. Such a family history of chronic venous insufficiency is a risk factor for the development of CVI in an individual. Marfan's syndrome only affects the arterial system and as such is not implicated in the development of chronic venous insufficiency.

Due to this, the approach to chronic venous insufficiency is largely symptom based, most commonly classified using CEAP scoring, which qualitatively grades the level of venous disease based on external symptoms, etiology, anatomic distribution, and pathophysiology.

Patients presenting with edema are by definition C3 patients.

11.4 Diagnosis of CVI in Patients Presenting with Lower Leg Edema

The general symptoms of chronic venous insufficiency include leg pain or cramps, fatigue, pruritis, and heaviness. When present, edema has a tendency to occur in the evening and decrease with walking or elevation above the level of the patient's heart (e.g., when supine and resting their leg on a pillow). Its likelihood may be further assessed with questioning directed at the risk factors related to the pathophysiology of CVI discussed previously. Risk factors for the development of venous insufficiency include pregnancy, smoking, obesity, trauma, DVT, superficial thrombophlebitis, and inactivity. Finally, chronic venous insufficiency is positively correlated with age, as are a multitude of other medical conditions that may present with lower limb edema [16]. Therefore, it is important to consider the individual holistically and thoroughly assess for comorbid conditions that may contribute to lower limb edema.

The signs of chronic venous insufficiency in the lower limbs manifest as a spectrum, from telangiectasias and spider veins, to edema and varicose veins, lipodermatosclerosis, and finally venous ulcers. Edema is a constant presentation of C3-6 venous insufficiency.

Edema due to chronic venous insufficiency presents as a pitting edema. If the disease has been present for a long time however, the edema may be non-pitting or brawny as lymphatic obstructive elements get involved with subcutaneous inflammatory changes. It can be elicited by palpating the skin over distal shaft of the tibia and over medial malleolus of the tibia and compressing the area for 15 s with the thumb. Tenderness may be present, so it is important to take patient comfort into consideration. Edema due to hypoalbuminemia, which also presents with pitting edema, generally refills more quickly than edema due to CVI. It is important to note the presence and characteristics of any ulcers, varicosities, or skin changes present, as these give important indicators of the sevcrity and possible etiology of the disease. If chronic venous insufficiency is the cause of lower limb edema, it is almost certain that varicosities (a less severe manifestation of the disease) will be present.

Clinically, there are three special tests to assess the competence of a patient's lower venous system: the sapheno-femoral and sapheno-popliteal junctional cough impulse test, the Trendelenburg (or Brodie-Trendelenburg) test, and Perthes' test. The cough impulse test can uncover an incompetent sapheno-femoral junction if a fluid thrill is felt in the proximal great saphenous vein (medial to the femoral vein) after a patient is prompted to cough. The Trendelenburg test may be useful in indicating the locations of superficial venous reflux points that result in varicose veins. The Trendelenburg test involves elevating a patient's affected leg while they are lying supine and applying pressure to the great saphenous vein just distal to the SFJ. The patient is then asked to stand up with the practitioner continuing to apply constant pressure to the area. If the sapheno-femoral junction is incompetent but the rest of the distal deep venous system is fine, the varicose veins would not re-engorge with blood as the practitioner will have occluded the area of reflux. However, if the varicose veins fill up with blood while the proximal great saphenous is occluded, it indicates that there is reflux in the more distal regions of the superficial venous system.

Perthes' test is an extension of the Trendelenburg test which tests the function of the musculo-venous pump in the legs. While standing, some pressure is released from the GSV allowing for more blood flow in the limb. The patient is then asked to perform several leg raises. If the perforating veins of the leg have competent valves, the pump will function effectively and superficial veins of the leg will appear less rigid compared to baseline [17].

Note that these tests may also be referred to as "tourniquet tests" as tourniquets can be used to occlude patient's superficial veins instead of manual occlusion. In practice however, these tests have largely been supplanted by venous duplex scans that provide more objective information.

11.4.1 Deep Vein Thrombosis in the Context of CVI and Leg Edema

Thrombotic etiologies of CVI result in symptoms ranging from mild edema to the classical red hot and swollen cellulitic limb with or without leg tenderness on exam ination. Lack of signs and symptoms of a current or past DVT should not preclude a thorough history for symptoms or risk factors of DVT. Previous DVT causing scarring and valvular dysfunction is a common cause of CVI known as post-thrombotic syndrome. Secondly, patients with past DVT are at increased risk of future DVT due to altered blood flow and endothelial injury in the recanalized segment of the vein [18]. Hence, there must always be a high index of suspicion for DVT.

11.4.2 Investigations

The preferred method for diagnosis of CVI is color flow venous duplex ultrasound. It is effective in evaluating venous reflux times and has a sensitivity and specificity of 91 and 99%, respectively, for diagnosing proximal DVTs using venous compression criterion. A reflux time of greater than 1 s in deep veins or greater than 0.5 s in superficial veins is diagnostic of reflux. Individual efficacy, however, is operator dependent, and a number of caveats must be taken into consideration. The patient must stand upright during ultrasound in order to elicit maximal reflux using gravity. The angle of insolation must be continuously adjusted in correspondence with the tortuous course of veins and kept under 60 degrees to ensure the accurate detection of doppler shift. Continuous wave doppler can be used to screen and mark varicose veins, however. If a definitive etiology is doubtful on duplex ultrasound, further investigations may be employed.

Air plethysmography testing is similar to Trendelenburg and Perthes' tests mentioned previously but now with a quantitative way of measuring venous volume. Specifically, an inflated cuff around the patient's calf can detect changes in pressure exerted by veins on the cuff and uses this information to calculate changes in volume. The rate of vein refill is known as the venous filing index. If, when a limb is moved from an elevated to a dependent position, the venous filling index is greater than >4 mL/s per second, the vein is incompetent and refilling too fast. A healthy vein has a maximum venous filling index of 2 mLs per second. Occlusion of superficial veins at different levels of the leg can indicate where the reflux is occurring. Similar to Perthes' test, changes in lower limb venous volume after activation of the musculo-venous pump of the calf can also be quantified using air plethysmography.

While largely given up except for research purposes, ambulatory venous pressure (AVP) can be measured by inserting a needle connected to a pressure transducer into the foot. As with previous tests and investigations, the use of gravity, cuffs or occlusion, and exercise or activation of the musculo-venous pump are used in conjunction with the investigation to ascertain the nature of the underling CVI [4, 9].

Air plethysmography is also mainly used as a research tool and for evaluating outcomes of treatments for venous reflux and obstruction.

Computed tomography (CT) and magnetic resonance (MR) contrast venography can be utilized in patients with suspected iliac vein and inferior vena caval pathology. They are ideal to screen for extrinsic etiologies of deep venous obstruction including May-Thurner syndrome, tumors, and cysts. Furthermore, they are useful in visualizing the venous system in patients with complex anatomical variants.

Invasive testing can be used to further visualize an individual's venous system and inform management. Digital subtraction ascending venography visualizes the flow of contrast and provides anatomical clarity and may help distinguish primary and secondary venous disease. Descending venography again can be used to define the anatomic extent of the reflux (Kistner classification) and can be used as a quantitative version of the "cough impulse test" in which the patient performs a valsalva maneuver to identify reflux in the deep venous system.

Intravascular ultrasound (IVUS) has a superior functionality to ascending and descending venograms, allowing 2- and 3-dimensional accurate measurement of deep vein venous stenosis and intraluminal anatomy and pathology.

11.5 Classification of CVI in the Context of Lower Limb Edema

The CEAP classification was developed by the American Venous Forum and is the most commonly used classification system for chronic venous disorders. The name is an acronym for "clinical manifestations," "etiology," "anatomy," and "pathophysiology." Spider veins have already been discussed as C1. C2 denotes the presence of varicose veins—>4 mm diameter palpable tortuous dilations of the superficial veins of the lower limbs in which retrograde flow and blood stasis may occur. Patients presenting with edema are classified C3 (Fig. 11.1). If patients have pigmentation or eczema in their lower limbs they are classified as C4a. C4b is for lipodermatosclerosis, the chronic inflammation and fibrosis of skin and subcutaneous tissues of the lower leg, or atrophie blanche, which present as white coin-sized to palm-sized atrophic plaques. C4c is corona phlebectatica; abnormally visible cutaneous blood vessels at the ankle with nous cups, blue and red telangiectasias, and capillary "stasis spots." Patients with healed venous ulcers are C5, C6 represents an active venous ulcer, and C6r denotes a recurrent active venous ulcer. Observe how CEAP classification system directly corresponds to the pathophysiologic "march" of chronic venous insufficiency. Varicose veins lead to edema, and edema contributes to pathologic skin changes.

In the etiological diagnosis, E_p denotes a primary etiology, where a degenerative process of the venous valves or wall leading to weakness and dilatations results in pathologic reflux. This does not involve scarring or post-thrombotic syndrome, which is a secondary intravenous cause. E_{si} refers to any intravenous secondary cause of venous disease. These include DVT, arteriovenous fistulas, and primary intravenous sarcomas. E_{se} on the other hand refers to extravenous secondary causes of CVI, such as central venous hypertension from obesity, congestive heart failure nutcracker syndrome, or extrinsic compression such as from tumors, fibrosis, May-Thurner syndrome, or poor musculo-venous pump function. Congenital conditions like Klippel-Trenaunay syndrome or arteriovenous malformations are classified as E_c, and finally, E_n is used for apparently idiopathic chronic venous insufficiency.

Anatomical classification is A_s, A_D, or A_p for disease in superficial, deep, or perforator veins, respectively. Disease may occur in novel combinations of the superficial, perforating, and deep venous systems in which case their corresponding subscripts can be combined.

Note that the limb affected should also be recognized with [L] or [R] [4, 9, 19].

Further detailed classification can be made using abbreviations for the specific veins in which there is pathology. While too numerous to all be listed here, 3 important ones that inform appropriate use criteria for management are whether the pathology is in the small saphenous vein (SSV), great saphenous vein above the knee (GSVa), or great saphenous vein below the knee (GSVb) [5, 20].

Finally, the pathophysiologic classification is separated into P_r, P_O, $P_{R,O}$, and P_n for "reflux," "obstruction," "reflux and obstruction," and "no pathophysiology identified," respectively [4, 9, 19].

While CEAP is best used to describe the severity of chronic venous insufficiency, the revised venous clinical severity score (rVCSS) is a more sensitive measure of the change in severity of CVI over time. It is calculated using parameters, viz. pain, varicose veins, venous edema, pigmentation, inflammation, induration, number of active ulcers, duration of active ulceration, active ulcer size, and use of compressive therapy. Calculators of this score are available for free from various sources on the Internet.

11.6 Conservative Management

Initial treatment is conservative and symptomatic. Elevation of the legs above the level of the heart for 30 min 3-4 times per day can reduce edema caused by CVI. The reduction in pressure in superficial tissues increases perfusion and hence also promotes the healing of venous leg ulcers if present.

Exercise in the form of daily walking and plantar flexion exercises to strengthen calf musculo-venous pump have been shown to improve hemodynamic parameters in patients and improve edema and ulcer healing rates.

There is mixed evidence for using compression therapy in patients with symptomatic varicose veins; however, in patients with more severe CVI such as edema or ulcers, long-term compression therapy has been shown to be beneficial. Elastic compression therapy results in faster ulcer healing compared with inelastic compression therapy. High compression is more effective than low compression, and multilayer bandages are more effective at providing desired compression pressures. An external pressure of 35–40 mmHg at the ankle is necessary to prevent capillary exudation in legs affected by venous disease. Compression stockings used for treating CVI need to exert a minimum of 20–30 mmHg (class II compression garments) at the ankle to be effective, with higher grades of compression stockings used for more severe venous disease. Knee-high stockings are sufficient for most patients. They should not, however, be pulled up into the popliteal fossa where they can cause skin irritation, strictures, and discomfort. Compression therapy should not be used in the presence of active infection or cellulitis. Furthermore, an ankle-brachial index ≤0.5 is an absolute contraindication to compression therapy. Compression therapy may also put extra stress on the heart in patients with chronic heart failure [21–23].

Pharmacological therapy can be used as an adjunct to therapy or in those with contraindications to or unaccepting of compression therapy. Venoactive agents which increase venous tone such as rutin and rutosides have been used, as well as medications such as stanozolol and prostacyclin analogues which affect blood flow properties. Hydroxyethylrutoside, a mixture of semisynthetic flavonoids, is effective in reducing leg volume and edema through reducing permeability of the microvascular endothelium. However, its effects have not been assessed in the past 6 months after follow-up. Escin, which is "horse chestnut seed extract," induces vasoconstriction through the release of prostaglandins and reduces leg volume and edema in CVI patients. Micronized purified flavonoid fraction (MPFF) is another flavonoid-based medication which has been shown to reduce ankle circumference, erythema, skin changes, ulcer healing, and overall quality of life. A meta-analysis showed that MPFF reduced lower leg edema more than hydroxyethylrutoside.

Stanozolol is an oral anabolic steroid which has shown efficacy in the treatment of lipodermatosclerosis and venous ulcers. Defibrotide is a DNA derivative with profibrinolytic and antithrombotic properties that was found to significantly reduce ankle circumference over one year of use.

Diuretics have no role in the treatment of lower leg edema but may be used to treat comorbid conditions which may be worsening the edema. Antibiotics are only indicated in the presence of infection.

Basic management of other symptoms of chronic venous insufficiency should also be understood in order to optimize patient care and minimize complications. Stasis dermatitis which has symptoms of pruritis, pigmentation, erythema, and scaling can often be present in patients with advanced venous disease. Patient education of proper skin care techniques including skin cleaning, the use of emollients, and the avoidance of itching or scratching is very important. Moderate use of topical corticosteroids may be considered in patients with difficult to manage symptoms. Allergic contact dermatitis and irritant contact dermatitis often develop in patients with CVI and present as a failure of skin symptom improvement with standard treatment. Diagnosis and avoidance of the offending substances is the main preventive measure.

Any venous ulcers present should be debrided. Surgical, enzymatic, or biological methods may be used. Autolytic agents such as hydrogel, EUSOL, and bio cellulose have been shown to increase wound debridement rates. The presence of bacteria is common, and unless signs of inflammation or lymphangitis are present systemic antibiotics and wound swabbing should be avoided. The use of antibiotics in patients with asymptomatic leg ulcers is associated with the development of resistant strains in individuals. Ulcer dressings come in various forms, and a systematic review found no dressing to be more efficacious than any other. As such decisions regarding their use may be centered on individual patient preferences and managing individual symptoms such as exudate, odor, comorbid skin conditions, and pain. There is insufficient evidence for the use of hyperbaric oxygen, electromagnetic therapy, and therapeutic ultrasound in ulcer care [21, 22].

11.7 Operative Management

In the context of edema, the rationale behind the ablation of superficial veins is that removing or collapsing the superficial venous reflux system, which is responsible for the pathological fluid extravasation, will lead to a reduction in oedema. Furthermore, by reducing venous volume in the limb, the effects of venous hypertension in the superficial tissues may be alleviated. However, if there is an underlying pathology in the deep venous system leading to the cause of varicose veins and edema, then edema and varicose veins may recur over time following surgery.

In general, candidates for venous ablation must be symptomatic and show >0.5 s retrograde flow in superficial axial veins. Axial reflux is defined as uninterrupted reflux from the groin to the calf, whereas segmental reflux is localized retrograde flow anywhere in the venous system of the lower limbs. In mild disease (C2–C3), saphenous reflux is treated with reflux in perforators often resolving naturally as a consequence. However, if persistent and large diameter >3 mm, perforator vessels may need to be ablated as well.

The precise indications for surgical correction in patients with edema in CVI are the most uncertain. In 2020, the American Venous Forum, together with the Society for Vascular Surgery, the American Vein and Lymphatic Society, and the Society of Interventional Radiology, developed appropriate use criteria for surgery of lower extremity venous disease in response to reports of inappropriate venous procedures. 119 scenarios of CVI were rated for appropriateness by an expert panel and the widest distribution of scores was observed for the indication of edema, especially edema in the context of segmental saphenous reflux or when considering proximal deep venous stenting for the relief of edema. This is because of the wide and often multifactorial cause of edema in the lower limbs. Hence when there is only mild evidence of venous pathology in the context of edema, clinical judgment based on unique features of the case must be taken into account in order to discern the best method of management. Ablation of below knee GSV, segmental GSV without SFJ reflux, or AAGSV (anterior accessory great saphenous vein) in patients with edema "may be appropriate" in that treatment may be acceptable or reasonable, but more research or patient information is necessary to classify the appropriateness of the intervention. Ablation of an SSV with evidence of reflux is always appropriate in the context of edema.

Note that this "gray zone" of management only exists at C3. If a patient has edema with any features of C4a-C6 disease, ablation of the GSV is almost always appropriate and is likely to lead to improved outcomes for the patient [20].

Superficial veins are known to display anatomical variance among individuals. These can present challenges in the management of chronic venous insufficiency. In the thigh, the GSV can have a large subcutaneous tributary running in the superficial fascia or have a twin lying in the same plane. These duplications can have a common junction with the femoral vein, join separately into the femoral vein, or be "insula" and merge proximally and distally to form a single GSV [24]. Orsini et al. found collaterals which flow underneath the sapheno-femoral junction which can be difficult to identify and cause sure relapse if ignored during surgery [25]. At the level of the knee, the long saphenous may once again be seen alone or alongside a large superficial tributary. In 29% of the population, it is absent at the level of the knee. This occurs when the GSV pierces the superficial fascia in the distal thigh. The now subcutaneous vessel now runs down past the knee and only reenters the "saphenous compartment" between the superficial and deep fascia distally in the leg. This variation can also be seen with a superficial branch that continues to run down the leg in superficial fascia near the distal GSV. There are also tributaries of the GSV in the leg that are large enough to look like duplications of the GSV [24]. There is also significant variability in deep veins, where classical anatomy may be present in as few as 16% of limbs [5].

There are a multitude of techniques available for vein ablation, with the field constantly moving toward therapies that are minimally invasive and maximally efficacious. Endovenous ablation is the most common format used, with multiple subcategories existing.

Thermal ablation involves denaturing the proteins of the vessel wall, causing collapse. Both laser ablation (Fig. 11.4a) and radiofrequency ablation (Fig. 11.4b) are modes of thermal ablation. Due to the high temperatures used, a large volume of dilute local anesthetic must be administered along the length of the vein being ablated to create a "heat sink." However, this in itself, known as tumescent infiltration, may be uncomfortable for the patient.

Various forms of non-thermal ablation are also in use, with advantages of a decreased likelihood of surrounding structure injury such as nerve injury and a decreased requirement for anesthesia. Mechanical occlusion chemically assisted (MOCA) ablation uses a rotating wire to damage the vein wall from inside with simultaneous application of a liquid sclerosant. In cyanoacrylate embolization (Fig. 11.5a, b), "glue" is introduced to the diseased vein and triggers an innate immune response that results in fibrotic occlusion of the vein.

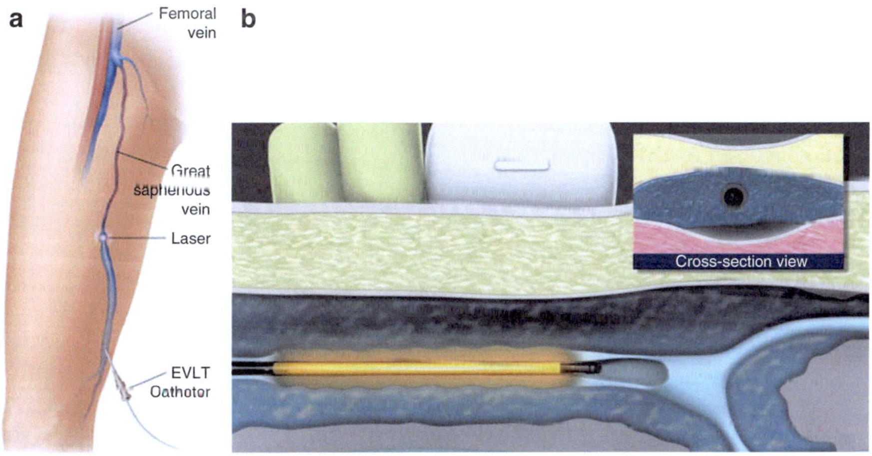

Fig. 11.4 (**a**) Endovenous laser ablation of varicose veins; (**b**) Endovenous radiofrequency ablation of varicose veins

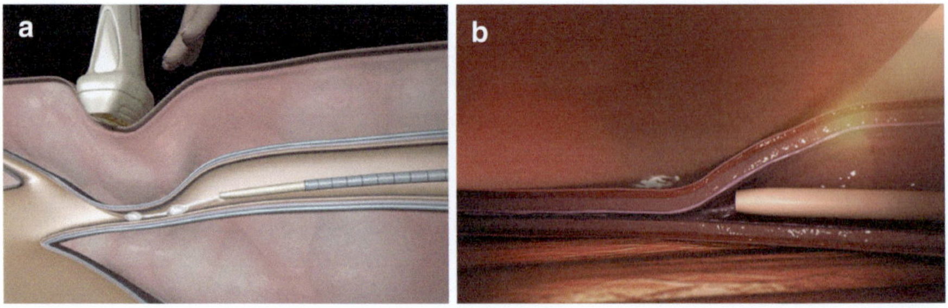

Fig. 11.5 (**a**, **b**) Endovenous cyanoacrylate glue ablation of varicose veins

Another example of endovenous ablation is polidocanol endovenous microfoam, where a mixture of oxygen, carbon dioxide, and 1% polidocanol solution is delivered into the diseased vein causing the formation of microfoam bubbles.

Despite being less invasive and achieving lower rates of recurrence than surgery, endovenous ablation is not always possible. Chronic phlebitis can result in the formation of fibrous adhesions known as synechiae. These can obstruct the passage of a catheter, making endovenous ablation impossible. Similarly, severe tortuosity of a vessel may have an obstructive effect on endovenous surgery. There are also specific contraindications to thermal ablation as the ablation of veins too close to the skin surface may result in burns. As such, target veins that are not at least 1 cm deep to the skin after tumescent anesthesia is administered should not be ablated. Veins over 1cm in diameter have an increased risk of non-closure so more advanced techniques may have to be used in order to ensure adequate closure. Saphenous veins with very large diameters at the sapheno-femoral junction may be at risk for heat-induced thromboembolism. Acute deep vein thrombosis and superficial vein thrombophlebitis are a contraindication to endovenous ablation for similar reasons. Pregnancy also puts patients in a prothrombic state and as such venous interventions should be delayed to at least 6 weeks after delivery.

Saphenous stripping and ligation have been virtually replaced by endovenous ablation techniques.

Great saphenous vein stripping at the level of knee or below it is rarely performed in order to avoid saphenous nerve injury. If peripheral artery disease is present and of a severity that would impede wound healing (ABI<0.5, absolute ankle pressure <60 mHg), it should first be treated before performing any venous intervention or surgery. Patients with genetic or congenital venous abnormalities such as Klippel-Trenaunay syndrome should generally not undergo venous surgery [21, 22].

11.8 Management of Deep Vein Obstruction in the Context of Oedema

In patients with known deep venous insufficiency, the incidence of varicose vein, leg ulceration, and recurrent ulcer recurrence rates are much higher.

Primary investigation of deep venous obstruction utilizing venous duplex ultrasound at 2–3 MHz to evaluate the iliac veins and IVC, CT, and MR venography is useful for estimating the location and severity of obstruction as outlined above. Intravascular ultrasound (IVUS) is the most sensitive diagnostic test and is performed during diagnostic venography or therapeutic intervention to confirm obstruction and select the location of the lesions and size of stents prior to proceeding with angioplasty and stenting (Fig. 11.6a, b).

Similar to operative management of the superficial venous system, the American Venous Forum is cautious with its recommendation for iliac vein or IVC stenting as a first-line therapy for a patient with C3 venous disease. 24% of patients with no history of lower extremity DVT or any other associated symptoms have at least 50% obstruction of the left common iliac vein [26]. Therefore, the presence of significant deep vein obstruction in a patient with lower limb edema does not necessarily imply causation. As such, other causes of edema and the relative impact of deep vein obstruction on the patient's edema must be considered. Treatment may improve the outcome, but the risks of surgery must be weighed against uncertain reward. If edema is present with lipodermatosclerosis, atrophie blanche, or ulceration, stenting is indicated (>C4a-6) for both NIVL and post-thrombotic obstructions of ilio-caval system (Fig. 11.7a, b).

For patients with superficial venous reflux and deep vein reflux, iliac vein obstruction correction is necessary to prevent superficial venous reflux recurrence—which could lead to a recurrent edema. In a 207-patient cohort with deep vein obstruction, patients who only received endovenous laser ablation had a high rate of superficial venous reflux recurrence when compared to patients who received both endovenous laser ablation and iliac stent placement [27].

If endovascular stenting fails, open surgery may be required to relieve symptoms of edema associated with c4a-C6 disease. This may include sapheno-femoral cross-over bypass, cross-pelvic venous bypass, femorofemoral or ilioiliac prosthetic bypass, and femorocaval and aortic elevation. Postoperative management is comprehensive with long-term anticoagulation and compression therapy.

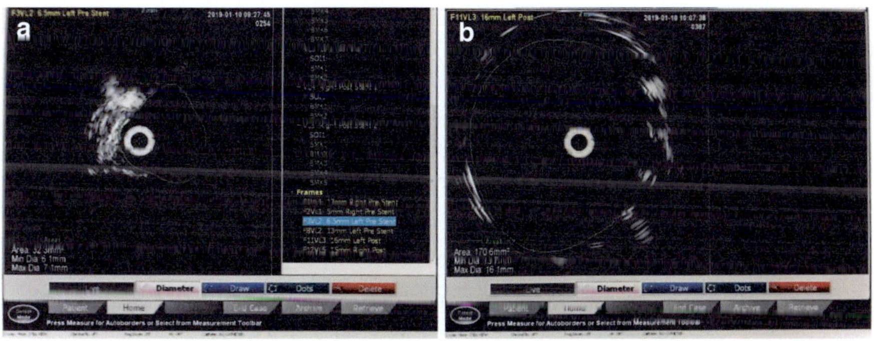

Fig. 11.6 (**a**) Intravascular ultrasound showing narrowed iliac vein; (**b**) Intravascular ultrasound showing widely open stented iliac vein

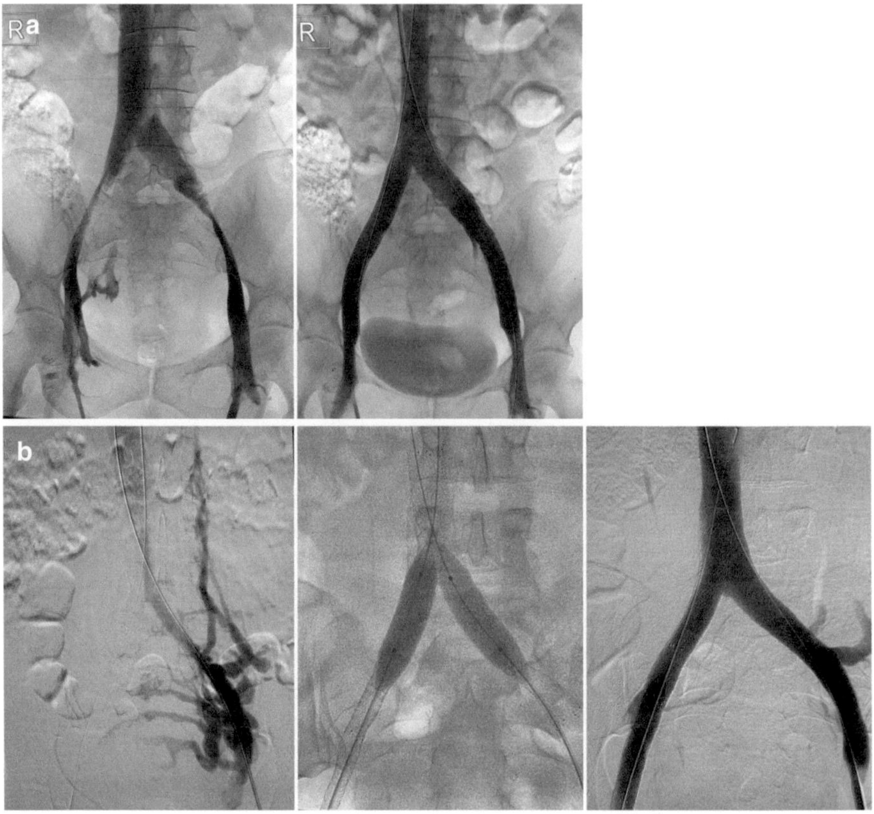

Fig. 11.7 (**a**) NIVL obstruction of bilateral Iliac veins Fig. 11.5b. After Iliac vein stents; (**b**) Post-thrombotic obstruction of left common iliac vein; (**b** and **c**) After Iliac vein balloon angioplasty and stents

Finally, in the case of more novel causes of deep vein obstruction like tumors, cysts, and osteophytes, conservative symptomatic treatment of chronic venous insufficiency should occur in tandem with treatment of the primary etiology.

Conflict of Interest None.

References

1. Beebe-Dimmer JL, Pfeifer JR, Engle JS, Schottenfeld D. The epidemiology of chronic venous insufficiency. Ann Epidemiol. 2005;15:175–84.
2. Kabnick LS, Scovell S. Overview of lower extremity chronic venous disease 2020, viewed 15 November 2020, UpToDate.
3. Gilroy AM. Anatomy an essential textbook. 1st ed. New York: Thieme Medical Publishers; 2013.
4. Eberhardt RT, Raffetto JD. Chronic venous insufficiency. Circulation. 2014;30:333–46.
5. Meissner M. Lower extremity venous anatomy. Semin Intervent Radiol. 2005;22:147–56.

6. Bell DJ, Knipe H. Great saphenous vein, viewed 14 November 2020, < https://radiopaedia.org/articles/great-saphenous-vein?lang=gb>.
7. van Vuuren TMAJ 2019 Deep venous obstruction: towards optimizing treatment strategies, PhD thesis. Maastricht: Maastricht University.
8. Labropoulos N, Volteas N, Leon M, Sowade O, Rulo A, Giannoukas AD, Nicolaides AN. The role of venous outflow obstruction in patients with chronic venous dysfunction. Arch Surg. 1997;132:46–51.
9. Santler B, George T. Chronic venous insufficiency – a review of pathophysiology, diagnosis, and treatment. Jounal der Deutschen Dermatologischen Gesellschaft. 2017;15:538–56.
10. Willenberg T, Schumacher A, Amann-Vesti B, Jacomella V, Thalhammer C, Diehm N, Baumgarter I, Husmann M. Impact of obesity on venous hemodynamics of the lower limbs. J Vasc Surg. 2010;52:664–8.
11. Tostes RC, Nigro D, Fortes ZB, Carvalho MHC. Effects of estrogen on the vascular system. Braz J Med Biol Res. 2003;36:1143–58.
12. Alkhater M, Jockenhöfer F, Stoffels I, Dissemond J. May-Thurner syndrome: an often overlooked cause for refractory venous leg ulcers. Int Wound J. 2017;14:578–82.
13. Khan TA, Rudolph KP, Huber TS, Fatima J. May-Thurner syndrome presenting as pelvic congestion syndrome and vulvar varicosities in a nonpregnant adolescent. J Vasc Surg Cases Innov Techniq. 2019;5:252–4.
14. Mako K, Puskas A. May-Thurner syndrome – are we aware enough? Eur J Vasc Surg. 2019;48:381–8.
15. Boisseau M. Chronic venous disease and the genetic influence. Phlebolymphology. 2014;21:100–11.
16. Musil, D, Kaletova M, Herman, J. Age, body mass index and severity of primary chronic venous disease Biomedical Papers of the Medical Faculty of the University Palacky, Olomouc, Czechoslovakia, 2011; 155:367–71.
17. Talley NJ, O'Connor S. Clinical examination a systemic guide to physical diagnosis. 8th ed. Sydney: Elsevier; 2018.
18. Farzamnia H, Rabiei K, Sadeghi M, Roghani F. The predictive factors of recurrent deep vein thrombosis. ARYA Atherosclerosis. 2011;7:123–8.
19. Lurie F, Passman M, Meisner M, Dasling M, Masuda E, Welch H, Bush RL, Blebea J, Carpentier PH, Maeseneer MD, Gasparis A, Labropoulos N, Marston WA, Rafetto J, Santiago F, Shortell C, Uhl JF, Urbanek T, van Rij A, Eklof B, Gloviczki P, Kistner R, Lawrence P, Moneta G, Padberg F, Perrin M, Wakefield T. The 2020 update of the CEAP classification system and reporting standards. J Vasc Surg Venous Lymphatic Disord. 2020;8:342–52.
20. Masuda E, Ozsvath K, Vossler J, Woo K, Kistner R, Lurie F, Monahan D, Brown W, Labropoulos N, Dasling M, Khilnani N, Wakefield T, Gloviczki P. The 2020 appropriate use criteria for chronic lower extremity venous disease of the American Venous Forum, the Society for Vascular Surgery, the American Vein and Lymphatic Society, and the Society of Interventional Radiology. J Vasc Surg Venous Lymphatic Disord. 2020;8:505–25.
21. Alguire PC, Mathes BM. Medical management of lower extremity chronic venous disease 2020, viewed 17 November 2020, UpToDate.
22. Passman MA. Approach to treating symptomatic superficial venous insufficiency 2019, viewed 17 November 2020, UpToDate.
23. Armstrong DG, Meyr A. Compression therapy for the treatment of chronic venous insufficiency 2019, viewed 17 November 2020, UpToDate.
24. Chen SS, Prasad SK. Long saphenous vein and its anatomical variations. Aust J Ultrasound Med. 2009;12:28–31.
25. Orsini A, Molfetta S, Pagani C. The importance of anatomical variants of the sapheno femoral junction in lower-limb varicose vein surgery. Minerva Cardioangiologica. 2001;49:257–62.
26. Singh D, Alshareef S, Meka M. Deep vein thrombosis secondary to extrinsic compression, a case report. Cureus. 2020;12:160.
27. Mousa AY. Overview of iliocaval venous obstruction, 2020 viewed 17 November 2020, UpToDate

Compression Stockings

12

Matthew Machin, Ankur Thapar, and Alun H Davies

12.1 History of Compression Therapy

Historians have dated compression therapy back to the Neolithic period 5000–2500 BC from paintings illustrating soldiers with leg ulcers treated with tight bandaging [1]. It is known that Hippocrates described the use of compression bandaging to treat ulceration of the lower limb in *Corpus Hippocraticum* (350 BC) [2]. Furthermore, he is reported as describing how to obtain an eccentric (focal) compression by placing sponges underneath the bandages [3].

However, the first reports of bandaging being used to prevent reflux of blood in the lower limbs were from the Galen c.130–200 BC which could be viewed as comparable to today's use of compression bandaging. An example of the utility of compression therapy was mentioned by Henry de Mondeville, a medieval French surgeon, who stated *"...compression expels bad humors that infiltrate legs and ulcers..."* (1260–1320) [3].

Compression for venous ulceration was classically achieved using bandaging techniques which applied a gradual concentric (uniform) pressure while being a suitable dressing for an exudative ulcer. This was historically in the form of single-layer bandaging, two-layer bandaging with an elastic material, or three-layer bandaging with an elastic material. Elastic stockings were first patented by William Brown in 1848 after the advent of rubber vulcanization in 1839 [3]

More recently, four-layer bandaging technique was developed at Charing Cross Hospital, London, UK [4]. This technique developed after conventional bandaging failed to apply sustained external pressure. The four-layer technique was thought to

M. Machin · A. Thapar · A. H. Davies (✉)
Academic Department of Vascular Surgery, Department of Surgery and Cancer, Imperial College London, London, UK
e-mail: a.h.davies@imperial.ac.uk

S. K. Tiwary (ed.), *Approach to Lower Limb Oedema*,
https://doi.org/10.1007/978-981-16-6206-5_12

provide lasting graduated pressure—the results of which were published in 1988 achieving ulcer healing rates of 75% at 12 weeks [5].

During this time, efforts also turned to utilizing other technologies to provide compression that could be applied by the patient at home. As early as 1982, studies assessing differing pneumatic compression devices were underway [6]. By 1985, randomized-controlled trials were conducted investigating intermittent pneumatic compression which utilized short duration high-pressure cycles [7].

Newer products have aimed at replicating this sustained pressure without the need for bandaging, which is labor intensive. CircAid Medical Products™ published a patent in 2008 for its "Limb encircling therapeutic compression device" which is discussed below.

12.2 Types of Compression Stockings and Devices

There are a variety of differing designs and sizes of compression devices available. These are discussed in turn.

Compression stockings, also known as graduated compression stockings, are an elastic stocking that apply the greatest amount of pressure at the ankle which reduces gradually up the limb. This provides graduated concentric pressure encouraging blood and lymph to flow from distal to proximal. It is important to note that graduated compression stockings differ from anti-embolism stockings, commonly known as thromboembolic deterrent stockings (TEDS). Thromboembolic deterrent stockings apply a level of graduated pressure but are **not** designed to achieve this graduation in an **ambulant** individual—they are designed for immobile patients at risk of venous thromboembolism, not for the management of deep venous/lymphatic insufficiency in ambulant patients.

Compression stockings can be classified by size and grade, i.e., the pressure the stockings apply to the limb. Compression stockings are available in a range of sizes and styles. For effective graduated compression, an above-knee size or thigh-length stocking is used depending on leg shape and patient preference.

The differing grades of compression stockings across the world are shown in Table 12.1. Within the UK, class II compression stockings are commonly prescribed for chronic venous disease and lipedema with an increase in class if symptoms persist, and if tolerated by the patient (see *Adherence*). Class III stockings are more commonly required for the more severe edema found in post-thrombotic syndrome and lymphedema (in combination with manual lymphatic drainage).

Table 12.1 Graduated compression classes across different countries [8]

Compression Class	USA (mmHg)	UK (mmHg)	France (mmHg)	Germany (mmHg)
ILight/moderate	15–20	14–17	10–15	18–21
IIMedium	20–30	18–24	15–20	23–32
IIIStrong	30–40	25–35	20–36	34–46
IVVery strong	40+		>36	>49

Compression bandaging involves the application of sequential bandaging which is usually changed bi-weekly by a trained specialist.

The four-layer bandaging system, which is now considered as the standard of care, consists of (see Fig. 12.1):

- Application of a non-adherent, inert dressing to the area of ulceration.
- Layer 1: wool applied in a spiral fashion without tension—this absorbs exudate and protects the bony prominences around the ankle.
- Layer 2: crepe applied in a spiral fashion—this further absorbs exudate and smooths the wool preserving the compression applied from the subsequent main layers.

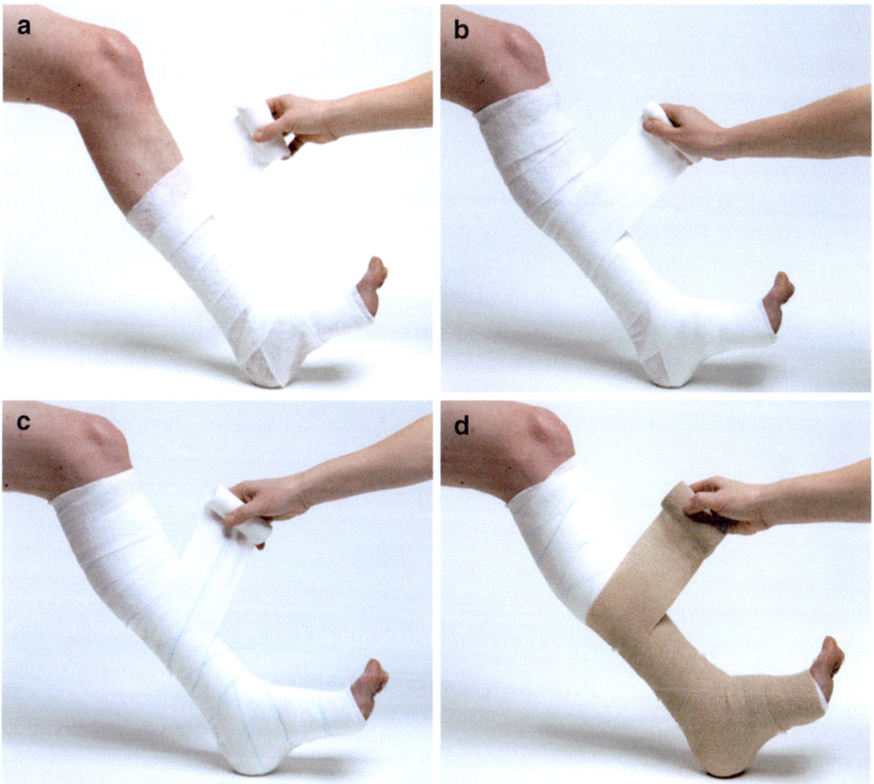

Fig. 12.1 Layers of four-layer compression bandaging, provided by Urgo Medical®, Urgo K-Four compression bandaging system©. (**a**) Layer 1: K-SOFT (sub-compression wadding, viscose, polyester); (**b**) Layer 2: K-LITE light support bandage type 2 (viscose, polyester, elastane); (**c**) Layer 3: K-PLUS: light support bandage type 3a (viscose, elastane); (**d**) Layer 4: KO-FLEX: cohesive long-stretch bandage (acrylic, cotton, elastane, cohesive material containing low levels of natural latex)

- Layer 3: elastic layer applied at mid-stretch in a figure-of-eight fashion with a 50% overlap, achieving 17 mmHg of pressure for an ankle circumference of 18—25 cm.
- Layer 4: light-weight cohesive bandage applied at mid-stretch with a 50% overlap—this will increase the ankle pressure applied to 23 mmHg.

Importantly, the bandaging combination is determined by the diameter of the ankle and hence will change from patient to patient. Furthermore, ulcer position will also affect the bandaging technique with some ulcers, such as those situated just posterior to the malleoli, requiring application of an additional pressure pad. In patients with bony prominences or peripheral arterial disease, pressure necrosis can easily develop. Hence, regular review is necessary when using compression therapy, with bi-weekly changes recommended. Pain after application of a bandage is a good indicator that the level of compression needs to be reduced.

Intermittent pneumatic compression therapy consists of a pneumatic pump and an inflatable sleeve worn on the limb. Different devices are available for venous thromboembolism and for the management of chronic venous or lymphatic insufficiency. The segments of the inflatable sleeve are inflated up to a desired pressure, pressurizing the osteofascial compartment, deep venous system, and lymphatics. In the application of pneumatic compression in preventing venous thromboembolism, the pressure is then released entirely prior to re-inflation. However, when used in deep venous or lymphatic insufficiency, a more complex arrangement is applied in which sequential inflation of the device applies a graduated pressure to "milk" the limb, encouraging venous and lymphatic return (Fig. 12.2). Devices are available to fit both the upper and lower limbs.

CircAid devices are an inelastic sleeve that is tightened around the limb consisting of an ankle compression stocking, a lower limb liner, and an inelastic

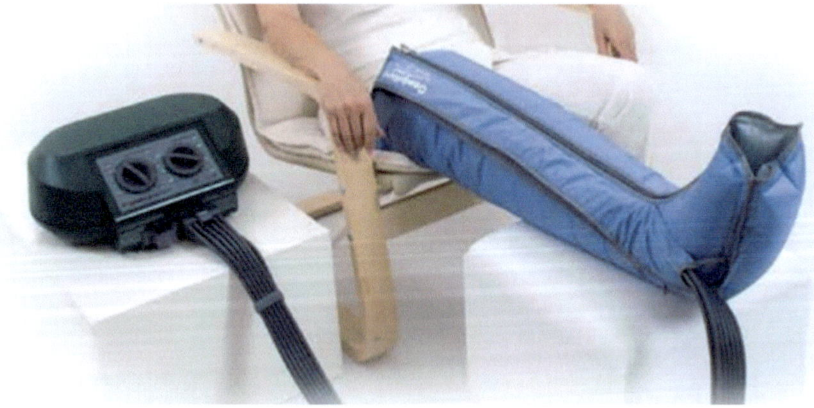

Fig. 12.2 The Lympha Press® Mini intermittent pneumatic compression device

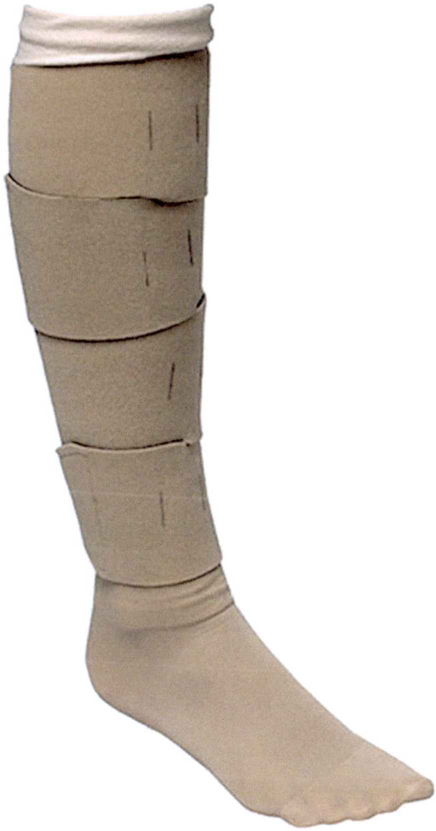

Fig. 12.3 The Juxta-Lite™ CircAid® below-knee compression device

Velcro-secured calf-compression band (Fig. 12.3). The ankle compression sock and liner are worn first prior to the band being tightened around the lower limb. A separate component is applied to the foot and thigh to provide compression to the full length of the limb if required. The CircAid is adjustable to provide differing grades of compression; this can be changed and managed by the patients themselves using a supplied gauge. CircAid products are also available for upper limb edema (commonly lymphedema or post-thrombotic syndrome).

Lastly, support hosiery such as "flight socks" available from commercial, non-medical suppliers are sometimes worn by patients for symptomatic relief. These socks/tights are made from elastic material and provide a low level of **non-graduated** pressure. Hence, they are not a substitute for graduated compression stockings and are not provided in the clinical setting. They are generally constructed of a much thinner weight material and are easily tolerated; hence they are commonly found on patients attending the outpatient clinic.

12.2.1 Pathophysiology

Chronic venous disease is a spectrum from asymptomatic telangiectasia and reticular veins to recurrent venous ulceration. The pathophysiology of chronic venous disease will be covered briefly to enable discussion of the mechanism of graduated compression stockings. Venous insufficiency can be caused by congenital venous malformation, post-thrombotic thrombotic obstruction or stenosis of the deep venous system, valve failure leading to reflux, calf-pump failure, morbid obesity, right heart failure, or a combination.

Post-thrombotic syndrome is thought to be due to sustained venous hypertension, as a result of venous outflow obstruction and valvular incompetence that occurs after deep vein thrombosis. Recent research has demonstrated that inflammatory cell signaling pathways occur in response to in situ thrombus with subsequent activation of inflammatory cells and matrix metalloproteinases, resulting in scarring and reduced compliance of the vein wall [9].

Primary superficial venous insufficiency is a term used to describe reflux and valve failure in the superficial system without another cause. Primary venous insufficiency is common, with many reported associations in the literature. Less commonly, there is primary reflux in the valves of the deep venous system.

12.3 Mechanism

The fundamental concept of how compression stockings work is that to narrow the superficial and deep leg veins, the external compression pressure applied should be higher than the intravenous pressure [10]. The pressure applied to the compartment is governed by Laplace's law.

$$P \propto \frac{T}{r}$$

The pressure will be zero over the horizontal areas (in principle), while it will be high over curved/acute angles. The pressure (***P***) is directly proportional to the tension of the textile (***T***). However, the pressure is inversely proportional to the radius ***r*** of the curvature to which it is applied [10]. Hence, this explains why the pressure applied to the ankle is greater than that at the calf.

Compression stockings act as an adjunct to the calf pump to empty osteofascial compartments and to more closely oppose widely separated valves (Fig. 12.4). The degree as to which this is required is dependent on the therapeutic intent. In order to prevent edema in the sitting position, pressures of around 20 mmHg are required. However, in order to improve venous return in the ambulant individual with deep venous insufficiency, higher pressures are required to overcome the intravenous pressure.

For an individual to tolerate this therapy, it is important that these applications of higher pressure, e.g., 50–80 mmHg, are intermittent. A resting pressure as high as this would be painful and hamper arterial inflow. Compression therapy achieves intermittent high pressure during ambulation; however, a stiff material is required.

There have been attempts to quantify the different compression properties between lying and standing for a compression modality using the static stiffness index (SSI), with elastic stockings having a lower index in comparison to inelastic bandaging or Velcro-assist wraps [12]. This means that the compression pressure provided by elastic stockings does not increase as much as inelastic wraps. As an individual walks with inelastic wraps, the movement of the muscle (change in radius) and the compression from the high-tensile wrap causes intermittent high compression forces.

Overall, the change in venous parameters is summarized in Table 12.2. The resting pressure of a graduated compression stocking helps to prevent edema in the sitting position. The intermittent high pressures exerted during ambulation help to reduce edema and improve venous insufficiency.

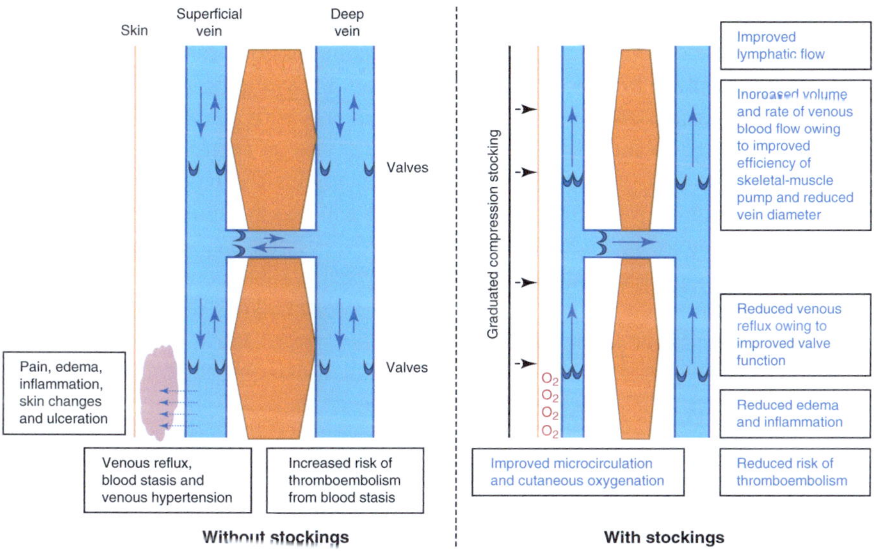

Fig. 12.4 The mechanisms of action of graduated compression stockings, Lim et al. [11]

Table 12.2 Effect of compression stockings on lower limb properties, the Vein Book [3]

Lower limb property	Direction of effect
Venous reflux	Decrease
Volume of deep veins	Decrease
Venous pump	Increase
Lymphatic return	Increase
Edema	Decrease
Arterial flow	Increase (intermittent compression only)

12.4 Safety

Individuals with arterial insufficiency have reduced arterial pressures in the lower limb. It is common for those with chronic limb-threatening ischemia to have arterial ankle pressures of <50 mmHg. Therefore, if a compression stocking is applied, which would apply ~24 mmHg to the ankle, this effectively halves perfusion to the foot and can result in limb loss. Hence, compression bandaging is contraindicated in those with peripheral arterial disease.

Absence of both foot pulses is a clear contraindication to compression therapy. In the UK, the National Institute for Health and Care Excellence (NICE) guidelines for compression therapy recommend that all individuals have an ankle-brachial pressure index measurement prior to commencing compression therapy [13]. Compression stockings are safe to wear with an ankle-brachial pressure index between 0.8 and 1.3.

This can be complicated by calcification of the arteries seen in those with diabetes and chronic renal failure. In this case, toe pressures (ideally >60 mmHg) and ankle Doppler waveforms (ideally biphasic or triphasic) can be substituted.

If there is a contraindication to graduated compression stockings, alternative strategies attempting to improve venous function are available. Most novel is the use of neuromuscular electrical stimulation in patients with chronic venous disease which is believed to increase arterial inflow and venous return [14]. The device comes in the form of an endplate that the user applies the base of their feet on (Fig. 12.5) which uses electrical stimulation to activate the muscles of the lower limb and calf pump. In a recent RCT, the REVITIVE device has been shown to improve disease-specific quality of life in comparison to a sham device. Furthermore, other technologies such as the wearable transcutaneous Geko™ device provide neuromuscular stimulation along the common peroneal nerve activating the calf pump [15]. Simpler devices, such as the calf-pump rocker, exist in which the user dorsiflexes and plantarflexes their feet in order to activate their calf pump.

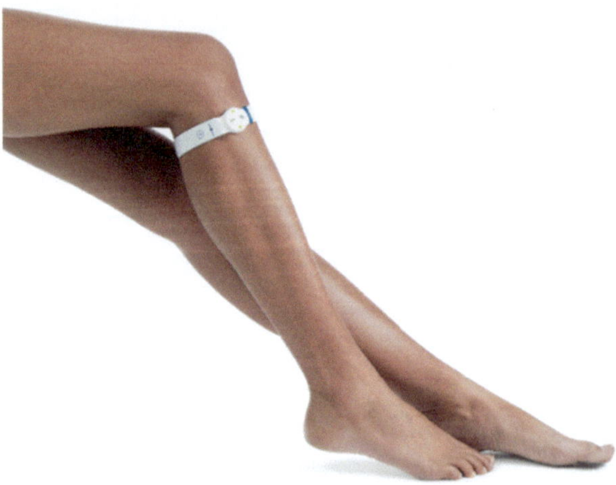

Fig. 12.5 Illustration demonstrating the use of the Geko™ transcutaneous neuromuscular stimulation worn over the common peroneal nerve

12.5 Fitting of Compression Stockings

Graduated compression stockings are constructed of an elastic material that can be difficult to manipulate onto the lower limbs and cause adherence problems if the correct fitting guidance is not followed.

12.6 Instructions to the Wearer

Graduated compression stockings should be fitted in the morning after waking when the lowers limbs are at their smallest diameter, to avoid them slipping down.

Furthermore, the stockings should be fitted so that there are no points of constrained or "rolled-up" material. If the elastic material is more concentrated around one part of the limb because the stockings have not been applied correctly, this can cause a constricting band and subsequent ischemia [16].

In a large RCT, CLOTS 1, which assessed the use of graduated compression stockings in the prevention of stroke, 5% of those wearing stockings suffered from skin breaks, ulceration, blisters, or skin necrosis [16].

Compression stockings should be taken off prior to sleep, both to rest the microcirculation in the skin and because the venous pressure at the ankles naturally reduces when in bed. If for some reason this is not possible, they should not be worn for any longer than 7 days continually. If there are any defects or holes in the stockings, then they need to be replaced. Furthermore, the elastic compression reduces with time as the stockings degenerate; current UK guidance is to replace the stockings at least every 6 months on the basis of having two sets of stockings in circulation at one time. When replacing stockings, it is recommended to have the stockings re-fitted as changes in lower limb size occur with successful compression.

12.7 Considerations When Fitting and Supplying Compression Stockings

When measuring an individual's limb for compression stockings, each manufacturer may vary. In the UK, the NICE guideline recommends the following for below-knee stockings: measurement should be taken with the person seated, and feet flat on the floor, measure the circumference of the ankle at the narrowest point just above the malleoli, measure the circumference of the widest part of the calf (usually the mid calf area), and measure the length of the foot from the heel to the tip of the longest toe (if a closed-toe stocking is required).

As an example of how to measure to size compression stocking, see Fig. 12.6; the Sigvaris© stockings require measurement of the following:

- Ankle circumference
- Calf circumference
- Calf length

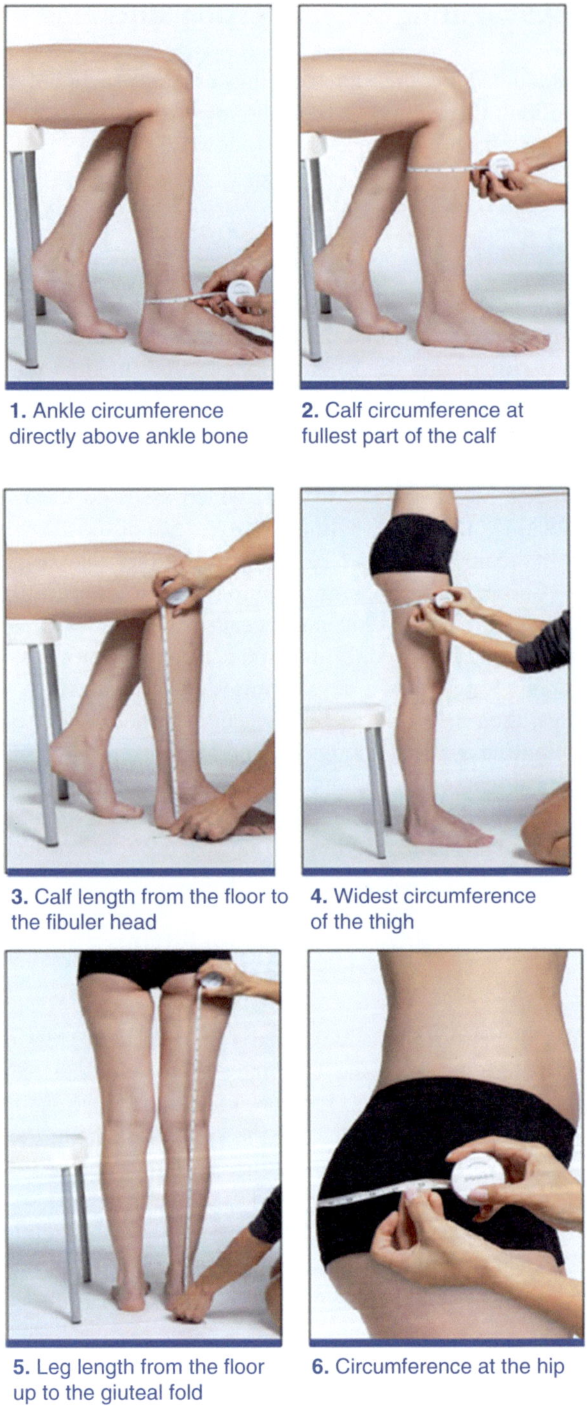

Fig. 12.6 Sigvaris© measurement guidelines for sizing compression stockings [17]

- Thigh circumference
- Leg length

The sizes available from Sigvaris© cater for an ankle circumference of 18 cm up to 36 cm.

12.8 Compression Stockings: Fabrics and Design

Graduated compression stockings are available in a range of fabric compositions and colors. Stockings are commonly made from a synthetic composite of polyamide and elastane in a 2 to 1 ratio. Addition of cotton to the composite is often added to change the properties of the material, making them easier to wear in hotter climates. Furthermore, some stocking manufacturers such as Sigvaris© add zinc to the sole of the stocking to combat odor [17].

Stockings are available in a range of colors and designs which is an important consideration for adherence, particularly in encouraging patients to remain socially active.

Both closed-toe and open-toe variations are available. Open-toe stockings are usually preferred by those with arthritic or deformed toes, or fungal infection of the forefoot or a relatively longer foot size compared with their calf dimeter [13]. Closed-toe stockings prevent the toe swelling that can, for example, trouble those with lymphedema.

The length of the graduated stocking prescribed will depend on if there is venous insufficiency or lymphoedema in the thigh. Regarding the prevention of PTS, it has been shown that there is no difference in prevention of PTS after acute proximal DVT when wearing thigh-length in comparison to knee-length stockings. However, knee-length stockings are better tolerated [18].

12.8.1 Donning Aids

Donning aids are devices designed to facilitate the application and subsequent removal of the graduated compression stocking to the upper or lower limb [19]. Donning aids are available in a range of designs including low-friction materials that allow manipulation of the stockings over it, fixed step-in cages which hold the stocking open as it is applied, and roller devices that apply the stockings as it rolled up the limb [19]. Figure 12.7 demonstrates the step-in Medi Valet frame type donning aid and the Sigvaris© roller ball applicator.

Other readily available aids, such as a plastic bag, can also be used to decrease friction over the foot.

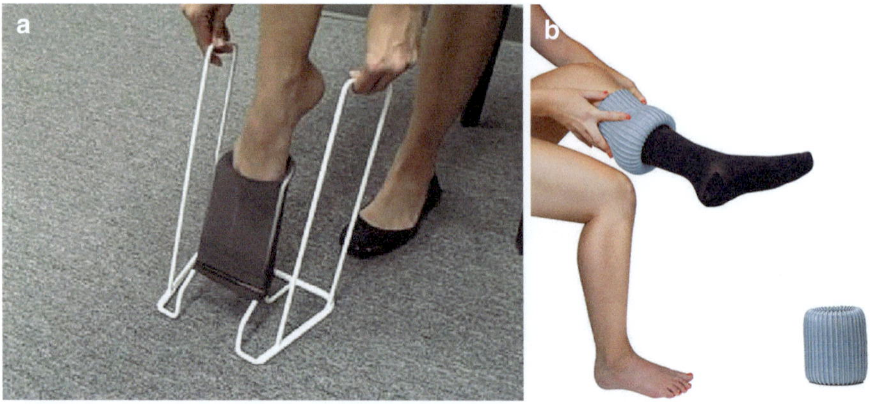

Fig. 12.7 (**a**) demonstrates the step-in Medi Valet frame type donning aid which can be held in place using the metal arms; (**b**) the Sigvaris© roller ball applicator which is shown as it is used and alone

12.8.2 Indications for Compression Therapy

The clinical indications for graduated compression therapy include:

1. Prevention of thromboembolic events (TEDS), although this benefit is marginal [20].
2. Prevention of post-thrombotic syndrome.
3. Symptomatic relief in post-thrombotic syndrome.
4. Symptomatic relief in chronic venous disease.
5. Management of venous ulceration.
6. Management of lymphedema and lipedema.

See Table 12.3 for summary of American and European clinical practice guidelines.

12.9 Thromboembolic Deterrent Stockings in the Prevention of Hospital-Acquired Thrombosis

The CLOTS-1 RCT assessed their use in hospital-acquired thrombosis prevention for stroke in patients who had a contraindication to low-molecular-weight heparin and demonstrated no difference in the rate of hospital-acquired thrombosis [16]. They did, however, cause a significant number of adverse skin events such as ulceration and necrosis. Furthermore, the large multicenter GAPS RCT demonstrated no additional benefit in reduction of hospital-acquired thrombosis when applying graduated compression stockings to surgical inpatients receiving low-molecular-weight heparin [16]. NICE guidelines currently still recommend their use in the prevention of hospital-acquired thrombosis [21].

12.10 Prevention of Post-Thrombotic Syndrome

Current NICE guidelines published in 2018 advise against the use of compression stockings in the prevention of post-thrombotic syndrome after acute ilio-femoral/proximal deep vein thrombosis [21]. Previous NICE guidelines had recommended compression stockings, but subsequent publication of the SOX trial promoted a change in recommendations [22].The SOX trial was a placebo-controlled double-blind RCT which assigned 803 participants to receive graduated compression stockings (30–40 mmHg) or placebo stockings. The cumulative incidence of PTS as defined by the Villalta scale did not differ between the two groups, with 53% in the graduated compression stocking arm and 52% in the placebo stocking arm (HR 1·00, 95% CI 0·81–1·24, $p = 0.96$).

The American Heart Association guidelines echo this, suggesting that the evidence for compression therapy in reducing post-thrombotic syndrome is uncertain and hence not recommended [23]. A systematic review and meta-analysis on the use of graduated compression stockings in prevention of PTS revealed high heterogeneity in the three pooled RCTs, the results of which are illustrated in Table 12.4 [24].

Table 12.3 Illustrative summary of American and European clinical practice guidelines

Recommendation for compression therapy	American Venous Forum	American College of Phlebology	European Society for Vascular Surgery	International Union of Phlebology
To increase venous leg ulcer healing rate	1A		1A	1A
Against their use for symptomatic venous reflux disease when other definitive treatments are appropriate	1B	1A		
Management of symptoms related to superficial disease	2C	2C	1B	

Class of evidence: level I–III
Grade of evidence: A–C

Table 12.4 Cumulative incidence of PTS in the three RCTs comparing graduated compression stockings to control stockings [24]

First author (study)	System used to define PTS	Incidence of PTS in graduated compression stockings arm	Incidence of PTS in control arm
Kahn et al.	Villalta	53%	52%
Prandoni et al.	Villalta	26%	49%
Brandjes et al.	Brandjes	31%	70%

However, it did suggest a trend between increased baseline risk of PTS and increasing benefit with stockings, for example in those in whom anticoagulation is ineffective.

12.11 Symptomatic Relief in Post-Thrombotic Syndrome

The use of class II compression stockings for symptomatic relief is widespread. This is reflected in clinical practice guideline recommendations; however, there is little evidence to support their use [9, 25]. A recent systematic review identified only two studies investigating the use of graduated compression stockings in the management of established PTS [25]. The first trial was published by Ginsberg et al. reporting a double-blind RCT of 35 participants with PTS randomized to either graduated compression stocking (30 to 40 mmHg) or a placebo stocking. At 2 years follow-up, there was no significant difference in the treatment success between the two arms.

The second study was a non-randomized prospective trial that allocated 34 consecutive patients with PTS (median Villalta score of 10) to four different compression stockings. Each participant wore each stocking for 60 min and underwent venous duplex and air plethysmography and subsequently offered a participant preference [26]. The venous volume and time to fill the venous volume significantly improved with use of all types of stocking versus no compression.

However, the reported results did not include long-term symptom control or quality of life, and limited conclusions regarding their efficacy could be drawn.

However, as compression represents a low-risk and low-cost intervention, a trial of stockings is often considered appropriate. This is mirrored in both the NICE and American Heart Association guidelines [21, 23].

12.12 Symptomatic Relief in Acute DVT

Kahn et al. undertook a large multicenter RCT investigating the use of graduated compression stockings in the treatment of acute leg pain in patients suffering from acute proximal DVT [22]. A total of 803 participants with acute proximal DVT were randomized to either graduated compression stockings or placebo stockings. There was no significant difference in pain score at any point up to the 60-day follow-up, and it was concluded that compression stockings failed to reduce pain in acute DVT.

12.13 Symptomatic Relief in Chronic Venous Disease

Class II compression stockings are often used for symptomatic relief in chronic venous disease; however, the evidence to support this is lacking. For superficial varicose veins, three RCTs have investigated the use of compression stockings in disease/symptom control [27–29]. The pooled analysis from the NICE evidence summary revealed that compression stockings were associated with a relative reduction in pain experiences and the feeling of "heavy"/tired legs; however, the uncertainty in evidence rendered the analysis low quality. UK NICE guidelines recommend endovenous intervention for incompetent varicose veins leading to venous insufficiency. NICE recommend against graduated compression stockings in these patients unless interventional treatment is unsuitable [30]. However, if there is evidence of skin changes such as lipodermatosclerosis or persistent venous eczema, these recommendations differ slightly. In addition to treatment of superficial venous insufficiency, NICE recommend class II graduated compression therapy. However, this is largely based on expert opinion [31].

12.14 Treatment of Venous Ulceration

The use of compression therapy in the treatment of venous ulceration was examined by a 2012 Cochrane systematic review. This identified 48 RCTs assessing the use of compression bandaging/stockings and wound dressings for the management of venous ulceration [32]. Overall, it was found that compression bandaging reduced time to ulcer healing. Importantly, pooled analysis from 3 RCTs demonstrated that three-component systems containing an elastic component, i.e., the Charing Cross four-layer bandaging healed more ulcers than those without elastic. The VenUS1 trial is known for demonstrating that four-layer bandage (multilayer elastic compression) is superior to the short-stretch bandage (multilayer, inelastic compression) with significant improvement in ulcer healing while being more cost-effective [33].

Furthermore, a systematic review assessing the use of four-layer bandaging in comparison to short-stretch bandaging identified 7 RCTs; pooled analysis revealed that four-layer bandaging was associated with a significantly shorter time to venous ulcer healing [32]. Interestingly, a recent multicenter RCT (the VenUS IV trial) comparing 4-layer bandaging to two-layer hosiery therapy found no difference in time to ulcer healing and suggested that two-layer hosiery therapy may be more cost-effective [34]. However, more research on this comparison is required.

It is important to note the isolated use of compression bandaging in venous ulceration is not recommended. The recent EVRA RCT demonstrated that early endovenous ablation of superficial venous reflux at the time of ulceration resulted in faster healing of venous leg ulcers and was subsequently found to be more cost-effective than compression alone [35].

Regarding deep venous insufficiency, Raju et al. report impressive results from a prospective cohort study of 504 patients with C2–C6 disease and deep venous incompetence undergoing intravascular ultrasound-guided iliac vein stent placement [36]. For patients with C5 disease, the rate of limbs with healed active ulcers and freedom from ulcer recurrence were 54% and 88%, respectively. Improvement in pain experienced at 5 years was reported in 78% of participants with a corresponding significant increase in quality of life.

Furthermore, Black et al. reported early results that the use of deep venous stent in chronic iliac vein occlusion may improve the healing of venous ulcers; however, this is an evolving area of research [37].

Adjunctive therapies such as pentoxifylline, micronized purified flavonoid fraction, skin care, and wound dressing also play an important role but are outside the scope of this chapter [38]. The UK NICE guidelines recommend multilayer bandaging in the management of venous ulceration [38]. This is also reflected in the Scottish Intercollegiate Guidelines Network publication [39].

12.15 Treatment of Acute Leg Pain Post-Endovenous Ablation

Graduated compression stockings are commonly used after endovenous ablation or manual avulsion of varicose veins. The best evidence that graduated compression stockings are beneficial in the reduction of postoperative pain comes from the RCT Compression After Endovenous Thermal Ablation of Varicose Veins (COMETA Trial) [40]. A total of 206 participants who underwent endothermal ablation, with or without concurrent phlebectomies, were allocated to receive either 7 days of graduated compression stockings or no stockings at all. Median pain scores in the graduated compression group were significantly lower within the first few days after the procedures suggesting that compression stockings are beneficial in the reduction of postoperative pain. There was also no difference in the degree of ecchymosis.

12.16 Treatment of Lipedema

Lipedema is a symmetrical and abnormal increase of adipose tissue in the gluteal region, hips, thighs, and calves [41]. This increase in adiposity is disproportional to the trunk and upper limbs. Nonsurgical treatment consists of manual lymph drainage, physical exercise, and multilayered/multicomponent compression bandaging; however, very little evidence exists in the literature. A randomized comparative study of 11 patients allocated participants to complete decongestive physiotherapy (including multilayered compression bandaging and manual lymph drainage) alone or combined with intermittent pneumatic compression for 5 days [42]. The reduction in limb diameter was significant (although relatively small) in the control arm and the intermittent pneumatic compression arm at 6.2% and 8.9%, respectively. Further research in this area is required in order to provide evidence-based recommendations.

12.17 Treatment of Lymphedema

The use of class II/III compression stockings in lymphedema is common practice. However, there is a lack of evidence to support their use [43, 44]. This could be due to RCTs using compression therapy as the control arm and then investigating additional treatment modalities as the intervention. Often lymphedema is approached with a treatment phase using manual lymphatic drainage and multilayer bandaging to reduce the size of the limb, followed by a maintenance phase using class II/III graduated compression stockings. This two-stage approach comes as a result of an RCT assessing the use of multilayer bandaging followed by stockings in comparison to stockings alone in patients with upper or lower limb lymphedema of any cause [45]. Greater and sustained limb volume reduction was seen in the two-phase approach in comparison to compression stockings alone.

12.18 Adherence to Compression Stockings

The adherence to graduated compression stockings varies dramatically. In two large RCTs investigating the use of graduated compression stockings in the prevention of PTS, the adherence at 2 years ranged from 56% in the SOX trial to 87% reported by Prandoni et al. 2014 [22, 46]. There are a variety of factors that influence adherence with graduated compression therapy including hot climate, season, belief that they work, comfort, fashion, and ability to easily don and doff stockings. In a regression analysis of participants with venous ulceration, there were two factors that were found to be associated with adherence: a belief that wearing stockings was beneficial and the belief that stockings were uncomfortable to wear [47]. Other reports have highlighted that adherence was better in those with knowledge about their underlying condition and self-efficacy, with a lower adherence seen in those with depression [48].

The authors of this chapter have previously undertaken focus groups and online surveys addressing adherence to graduated compression stockings in patients with PTS.

When questioned regarding measures to improve adherence the responses were more choice of stocking colors and fabrics, a custom-fitted stocking, stockings that are easier to get on and off, and more information on the risk of reducing ulceration by wearing stockings.

Furthermore, other pragmatic issues were identified such as owning two pair of stockings may increase compliance as when one pair is in the wash, the other pair can be worn.

Adherence to compression stockings is complex, with a variety of environmental and patient-related factors. However, a belief that wearing the stockings is worthwhile seems to be key.

References

1. Lippi G, Favaloro EJ, Cervellin G. Prevention of venous thromboembolism: focus on mechanical prophylaxis. Semin Thromb Hemost [Internet]. 2011 [cited 2021 Jun 2];37(3):237–51. Available from: https://pubmed.ncbi.nlm.nih.gov/21455858/
2. DeWeese JA. Treatment of venous disease – the innovators. J Vasc Surg [Internet]. 1994 [cited 2021 Jun 2];20(5):675–83. Available from: https://pubmed.ncbi.nlm.nih.gov/7966801/
3. Bergan J. The Vein Book. 30 Corporate Drive, Suite 400, Burlington, MA: Elsevier; 2007.
4. Moffatt CJ, DD. The Charing cross high compression four-layer bandage system. J Wound Care. 1993;2:91–4.

5. Blair SD, Wright DDI, Backhouse CM, et al. Sustained compression and healing of chronic venous ulcers. Br Med J [Internet]. 1988 Nov 5 [cited 2021 Jun 2];297(6657):1159–61. Available from: http://www.bmj.com/
6. Kamm RD. Bioengineering studies of periodic external compression as prophylaxis against deep vein thrombosis—Part I: Numerical studies. J Biomech Eng [Internet]. 1982 [cited 2021 Jun 2];104(2):87–95. Available from: https://pubmed.ncbi.nlm.nih.gov/7078134/
7. Richmand DM, O'Donnell TF, Zelikovski A. Sequential pneumatic compression for lymphedema: a controlled trial. Arch Surg [Internet]. 1985 [cited 2021 Jun 2];120(10):1116–9. Available from: https://pubmed.ncbi.nlm.nih.gov/4038053/
8. Rabe E, Partsch H, Jünger M, et al. Guidelines for clinical studies with compression devices in patients with venous disorders of the lower limb. Eur J Vasc Endovasc Surg [Internet]. 2008 Apr [cited 2021 Jun 2];35(4):494–500. Available from: https://pubmed.ncbi.nlm.nih.gov/18249571/
9. Henke PK, Comerota AJ. An update on etiology, prevention, and therapy of postthrombotic syndrome. J Vasc Surg. Mosby Inc.; 2011;53:500–9.
10. Partsch H. Physics of compression.
11. Lim CS, Davies AH. Graduated compression stockings [Internet]. CMAJ. Can Med Assoc 2014;186[cited 2020 Dec 26]:E391–8. Available from: https://www.cmaj.ca/content/186/10/E391
12. Partsch H, Schuren J, Mosti G, et al. The Static Stiffness Index: An important parameter to characterise compression therapy in vivo. J Wound Care [Internet]. 2016 Sep 1 [cited 2021 Jun 2];25(9):S4–10. Available from: https://pubmed.ncbi.nlm.nih.gov/27608740/
13. Compression stockings | Health topics A to Z | CKS | NICE [Internet]. [cited 2021 Jun 2]. Available from: https://cks.nice.org.uk/topics/compression-stockings/
14. Ravikumar R, Williams KJ, Babber A, et al. Randomised controlled trial: potential benefit of a footplate neuromuscular electrical stimulation device in patients with chronic venous disease. Eur J Vasc Endovasc Surg. 2017 Jan 1;53(1):114–21.
15. Zhang Q, Styf J, Ekström L, et al. Effects of electrical nerve stimulation on force generation, oxygenation and blood volume in muscles of the immobilized human leg. Scand J Clin Lab Invest [Internet]. 2014 [cited 2020 Dec 28];74(5):369–77. Available from: https://www.tandfonline.com/doi/abs/10.3109/00365513.2014.898323
16. Dennis M, Cranswick G, Deary A, et al. Effectiveness of thigh-length graduated compression stockings to reduce the risk of deep vein thrombosis after stroke (CLOTS trial 1): a multicentre, randomised controlled trial. Lancet [Internet]. 2009 Jun 6 [cited 2021 May 11];373(9679):1958–65. Available from: www.thelancet.com
17. What is compression, what are compression levels? - Sigvaris US [Internet]. [cited 2021 Jun 2]. Available from: https://www.sigvaris.com/en/your-health/compression-therapy
18. Prandoni P, Noventa F, Quintavalla R, et al. Thigh-length versus below-knee compression elastic stockings for prevention of the postthrombotic syndrome in patients with proximal-venous thrombosis: a randomized trial. Blood. 2012;119(6):1561–5.
19. Wassall A. Compression hosiery: donning aids and garment removal. Br J Community Nurs. 2007;12(S10-S16)
20. Shalhoub J, Lawton R, Hudson J, et al. Graduated compression stockings as adjuvant to pharmaco-thromboprophylaxis in elective surgical patients (GAPS study): Randomised controlled trial. BMJ [Internet]. 2020 May 13 [cited 2021 Apr 7];369. Available from: https://www.bmj.com/content/369/bmj.m1309
21. The National Institute for Health and Care Excellence. Venous thromboembolism in over 16s: reducing the risk of hospital-acquired deep vein thrombosis or pulmonary embolism, NICE guideline [NG89] [Internet]. 2018. Available from: https://www.nice.org.uk/guidance/ng89
22. Kahn SR, Shapiro S, Wells PS, et al. Compression stockings to prevent post-thrombotic syndrome: a randomised placebo-controlled trial. Lancet. 2014;383(9920):880–8.
23. Kahn SR, Comerota AJ, Cushman M, et al. The postthrombotic syndrome: evidence-based prevention, diagnosis, and treatment strategies: a scientific statement from the American

heart association. Circulation [Internet]. 2014 Oct 28 [cited 2020 Dec 17];130(18):1636–61. Available from: https://www.ahajournals.org/doi/10.1161/CIR.0000000000000130

24. Skervin AL, Thapar A, Franchini AJ, et al. Systematic review and meta-analysis of utility of graduated compression stockings in prevention of post-thrombotic syndrome [Internet]. Eur J Vasc Endovasc Surg. W.B. Saunders Ltd; 2016; [cited 2021 Jun 2]51:838–45. Available from: https://pubmed.ncbi.nlm.nih.gov/27026391/
25. Azirar S, Appelen D, Prins MH, et al. Compression therapy for treating post-thrombotic syndrome. Cochrane Database Syst Rev [Internet]. 2019 Sep 18 [cited 2020 Dec 28];(9). Available from: https://www.cochranelibrary.com/cdsr/doi/10.1002/14651858.CD004177.pub2/full
26. Lattimer CR, Azzam M, Kalodiki E, et al. Compression stockings significantly improve hemodynamic performance in post-thrombotic syndrome irrespective of class or length. J Vasc Surg. 2013 Jul 1;58(1):158–65.
27. Anderson JH, Geraghty JG, Wilson YT, et al. Paroven and graduated compression hosiery for superficial venous insufficiency. Phlebology [Internet]. 1990 Jun 24 [cited 2021 Jun 2];5(4):271–6. Available from: https://journals.sagepub.com/doi/abs/10.1177/026835559000500408
28. Benigni J, Sadoun S, Allaert F, Vin F. Efficacy of class 1 elastic compression stockings in the early stages of chronic venous disease. Int Angiol. 2003;22:383–92.
29. Krijnen RMA, De Boer EM, Adèr HJ, et al. Compression stockings and rubber floor mats: do they benefit workers with chronic venous insufficiency and a standing profession? J Occup Environ Med [Internet]. 1997 Sep [cited 2021 Jun 2];39(9):889–94. Available from: https://pubmed.ncbi.nlm.nih.gov/9322173/
30. NICE. Varicose veins: diagnosis and management Clinical guideline [Internet]. 2013 [cited 2021 Jun 2]. Available from: www.nice.org.uk/guidance/cg168
31. NICE CKS. Scenario: Management | Management | Venous eczema and lipodermatosclerosis | CKS | NICE [Internet]. [cited 2021 Jun 2]. Available from: https://cks.nice.org.uk/topics/venous-eczema-lipodermatosclerosis/management/management/
32. O'Meara S, Tierney J, Cullum N, et al. Four layer bandage compared with short stretch bandage for venous leg ulcers: Systematic review and meta-analysis of randomised controlled trials with data from individual patients. BMJ [Internet]. 2009 May 2 [cited 2021 Jun 2];338(7702):1054–7. Available from: http://www.bmj.com/
33. Iglesias C, Nelson EA, Cullum NA, et al. VenUS I: A randomised controlled trial of two types of bandage for treating venous leg ulcers [Internet]. Vol. 8, Health Technology Assessment. National Co-ordinating Centre for HTA; 2004 [cited 2021 Jun 2]. Available from: https://pubmed.ncbi.nlm.nih.gov/15248939/
34. Ashby RL, Gabe R, Ali S, et al. Clinical and cost-effectiveness of compression hosiery versus compression bandages in treatment of venous leg ulcers (Venous leg Ulcer Study IV, VenUS IV): a randomised controlled trial. Lancet [Internet]. 2014 [cited 2021 Jun 2];383(9920):871–9. Available from: https://pubmed.ncbi.nlm.nih.gov/24315520/
35. Gohel MS, Heatley F, Liu X, et al. A randomized trial of early endovenous ablation in venous ulceration. N Engl J Med [Internet]. 2018 May 31 [cited 2021 May 17];378(22):2105–14. Available from: https://www.nejm.org/doi/full/10.1056/NEJMoa1801214
36. Raju S, Darcey R, Neglén P. Unexpected major role for venous stenting in deep reflux disease. J Vasc Surg [Internet]. 2010 Feb [cited 2021 Jun 2];51(2):401–8. Available from: https://pubmed.ncbi.nlm.nih.gov/20006920/
37. Black S, Gwozdz A, Karunanithy N, et al. Two year outcome after chronic iliac vein occlusion recanalisation using the vici venous stent®. Eur J Vasc Endovasc Surg. 2018;56(5):710–8.
38. NICE CKS. Scenario: Venous leg ulcers | Management | Leg ulcer - venous | CKS | NICE [Internet]. [cited 2021 Jun 2]. Available from: https://cks.nice.org.uk/topics/leg-ulcer-venous/management/venous-leg-ulcers/#when-to-refer [.
39. SIGN NQIS (NHS Q. Management of chronic venous leg ulcers [Internet]. 2010 [cited 2021 Jun 2]. Available from: www.sign.ac.uk.
40. Bootun R, Belramman A, Bolton-Saghdaoui L, et al. Randomized controlled trial of compression after endovenous thermal ablation of varicose veins (COMETA Trial). Ann Surg

[Internet]. 2021 Feb 1 [cited 2021 Jun 2];273(2):232–9. Available from: https://pubmed.ncbi.nlm.nih.gov/31850976/

41. Forner-Cordero I, Szolnoky G, Forner-Cordero A, et al. Lipedema: an overview of its clinical manifestations, diagnosis and treatment of the disproportional fatty deposition syndrome - systematic review. Clin Obes [Internet]. 2012 Jun [cited 2021 Jun 2];2(3–4):86–95. Available from: https://pubmed.ncbi.nlm.nih.gov/25586162/
42. Szolnoky G, Borsos B, Bársony K, et al. Complete decongestive physiotherapy with and without pneumatic compression for treatment of lipedema: a pilot study. Lymphology. 2008;40
43. Lee BB, Andrade M, Bergan J, et al. Diagnosis and treatment of primary lymphedema. Consensus document of the International Union of Phlebology (IUP)-2009. Int Angiol [Internet]. 2010 [cited 2021 Jun 2]. p. 454–70. Available from: https://europepmc.org/article/med/20924350
44. Rabe E, Partsch H, Hafner J, et al. Indications for medical compression stockings in venous and lymphatic disorders: an evidence-based consensus statement [Internet]. Vol. 33, Phlebology. SAGE Publications Ltd; 2018 [cited 2021 Jun 2]. p. 163–84. Available from: https://journals.sagepub.com/doi/full/10.1177/0268355516689631
45. Caroline MA, Badger PD, Janet L, Peacock PD, PSMMD. A randomized, controlled, parallel-group clinical trial comparing multilayer bandaging followed by hosiery versus hosiery alone in the treatment of patients with lymphedema of the limb. Cancer. 2000;88:2832–7.
46. Prandoni P, Lensing AWA, Prins MH, et al. Below-knee elastic compression stockings to prevent the post-thrombotic syndrome. Ann Int Med [Internet]. 2004 Aug 17 [cited 2020 Dec 28];141(4):249. Available from: http://annals.org/article.aspx?doi=10.7326/0003-4819-141-4-200408170-00004
47. Jull AB, Mitchell N, Arroll J, et al. Factors influencing concordance with compression stockings after venous leg ulcer healing. J Wound Care [Internet]. 2004 Sep 29 [cited 2021 Jun 2];13(3):90–2. Available from: https://www.magonlinelibrary.com/doi/abs/10.12968/jowc.2004.13.3.26590
48. Finlayson K, Edwards H, Courtney M. The impact of psychosocial factors on adherence to compression therapy to prevent recurrence of venous leg ulcers. J Clin Nurs [Internet]. 2010 May 1 [cited 2021 Jun 2];19(9–10):1289–97. Available from: https://onlinelibrary.wiley.com/doi/full/10.1111/j.1365-2702.2009.03151.x

13 Imaging Assessment of Lower Limb Swelling

Amit Nandan Dhar Dwivedi and Jyoti Dangwal

13.1 Introduction

Limb swelling, known as edema, is a common clinical problem encountered in both inpatient and outpatient department. It is a challenge to determine the cause and formulate a line of treatment. A wide spectrum of causes makes it difficult for clinicians to diagnose the exact etiology; therefore, imaging can play an important role in not only determining the cause but also in image-guided interventions and follow-up after treatment. Edema is defined as a palpable swelling caused by an increase in interstitial fluid volume. In order to be specific regarding the causes, limb swelling could be unilateral or bilateral as regarding the side of affection, but regarding the onset of condition, it could be acute or chronic. In acute edema, the timing of swelling is less than 72 h and may occur in conditions like (acute DVT, cellulitis, acute compartmental syndrome, ruptured Baker's cyst, etc.), but in chronic edema the timing should exceed 72 h and usually results from chronic fluid accumulation due to systemic conditions or lymphatic obstruction [1]. There are three types of leg edema: venous edema, lymphedema, and lipedema. Venous edema consists of excess low viscosity, protein-poor interstitial fluid resulting from increased capillary filtration that cannot be accommodated by a normal lymphatic system [2]. Lymphedema consists of excess protein-rich interstitial fluid within skin and subcutaneous tissue resulting from lymphatic dysfunction [3]. Lipedema is more accurately considered a form of fat maldistribution rather than true edema [4].

A. N. D. Dwivedi (✉) · J. Dangwal
Department of Radiodiagnosis and Imaging, Institute of Medical Sciences, Banaras Hindu University, Varanasi, India

S. K. Tiwary (ed.), *Approach to Lower Limb Oedema*,
https://doi.org/10.1007/978-981-16-6206-5_13

13.2 Causes

On the basis of laterality and duration of onset of edema, some important causes are listed below (Table 13.1).

13.3 Diagnostic Imaging Evaluation in Lower Limb Swelling

A multimodality imaging approach is required to overcome the clinical dilemma faced in the diagnosis of limb swelling. The main focus while imaging evaluation is to distinguish between acute DVT and its mimics. Imaging modalities to evaluate lower extremities include contrast venography, ultrasonography (B-mode and Doppler spectral analysis), MR venography, computed tomography (CT), and various radionuclide approaches (lymphoscintigraphy). A step-wise imaging work-up and keeping the anatomical spectrum of etiologies in mind while analyzing and performing different imaging techniques is a useful strategy for localizing and identifying the pathology. The examined extremity can be divided into following planes anatomically:

Table 13.1 Causes of lower leg swelling

Unilateral		Bilateral	
Acute (<72 h)	Chronic (>72 h)	Acute (<72 h)	Chronic (>72 h)
– Deep vein thrombosis	– Venous insufficiency	– Bilateral deep vein thrombosis	– Venous insufficiency
– Ruptured Baker's cyst	– Secondary lymphedema (tumor, radiation, surgery, bacterial infection)	– Acute worsening of systemic cause(heart failure, renal disease)	– Pulmonary hypertension
– Ruptured medial head of gastrocnemius	– Pelvic tumor or lymphoma causing external pressure on veins		– Heart failure
– Compartment syndrome	– Reflex sympathetic dystrophy		– Renal disease (nephrotic syndrome, glomerulonephritis)
– Acute superficial thrombophlebitis.			– Liver disease
			– Secondary lymphedema
			– Bacterial infection
			– Filariasis
			– Idiopathic edema
			– Lymphedema
			– Drugs (diuretics, etc.)
			– Premenstrual edema
			– Pregnancy

Table 13.2 Anatomical distribution of causes of lower limb swelling

1. Skin and subcutaneous tissue • Cellulitis (superficial and deep) • Closed traumatic injuries and contusions
2. Vascular system • Acute DVT • Acute superficial thrombophlebitis • Chronic venous insufficiency
3. Muscular and tendons • Injuries (hematomas, strains, tears) • Pyomyositis • Tenosynovitis • Ruptured tendons
4. Osseous and joint space related • Osteomyelitis • Fractures • Joint effusion • Septic arthritis • Baker's cyst
5. other miscellaneous causes

- Skin/subcutaneous tissues
- Vessel (mainly venous system)
- Muscles and tendons
- Joints and bones
- Other causes (systemic causes) (Table 13.2).

The key to a precise diagnosis is the definition of the imaging characteristics of various diseases that can be etiology for limb swelling.

13.4 Skin and Subcutaneous Tissue

13.4.1 Cellulitis

Cellulitis is an inflammatory condition resulting from skin or subcutaneous tissue infection usually affecting lower limbs more than upper limbs [5]. Its diagnosis is often suspected clinically and needs to be confirmed by imaging. However, imaging cannot differentiate septic from a septic fluid. **Ultrasound (US)** is an initial modality for evaluation of acute cellulitis, it is usually done first to exclude acute DVT, and then to define the ultrasound features of cellulitis which include diffusely swollen subcutaneous tissue with increased echogenicity in the affected area; further accumulation of the fluid in the subcutaneous fat gives "marbled fat appearance" or "cobble-stone appearance" (Fig. 13.1); however, this appearance is nonspecific and may exist in many other causes of edema. **Computed tomography (CT)** is particularly helpful to differentiate between the superficial (uncomplicated) type and deep

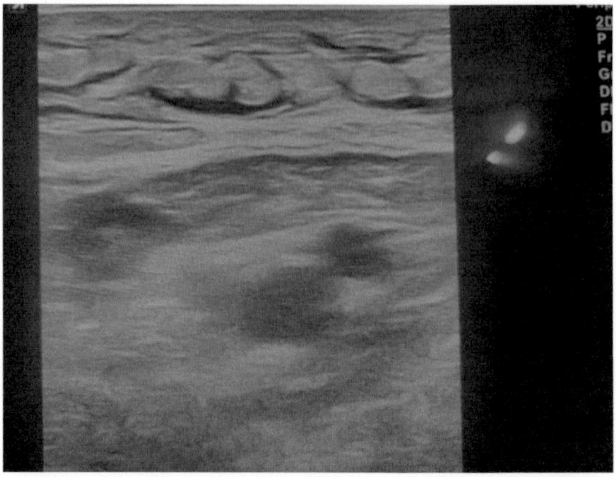

Fig. 13.1 Subcutaneous edema with cobble stoning

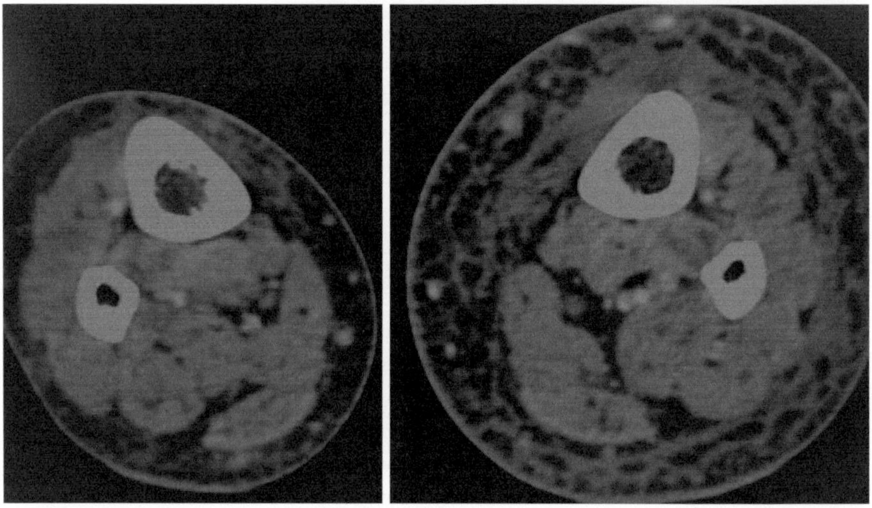

Fig. 13.2 A patient with left lower limb subcutaneous edema showing smudging and septation in subcutaneous fat

(complicated) type; the latter is usually associated with deep-seated soft tissue infections. In the superficial (uncomplicated) cellulitis, CT demonstrates thickening of the skin and superficial fascia with smudging and septation of the subcutaneous fat (Fig. 13.2). In the deep-seated cellulitis, the deep tissues are affected and may show abscess formation, myositis, and osteomyelitis, and sometimes, necrotizing fasciitis can occur caused by gas-forming pathogens with characteristic air densities that can be demonstrated in the CT examinations as well as USG (Fig. 13.3). **Magnetic resonance imaging (MRI)** in cellulitis has a nonspecific pattern similar to that of soft tissue edema; it may show thickened skin with subcutaneous fat reticulations and elicit intermediate signal intensity on T1-weighted images (T1WIs)

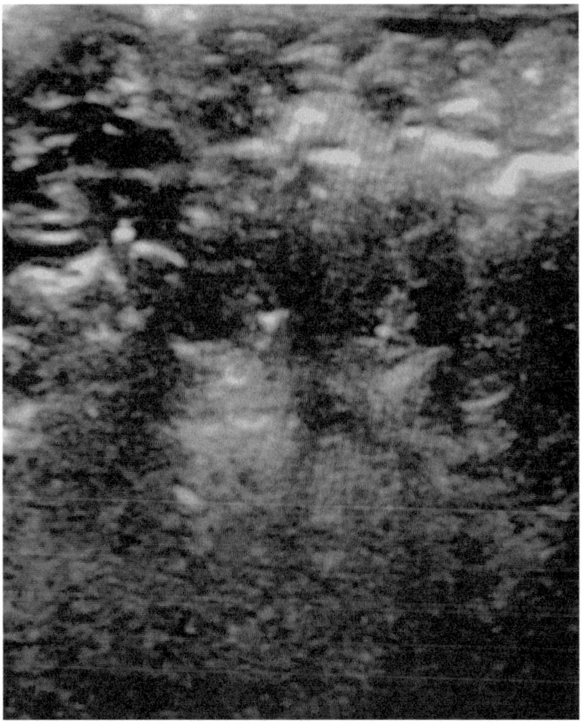

Fig. 13.3 Multiple air foci in a patient with necrotizing fasciitis

and high signal intensity on T2-weighted (T2WIs) or short tau inversion recovery (STIR) images; often the affected area has a poorly defined margin [6]. However, some differentiation can be done after contrast administration with some delay in image acquisition, where the enhancement can be detected in cellulitis but not present in nonspecific edema [7]. In some cases, associated reactive lymphadenopathy in the regional lymph nodes can be indicative of infective cause.

13.5 Vascular Disorders (Venous System)

13.5.1 Deep Venous Thrombosis

Deep venous thrombosis (DVT) is an extremely common medical problem worldwide with an estimated incidence of 120 per 100,000 person years. It is noted in both OPD and IPD, more so in patients who are sedentary. It is rarely noted in children. Some of the common predisposing factors are heart failure (prolonged), lower limb and pelvic surgeries, pregnancy, airplane travel, obesity, paraplegias, and coagulopathies [8]. The diagnosis of acute DVT is important as it may result in acute pulmonary embolism; therefore, early detection of DVT can prevent its development. Reported data suggest that in an untreated DVT, pulmonary embolism occurs in nearly 50% cases. Therefore, accurate sonographic assessment of lower limb venous system in clinically suspected cases of DVT can significantly reduce mortality due to embolism [9]. DVT is difficult to diagnose clinically because of discrepancy in location of pain and swelling to the extent and location of thrombus within the venous system. For example, symptoms present in the calf region may be due to thrombosis of femoral veins, and calf vein occlusion can result in thigh pain and swelling. Musculoskeletal and lymphatic etiologies can also mimic the symptoms of acute DVT. DVT can also be asymptomatic, and still can be severe enough to result in death by pulmonary embolism.

13.5.2 Diagnosis of DVT

D-DIMER is a clinically useful serological test. Almost all patients of acute DVT have raised D-dimer levels. It is sensitive (97%), but its specificity is less than 50%. Patients who have undergone recent surgery, recent trauma, malignancy, and sepsis also have raised D-dimer levels. However, it has a negative predictive value of 97%; hence, DVT can be excluded easily. D-dimer along with clinical assessment has been shown to reduce the need for noninvasive tests [10].

VENOUS DOPPLER with high sensitivity (95%) and specificity (100%), being simple and noninvasive with no ionizing radiation, plays an important role in the diagnosis of DVT [11]. **Further** imaging studies including CT venography (CTV) or magnetic resonance venography (MRV) are planned if there is clinical suspicion about the diagnosis or to exclude proximal obstruction either by intraluminal thrombosis or extrinsic venous compression [8]. However, CT and MR are relatively expensive than USG. They are reserved for evaluating the more proximal venous occlusions in cases where ultrasound examination is not satisfactory. Considering the overall cost, specificity, and sensitivity of different testing options, ultrasound turns out to be screening test of choice for deep venous thrombosis. ULTRASOUND examination should integrate B-mode imaging, compression by transducer, color flow Doppler imaging (CFDI), and spectral Doppler analysis to complete the study of the venous structures of the lower extremity. Contrast agents and harmonic imaging can be used in the near future, in cases having uncertainty regarding complete venous occlusion. The transducer choice depends upon the patient built and depth of vessel under evaluation. 5 to 10 MHz linear transducer is appropriate for an average patient. Linear array transducers are preferred for imaging long segments of vessels more rapidly.

13.5.3 Normal Findings

Four following parameters of normal veins are assessed using Doppler imaging:

- Respiratory phasicity
- Spontaneous flow
- Augmentation
- Transducer compression

The variation in venous flow during each respiratory cycle is termed respiratory phasicity. In inspiration, there is an increased intra-abdominal pressure resulting in compression of the inferior vena cava and a decrease in the color Doppler signal and vice versa during expiration (Fig. 13.4). In a normal venous system, augmentation can be demonstrated with distal mechanical compression and Valsalva maneuver. Increased venous diameter and increased Doppler signal indicate augmentation of flow in normal vessels (Fig. 13.5). Spontaneous venous flow can be easily detected in the large lower limb vessels using color flow Doppler imaging. A normal vein has unidirectional flow, is compressible, and has no internal echoes on B mode. The transducer is held transverse to the vein to demonstrate compressibility. An adequate amount of pressure sufficient is then applied with the transducer which causes the collapse of vein lumen (Fig. 13.6). Unidirectional flow can be best identified with color flow Doppler imaging (Fig. 13.7). Diagnosis of acute DVT depends on the presence of all or any of the following findings: incompressible and distended veins with an intraluminal obstructive material, lack of color filling of the vein in color Doppler, and absence of flow on spectral Doppler interrogation of the affected segment (Fig. 13.8). Fresh thrombus is anechoic or hypoechoic, and it becomes increasingly echogenic as it matures. In addition, fresh thrombus has a tendency to expand the vein and make it look rounder and fuller than a normal vessel [12]. Fresh thrombus is non-adherent to the vein wall; therefore, some blood may be seen around the periphery of the clot in the vein on color Doppler (Fig. 13.9). Another appearance which may be seen in early thrombosis is that of a thin tail of thrombus extending up the vein from its origin and lying free in the lumen of the vein. Older thrombus becomes increasingly echogenic, is adherent to the vein wall, and contracts as it becomes more organized and fibrotic. This may result in the vein being reduced to a relatively small echoic structure that may be difficult to locate

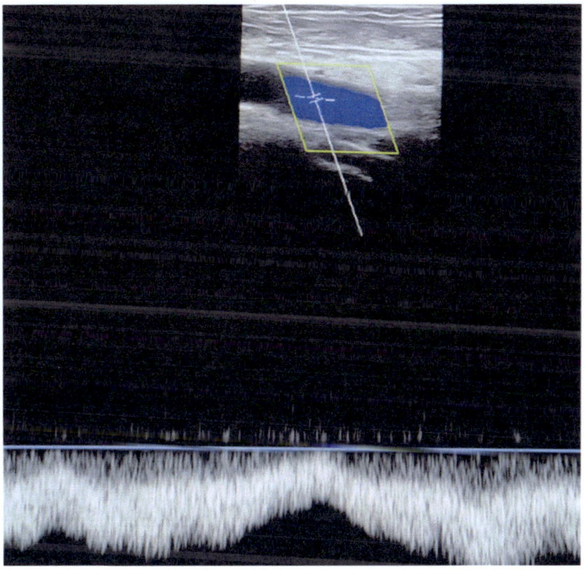

Fig. 13.4 Normal cardiac and respiratory phasicity

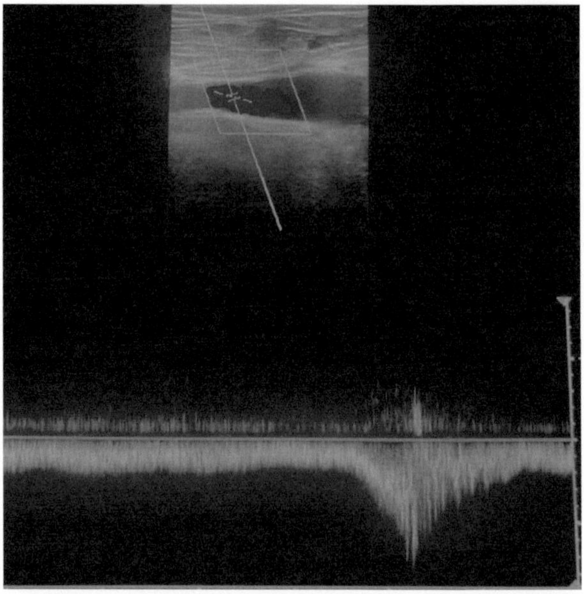

Fig. 13.5 Normal augmentation in deep veins on calf squeezing

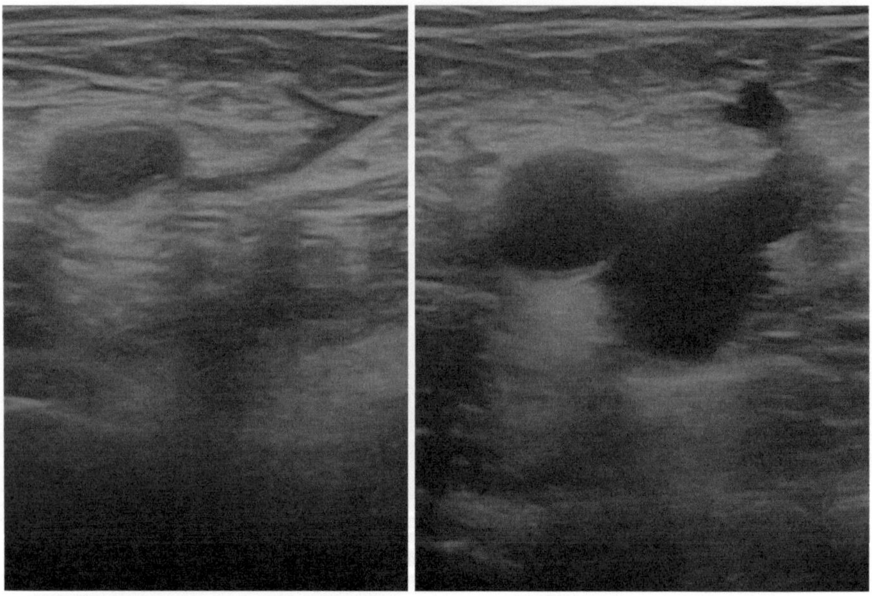

Fig. 13.6 Normal compressibility of veins

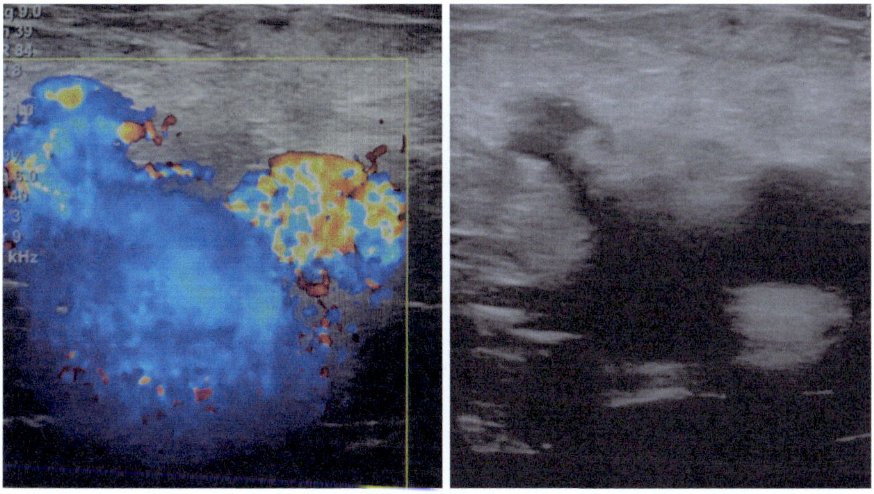

Fig. 13.7 Classic "mickey mouse" appearance of sapheno-femoral junction showing normal spontaneous color flow

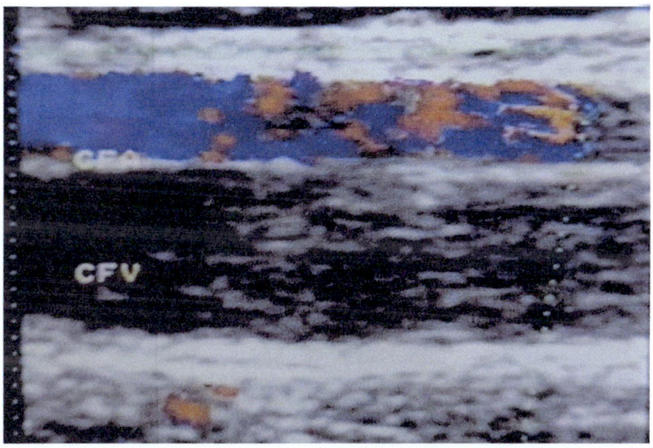

Fig. 13.8 Echogenic thrombus in lumen of common femoral vein

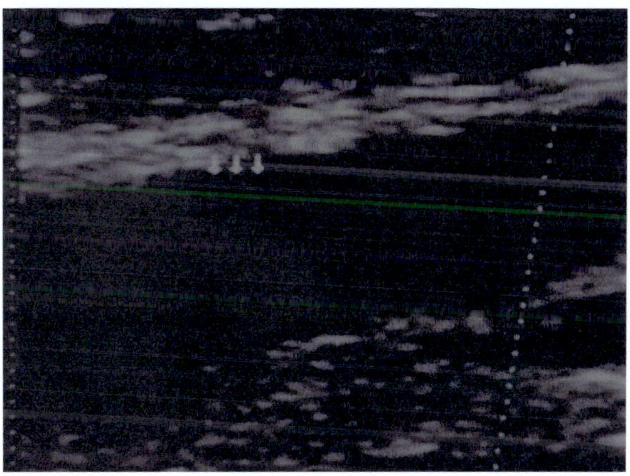

Fig. 13.9 Anechoic fresh thrombus in the lumen of vein. No color flow on Doppler study

(Table 13.3). Despite the high accuracy of the ultrasound in the detection of DVT in the thighs, some limitation could exist like the morbid obesity, marked edema, and the overlying limb casts in some patients (Table 13.4) Therefore one may require CT venography or MR venography if diagnosis is suspicious on USG. CT venography (CTV) has a wider view not only for the pathology but also regarding the complex anatomical details especially in the hardly accessible veins by ultrasound (like iliac, profunda femoral, and the central veins); moreover, it helps in detection of soft tissue and osseous abnormalities. Sources of extrinsic compression of the iliac veins can also be identified by CT. Recently, CT venography has been recommended as a quick and safe means to evaluate the deep venous system after multidetector row CT (MDCT) angiography of the pulmonary arteries (within the same examination), particularly if the patient is clinically unstable and requires immediate diagnosis. This method has a sensitivity between 71–100% and is 93–97% specific. The positive predictive value is 53–92% and negative predictive value is between 92 and 97%. However, the estimated median cumulative effective radiation dose is 8.26 mSv for all patients with an effective gonadal dose of 3.87 mSv. This dose is more than 300% of the median effective dose for CTA of the pulmonary arteries (2.5 mSv). Hence, the dose must be significantly reduced before this can be used as a routine clinical method to evaluate for DVT in clinically stable patients, particularly for those who are young [13]. MR venography is particularly useful in detecting femoral and iliac vein thrombi and can help in determining proximal extent of disease in these vessels [14] (Froehlich et al. 1997). Newer techniques like venous enhanced subtracted peak arterial (VESPA) MR venography, flow-independent MR venography, and direct thrombus MR imaging may allow MR to play a more significant role in DVT imaging in the future [15, 16].

Table 13.3 Distinction between acute and chronic thrombus

Acute	Chronic
Can be anechoic/hypoechoic	Echogenicity increases with time
Causes vein to expand	Causes vein to contract
Some compression of vein is possible	Vein is incompressible
Thrombus lies freely in the vessel lumen or is loosely adhered to the wall	Clot is adherent to the vessel wall
Collaterals are absent	Multiple collateral channels develop with time in the surrounding tissues

Table 13.4 Pitfalls in diagnosis of DVT by USG

• Dual thigh and popliteal vein
• Non-occlusive thrombus
• Swollen/edematous/fat legs
• Segmental calf and iliac vein thrombus
• Segmental iliac vein thrombus

13.6 Acute Superficial Thrombophlebitis

It usually affects the superficial veins or their tributaries either in normal or varicose veins and is more common in the lower extremities; however, it is usually a benign condition unless complicated or extended to involve the deep venous system. Key questions in cases of superficial thrombophlebitis concern the location and extent of the thrombosis, as well as its proximity to the deep venous system at the sapheno-femoral or sapheno-popliteal junction. Migratory thrombophlebitis, especially without good cause, may be an indication for a more detailed evaluation of the patient to determine whether a malignant lesion exists. This evaluation should include selective application of serum carcinoembryonic antigen (CEA) testing, prostate-specific antigen (PSA) testing, colonoscopy, computed tomography (CT), and mammography. All patients with superficial thrombophlebitis above the knee should undergo duplex US as the initial diagnostic modality of choice to rule out DVT. When the patient has superficial thrombophlebitis below the knee, duplex ultrasound is indicated for signs and symptoms consistent with DVT (e.g., asymmetrical swelling, erythema, pain). Superficial thrombophlebitis in lower-extremity varicose veins has an extremely low incidence of DVT. On ULTRASOUND, thrombosed veins may appear thickened or inflamed on US with echogenic content in lumen, but the most accurate diagnostic finding is a lack of compressibility of the vein.

13.7 Chronic Venous Insufficiency

In limbs affected by DVT, 50–80% will recanalize within months or years after the event. Sometimes previous thrombosis may not clear completely, resulting in chronic obstruction and damage to the valves [17]. This damage results in loss of the protective action of the valves so that a continuous column of blood is present between the heart and the tissues of the calf, ankle, and foot which exerts hydrostatic pressure on tissues and interferes with transfer of nutrients resulting in local inflammatory responses, which ultimately leads to development of reticular veins, eczema, skin discoloration, edema, and venous ulceration. The pattern of damaged and incompetent veins can be defined using Doppler ultrasound to examine the deep and superficial veins in order to identify thrombosed or partially recanalized veins. Incompetent venous segments together with incompetent perforating veins can be mapped out and appropriate surgical or medical techniques can be applied. Ultrasound apart from diagnosis also has a major role in the localization of catheters and ablation devices used in the treatment, as well as monitoring the progress of these treatments.

13.8 Technique of Examination

The patient is best examined standing, or with a large degree of head-up tilt if the couch can be elevated. Various techniques can be used to assess competence or incompetence of a venous segment. The most convenient method for general assessment is to squeeze firmly and then release the patient's calf, or lower thigh, to promote forward flow. Incompetent valves will allow reverse flow back through them after forward flow has ceased, whereas competent valves will stop any reverse flow. Alternatively, proximal compression may be applied to induce reverse flow. Getting the patient to perform a Valsalva maneuver will also show incompetent segments, but there are two disadvantages to this technique. Firstly, the effect will only demonstrate reverse flow as far as the first competent valve is considered, and any incompetent segments below this will not be demonstrated. Second, it is quite difficult to explain to many patients the exact nature and method for performing a Valsalva. Reflux can be defined as reverse flow occurring after the cessation of forward flow. It is significant if it lasts >0.5 s in the superficial, deep femoral, and calf veins [18]. For the femoro-popliteal veins, a cutoff of 1.0 s is used as their larger diameters and smaller number of valves are thought to contribute to slower valve closure rates. Shorter periods of reversed flow may be seen in normal veins and represent the short period as the valve cusps come together and blood in the venous segment settles under the influence of gravity. The patency and competence of the deep and superficial veins of the thigh are assessed down to the level of the knee. While examining the great saphenous vein the presence of incompetent perforators should be sought, especially if the vein becomes incompetent at a level below the sapheno-femoral junction. These can be identified most easily by scanning down the vein transversely while applying recurrent compression to the calf or lower thigh and looking for outward flow with color Doppler. The perforators are seen piercing the fascial layer. The commonest of these perforating veins is in the lower thigh at the level of the junction of the middle and lower thirds of the great saphenous vein and is called the mid-thigh perforator vein. The patient is then turned to examine the popliteal region. The veins in the popliteal fossa are assessed and the sapheno-popliteal junction is examined. The level of the sapheno-popliteal junction should be noted, especially if this is not in the expected location.

13.9 Muscular and Tendinous Disorder

13.9.1 Muscle Contusion or Hematoma

They occur as a result of direct trauma or spontaneously in patients treated with anticoagulants, precipitated by trivial trauma or even in the absence of any history of trauma. In **USG** contusion may appear as focal intramuscular swelling that may resolve with no residual abnormality over time. In mild cases, however significant lesions and hematomas may show variable appearance on ultrasound, they may present as cyst-like, hypoechoic, hyperechoic areas, or mixture of different echogenicities; then over a period of time, some hematomas may show more hypoechoic appearance with internal echoes, debris, and some septations and even fluid-fluid level may be seen; however, hematomas may resolve completely or show residual scarring [19]. On MRI, muscle edema may be diffuse or focal and the edematous muscles are swollen due to large fluid contents, so fluid-sensitive sequences (e.g., STIR sequence) are specifically used in the detection of muscle. In muscle contusion, a feathery pattern of a high T2 signal is identified, with possible edema signal in the overlying subcutaneous fat and in the deep portion of the affected muscle [20].

13.9.2 Muscle Strain and Tears

Muscle strain. It occurs when there is increased activity and is associated with tenderness and occasionally swelling. Muscle tears are commonly seen in the calves and occur as a result of suddenly forced contraction and typically at the myotendinous junction or at the muscle bellies and sometimes the tendon itself ruptures with or without gapping [21]. Muscle strain injuries are seen by USG and are graded according to the percent of the affected area to the whole muscle, starting from small hypoechoic muscle disruption foci not exceeding 5% of the whole muscle (grade I), then partial tear is diagnosed when the affected area exceeds 5% of the whole muscle (grade II), and complete tear occurs when bunching of the muscle with frayed edges on dynamic stress is identified (grade III) [19].

13.9.3 Tennis Leg

An isolated rupture of the medial head of the gastrocnemius muscle, usually at its distal musculotendinous junction, results in TENNIS LEG. Tears in this muscle and its tendon are also included under the term "tennis leg" [22]. A secondary DVT can occur as a complication. Tennis leg occurs more commonly in male athletes with poorly conditioned muscles. Secondary DVT is a common complication [23]. USG shows hypoechoic fluid collection deep to the medial gastrocnemius and superficial to the soleus muscle, prominent at the level of the myotendinous junction. There is disruption of the normal pennate pattern of the muscle close to its interface with the soleus and plantaris muscle. An anechoic collection representing hematoma can also be noted. Fluid-sensitive sequences in MRI show increased signal intensity deep to the medial gastrocnemius and superficial to the soleus muscles. Focal areas of muscular disruption in deep part of the medial gastrocnemius along with muscle edema can also be noted. It is important to distinguish tennis leg from acute DVT, as treatment with anticoagulation can increase the risk of bleeding within the affected muscle which can be grave for the patient [21].

13.9.4 Calcific Myonecrosis

It is a rare soft tissue disorder, which mimics the presentation of acute DVT. It is assumed to arise secondary to compartment syndrome or post-trauma-related necrosis and fibrosis, although the exact pathophysiology is unknown [25]. There is repeated intralesional hemorrhage with subsequent calcification and mass formation. The mass is expansive and can compress veins to mimic the symptoms of a DVT. The typical presentation is presence of a fusiform mass in the lower leg long time after a traumatic event [26]. **USG** of the site of the swelling demonstrates a relatively defined heterogeneous mass-like lesion with internal hyperechoic areas casting posterior acoustic shadow suggestive of calcifications and hypoechoic areas of necrosis. Soft tissue components can also be noted in the mass. Increased Doppler neo-vascularity may also be present. Fusiform masses with sheet-like calcification and pressure erosions are some of the features that can suggest diagnosis of calcific myonecrosis on MRI.

13.9.5 Pyomyositis

Muscle infection is caused by a bacterial pathogen that usually occurs in immunocompromised patients; thereby edema may affect a single muscle or may involve a group of muscles. However, the infection could affect the muscles from the deeper osseous structures or deep-seated (complicated) cellulitis [20]. In **USG** muscle abscesses appear as intra/intermuscular complex cystic collection with thick shaggy walls and internal debris; sometimes air echogenicity may be present. On power Doppler, a marginal vascularity in the abscess wall can be detected. CT and MRI may demonstrate rim enhancement pattern which is considered as a discriminative feature of pyomyositis and indicates abscess formation, but this finding may not be present in early stages of the disease process [20].

13.9.6 Tenosynovitis

It is an inflammatory condition affecting the synovial covering of the tendons. It may be infectious or noninfectious in origin. Ultrasound reveals distended tendon sheaths by hypoechoic fluid collection with possible synovial thickening and hyperemia on power Doppler. Subcutaneous edema of the affected region can be seen as well; however, when the fluid collection shows turbidity or associated gaseous echogenicity inside, the possibility of infectious causes is considered. MRI findings include tendon sheath distension with a fluid signal, associated synovial proliferation, and synovial enhancement on contrast administration. The main etiologic factor could not be determined by the MRI solely; however, bilateralism of condition may favor noninfectious causes. Small fibrinous bodies called "rice bodies" may be seen in certain inflammatory conditions (like rheumatoid arthritis, TB, and sarcoidosis) affecting the synovial lined structures like joints and tendon sheaths and are usually associated with focal swelling.

13.10 Osseous and Joint Space Related

13.10.1 Baker's Cyst

Baker's cysts, synovial cysts, or popliteal cysts are the most commonly encountered nonvascular popliteal masses. Classically, Baker's cysts do not contain a true synovial lining and are filled with synovial fluid which is gelatinous in consistency [27]. These cysts comprise of a fluid-filled sac and a neck which arises from the space between the medial head of gastrocnemius muscle and the semimembranosus tendon. They are located posteriorly in the popliteal fossa and present with knee pain, swelling, and knee joint stiffness. When these cysts rupture, the fluid contents track down in inter- and perimuscular fat planes inducing inflammation with mimicking clinical picture of acute DVT. These cysts can be incidentally found in up to 49% of patients on USG when performing a DVT scan of the lower extremity [28]. USG features include a well-defined anechoic cystic lesion in popliteal fossa with posterior acoustic enhancement. Some cyst may show internal echoes suggesting infection. A neck is noted arising from the space between the medial head of gastrocnemius and semimembranosus tendon. This looks like a "talk bubble" in the transverse plane. There is no Doppler flow unless there is an associated infective or inflammatory process. When there is Doppler flow, or some solid components are noted in the cyst, imaging with MRI is usually indicated for further evaluation. MRI features include a high signal intensity mass in the gastrocnemius/semimembranosus bursa on T2-W images. Presence of T2-W hyper-intense fluid in the intermuscular fat planes along with a Baker's cyst indicates rupture of cyst with leakage. Complicated Baker's cysts may have thickened walls, internal hemorrhage, and intracystic debris which can be misinterpreted for a complex lesion. An important feature in differentiating a Baker's cyst from a DVT is the presence of a neck between the medial head of gastrocnemius head and semimembranosus tendon. For simple cysts, approximately two-thirds of patients benefit from treatment through image-guided aspiration and injection of steroid [29].

13.11 Joint Effusion and Septic Arthritis

The synovial joints have a joint capsule that is lined by synovium which normally secretes minimal synovial fluid; when this fluid is secreted in excess amount in certain pathological conditions, then it is called joint effusion, but when this fluid became infected, the condition is called septic arthritis that may necessitate prompt arthrocentesis. Septic arthritis occurs at any age with a predilection to the extreme age groups (both elderly individuals and newborns) as well as in immunocompromised patients like diabetics. Large joints are often involved with the knee; hip and shoulder joints are the most commonly affected in a respective pattern [30] Ultrasound is particularly helpful in pediatrics as it can assess joint spaces for effusion and subperiosteal collections and even detects osteomyelitis earlier than plain radiography [31]. Color and power Doppler helps in assessing hyperemic changes in the inflamed soft tissues. MRI findings: MRI with contrast enhancement as well as the fat suppression sequences are proved to have high sensitivity and specificity (100% and 77%, respectively); the findings include joint effusion, synovial thickening, perisynovial edema, bone marrow changes, high signal in T2WIs, and underlying osteomyelitis if present, and on contrast-enhanced examination findings could be synovial enhancement; enhancing fluids with pockets of fluid outpouchings can be seen [32].

13.12 Miscellaneous Causes

There are other causes of edema that should be considered during clinical and radiological assessment of limb swelling. It includes edema due to underlying pathology in the heart, liver, and kidney. Apart from subcutaneous edema in limbs, USG can also demonstrate changes in the above mentioned organs. Idiopathic edema is common in young females due to pathologic fluid retention in upright position. Patients also complain of face and hand edema apart from leg edema. The diagnosis is usually clinical after ruling out systemic causes. Another etiology that one should keep in mind while performing radiological examination is lymphedema.

Secondary lymphedema is much more common than primary, and the cause is generally apparent from the history. The most common causes of leg lymphedema are tumor (e.g., lymphoma, prostate cancer, and ovarian cancer), surgery involving lymphatics, radiation therapy, and infection (filariasis or bacterial infection) [33]. Chronic lymphedema is usually distinguished from venous edema based on characteristic skin changes, absence of pitting, and history of an inciting cause. The skin becomes thickened and darkened and may develop multiple projections called lymphostatic verrucosis. The dorsum of the foot is prominently involved and may have a squared-off appearance [34]. Ultrasound features of lymphedema are volumetric changes (a minimal increase in the thickness of dermis) and an increase in the subcutaneous layer, and an increase, decrease, or no change in the muscle mass and structural changes (hyperechogenic dermis and hypoechogenic subcutaneous layer). It allows for an assessment of soft tissue changes but does not give information about anatomy [35]. Computed tomography (CT) scanning can be used not only to confirm the diagnosis but also to monitor the effect of treatment. The common CT findings in lymphedema include calf skin thickening, thickening of the subcutaneous compartment, increased fat density, and thickened perimuscular aponeurosis. A typical honeycomb appearance is seen in most patients.

Lymphoscintigraphy may be indicated to differentiate between early lymphedema and venous edema. It is done by injecting radioactive tracer into the first web space and monitoring lymphatic flow by gamma camera. The distinction cannot always be made because chronic venous insufficiency can lead to secondary lymphedema with abnormally delayed lymph drainage on lymphoscintigram [35]. MRI can aid in differentiating lymphedema, phlebedema, and lipedema of the lower limb. T1- and T2-weighted transaxial sequences can be performed before administration of gadolinium tetraazacyclododecane-tetraacetic acid (DOTA), and

T1-weighted spin-echo sequences are performed after administration of Gd-DOTA in each patient. Images of patients with lipedema will show homogeneously enlarged subcutaneous layers, with no increase in signal intensity at T2-weighted imaging or after Gd-DOTA administration. Patients with phlebedema will show areas containing increased amounts of fluid within muscle and subcutaneous fat. In lymphedema, a honeycomb pattern above the fascia between muscle and subcutis can be observed, with a marked increase in signal intensity at T2-weighted imaging. After Gd-DOTA administration, there will be only a slight increase in signal intensity in the subcutis in lymphedema and phlebedema and a moderate increase in signal intensity in muscle in phlebedema [36].

13.13 Summary

Leg swelling is common and may be caused by a wide variety of disorders. Causes may be both acute and chronic. Of the acute causes most important is to rule out DVT because of the risk of pulmonary embolism which can be life-threatening. Therefore, a quick and accurate diagnosis by proper selection of the imaging study of choice is important. Keeping the anatomical spectrum of causes in mind while evaluating patients can help a radiologist to reach a set of differential diagnosis. Ultrasonography is the initial preferred modality of choice in evaluating lower limb edema. It is inexpensive, simple, and non-ionizing radiation with a high sensitivity and specificity especially in diagnosing DVT. B-mode scan, color flow Doppler imaging, and spectral analysis should be used cohesively. Non-compressibility, lack of color flow, and loss of respiratory phasicity indicate the presence of thrombus in a vessel. MR and CT venography are indicated in cases where there are limitations to USG (obesity, segmental calf vein, and iliac vein thrombosis). Chronic venous insufficiency is usually a sequela to DVT that can be diagnosed on USG by demonstrating reflux at sapheno-femoral and sapheno-popliteal junction. Once DVT has been ruled out, one should focus on the other acute causes that can mimic DVT (ruptured Baker's cyst, muscle hematomas, cellulitis, acute superficial thrombophlebitis, ruptured muscles and tendons, myositis, septic arthritis in neonates, etc.). In cases of chronic edema systemic causes should be ruled out. Lymphedema should be taken into consideration. Ultrasound cannot differentiate between venous and lymphatic edema; therefore, lymphoscintigraphy is indicated. Recently, studies have shown that contrast and non-contrast sequences in MR can differentiate between lipedema, phlebedema, and lymphedema.

Disclaimers and Disclosure of Conflicts of Interest None.

Prior Presentations None.

Sources of Support that Require Acknowledgment None.

References

1. Trayes K, Studdiford J, Pickle S, Tully A. Edema: diagnosis and management. Am Fam Physician. 2013;88(2):102–10.
2. Gorman WP, Davis KR, Donnelly R. ABC of arterial and venous disease. Swollen lower limb 1: general assessment and deep vein thrombosis. BMJ. 2000;320:1453–6.
3. Mortimer PS. Swollen lower limb-2: lymphoedema. BMJ. 2000;320:1527–9.
4. Rudkin GH, Miller TA. Lipidema: a clinical entity distinct from lymphedema. Plast Reconstr Surg. 1994;94:841–7.
5. Dupuy A, Benchikhi H, Roujeau J, Bernard P, Vaillant L, Chosidow O, et al. Risk factors for erysipelas of the leg (cellulitis): case-control study. BMJ. 1999;318(7198):1591–4.
6. Moore T, Yuh W, Kathol M, el-Khoury G, Corson J. Abnormalities of the foot in patients with diabetes mellitus: findings on MR imaging. Am J Roentgenol. 1991;157(4):813–6.
7. Ledermann H, Morrison W, Schweitzer M. Pedal abscesses in patients suspected of having pedal osteomyelitis: analysis with MR imaging. Radiology. 2002;224(3):649–55.
8. Useche J, de Castro A, Galvis G, Mantilla R, Ariza A. Use of US in the evaluation of patients with symptoms of deep venous thrombosis of the lower extremities. Radio Graph. 2008;28(6):1785–97.
9. Perlin SJ. Pulmonary embolism during compression US of the lower extremity. Radiology. 1992;184:165–6.
10. Wells PS, Anderson DR, Rodgers M, et al. Evaluation of D-dimer in the diagnosis of suspected deep-vein thrombosis. NEJM. 2003;349:1227–35.
11. Hamper UM, DeJong MR, Scoutt LM. Ultrasound evaluation of the lower extremity veins. Radiol Clin N Am. 2007;45:525–47.
12. Hertzberg BS, Kliewer MA, DeLong DM, et al. Sonographic assessment of lower limb vein diameters: implications for the diagnosis and characterization of deep venous thrombosis. Am J Roentgenol. 1997;168:1253–7.
13. Thomas SM, Goodacre SW, Sampson FC, et al. Diagnostic value of CT for deep vein thrombosis: results of a systematic review and meta-analysis. Clin Radiol. 2008;63:299–304.
14. Froehlich JB, Prince MR, Greenfield LJ, et al. 'Bull's-eye' sign on gadolinium-enhanced magnetic resonance venography deter- mines thrombus presence and age: a preliminary study. J Vasc Surg. 1997;26:809–16.
15. Fraser DG, Moody AR, Davidson IR, et al. Deep venous thrombosis: diagnosis by using venous enhanced subtracted peak arterial MR venography versus conventional venography. Radiology. 2003;226:812–20.
16. Sampson FC, Goodacre SW, Thomas SM, et al. Accuracy of MRI in diagnosis of suspected deep vein thrombosis: systematic review and meta-analysis. Eur Radiol. 2007;17:175–81.
17. Nicolaides AN. Investigation of chronic insufficiency: a consensus statement. Circulation. 2000;102:e126–63.
18. Labropoulos N, Tiongson J, Pryor L, et al. Definition of venous reflux in lower-extremity veins. J Vasc Surg. 2003;38:793–8.
19. Woodhouse JB, McNally EG. Ultrasound of skeletal muscle injury: an update. Seminars in Ultrasound, CT and MRI. 2011;32(2). WB Saunders.
20. McMahon C, Wu J, Eisenberg R. Muscle edema. Am J Roentgenol. 2010;194(4):W284–92.
21. Hirsh J, Hull R, Raskob G. Clinical features and diagnosis of venous thrombosis. J Am Coll Cardiol. 1986;8(6):114B–27B.
22. Harwin JR, Richardson ML. "Tennis leg": gastrocnemius injury is a far more common cause than plantaris rupture. Radiol Case Rep. 2017;12:120–3.
23. Bright JM, Fields KB, Draper R. Ultrasound diagnosis of calf injuries. Sports Health. 2017;9:352–5.
24. Bianchi S, Martinoli C, Abdelwahab IF, Derchi LE, Damiani S. Sonographic evaluation of tears of the gastrocnemius medial head ("tennis leg"). J Ultrasound Med. 1998;17:157–62.

25. Ukon Y, Tanaka T, Nagata S, Hagizawa H, Imura Y, Tamiya H, et al. Calcific myonecrosis mimicking soft tissue sarcoma: a case report. Oncol Lett. 2018;15:7909–13.
26. O'Dwyer HM, Al-Nakshabandi NA, Al-Muzahmi K, Ryan A, O'Connell JX, Munk PL, et al. Calcific myonecrosis: keys to recognition and management. AJR Am J Roentgenol. 2006;187:W67–76.
27. Burk DL Jr, Dalinka MK, Kanal E, Schiebler ML, Cohen EK, Prorok RJ, et al. Meniscal and ganglion cysts of the knee: MR evaluation. AJR Am J Roentgenol. 1988;150:331–6.
28. Ward EE, Jacobson JA, Fessell DP, Hayes CW, van Holsbeeck M. Sonographic detection of Baker's cysts: comparison with MR imaging. AJR Am J Roentgenol. 2001;176:373–80.
29. Handy JR. Popliteal cysts in adults: a review. Semin Arthritis Rheum. 2001;31:108–18.
30. Ortega RR. Septic arthritis: a real emergency. Radiological manifestations. Advantages and disadvantages associated to the different types of tests based on images. Eur Congr Radiol. 2014:11.
31. Kaiser S, Rosenborg M. Early detection of subperiosteal abscesses by ultra- sonography. Pediatr Radiol. 1994;24(5):336–9.
32. Karchevsky M, Schweitzer M, Morrison W, Parellada J. MRI findings of septic arthritis and associated osteomyelitis in adults. Am J Roentgenol. 2004;182(1):119–22.
33. Szuba A, Rockson SG. Lymphedema: classification, diagnosis, and therapy. Vasc Med. 1998;3:145–6.
34. Ciocon JO, Fernandez BB, Ciocon DG. Leg edema: clinical clues to the differential diagnosis. Geriatrics. 1993;48(34–40):45.
35. Tiwari A, Cheng KS, Button M, Myint F, Hamilton G. Differential diagnosis, investigation, and current treatment of lower limb lymphedema. Arch Surg. 2003;138:152–61.
36. Duewell S, Hagspiel KD, Zubeidaa J, Schulthess GK, Bollinger A, Fuchs WA. Swollen lower extremity: role of MR imaging. Radiology. 1992;184(1):227–31.

Genetic Association in Lower Limb Swelling

14

Geeta Rai, Khushbu Priya, and Doli Das

14.1 Introduction

The majority of the medical appointments related to vascular medicine involve cases with leg swelling or edema due to the accumulation of fluid in the tissues [1]. The development may have happened abruptly or gradually which may also take months or years to subsidize. The physiological reason behind the occurrence of edema is the increased capillary filtration rate than that of the lymphatic drainage rate over a time period [2]. Increased capillary filtration may be due to increased capillary pressure, reduced plasma proteins, or increased capillary permeability (Fig. 14.1). Increased venous pressure may lead to right ventricular failure and deep vein thrombosis (DVT), whereas lower plasma proteins may cause nephrotic syndrome, protein-losing enteropathy, and cirrhosis. Increased capillary permeability may cause inflammation, infection, and dermatitis. Reduced lymph drainage causes primary (Milroy's and Meige disease) as well as secondary (recurrent cellulitis, filariasis, erysipelas) lymphatic insufficiency and dysfunctional lymphatics (dependency syndrome) [3]. Often this is not due to serious illness but due to some primary health issues. Genetics plays an essential role, to a larger extent in almost all diseased states, even in those that involve significant environmental factors. In certain conditions, single genetic mutation is sufficient for causing disease, whereas in others interaction between the genetic variants and environmental factors is evident. In medicine, the knowledge of genetics has improved the understanding of the impact of genetic predisposition and the epigenetic changes on the common diseases and the role of genetic modifications in response to medical treatment.

G. Rai (✉) · K. Priya · D. Das
Department of Molecular and Human Genetics, Institute of Science, Banaras Hindu University, Varanasi, India
e-mail: grai@bhu.ac.in

S. K. Tiwary (ed.), *Approach to Lower Limb Oedema*,
https://doi.org/10.1007/978-981-16-6206-5_14

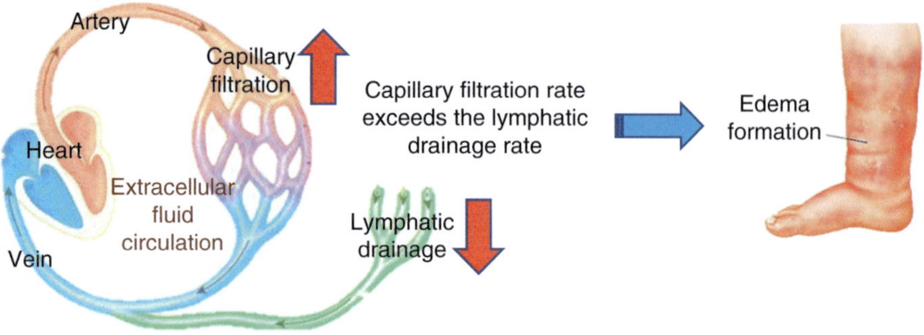

Fig. 14.1 Edema develops when the capillary filtration rate exceeds the lymphatic drainage rate for a sufficient period of time

For a better understanding of the cause of leg edema and the underlying genetic causes, it can be categorized on the basis of the swelling in—"both the legs" versus "one leg," and others involving "one or both legs" [1].

14.2 Edema of Both Legs

The main underlying cause of peripheral edema is congestive heart failure which is the consequence of activation of sequences of humoral and neurohumoral mechanisms which promote the reabsorption of sodium and water by the kidneys and increase in extracellular fluid [4]. In addition to these mechanisms, the increased capillary pressure and decreased osmotic pressure lead to fluid extravasation and, hence, edema formation. Patients with congestive heart failure may experience deteriorated heart activity and lowered blood pumping leading to reduced forward blood flow which results in the swelling of both the legs. Hence, pedal edema is one of the symptoms of congestive heart failure [5]. B-type natriuretic peptides (BNP) gene gets activated in cardiomyocytes due to the increased myocardial stress and volume/pressure overload condition. Consequently, BNP serves as the biomarker and the gold standard for heart failure diagnosis [6]. Both BNP and its amino-terminal propeptide equivalent (NT-proBNP [N-terminal proBNP]) are extensively used to confirm or exclude the diagnosis and to predict the patients at the risk [7].

Stress in the left ventricular wall causes a trigger for release of natriuretic peptides that include BNP and NT-proBNP. ProBNP, a 26-amino acid prepeptide, is released upon the induction of BNP gene which is a 134 prepro-peptide precursor [8]. Therefore, in normal heart during the non-stressed condition, the production of proBNP is less as compared to the congestive heart failure condition. Proteases like corin or furin, act upon proBNP and cleave it to form biologically active 32-amino acid peptide, BNP, and a biologically inert 76-amino acid peptide, NT-proBNP, within the cardiomyocytes and at peripheral sites [9]. The amino-terminal of proBNP undergoes glycosylation exposing the cleavage site for reduction [10]. Both BNP and NT-proBNP are released within minutes of their synthesis along with

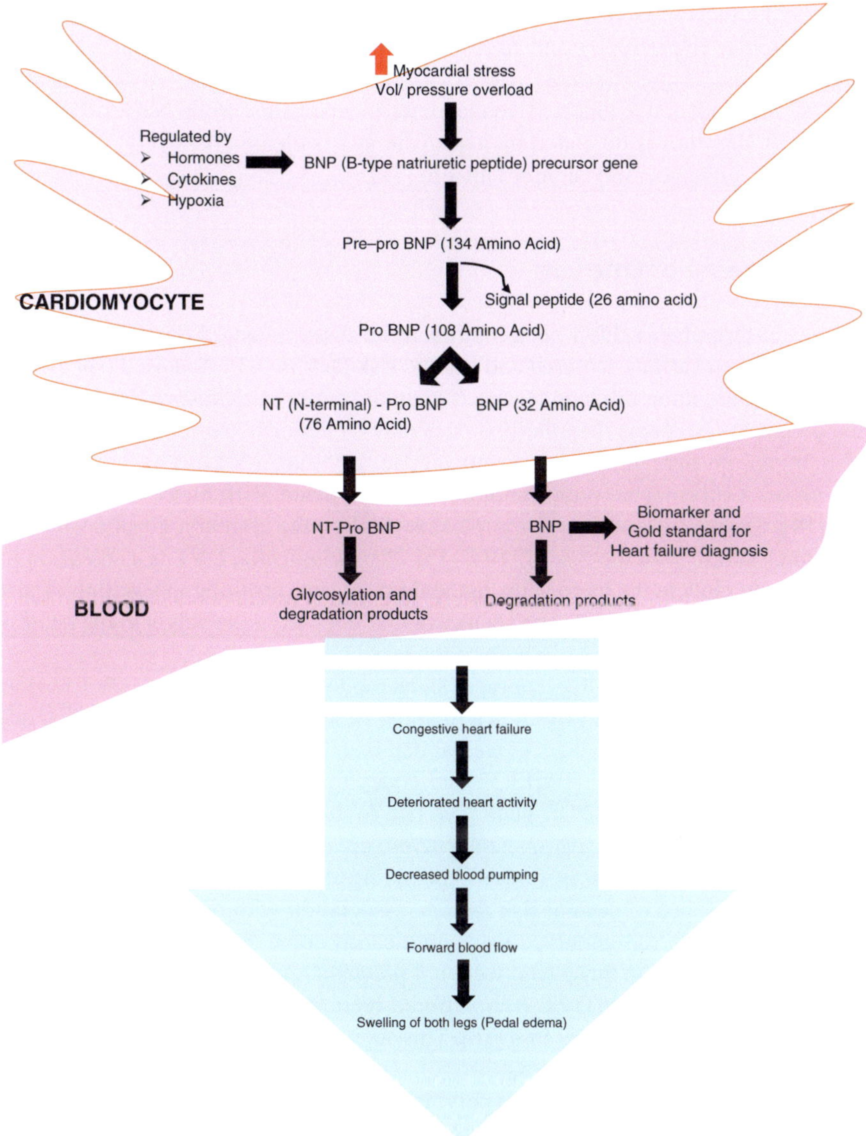

Fig. 14.2 Underlying mechanism leading to development of pedal edema which is one of the symptoms of congestive heart failure

uncleaved proBNP in varying amount (Fig. 14.2). Both BNP and NT-proBNP cross-react with circulating proBNP which contributes to the measured peptide values as they are a mixture of cleaved and non-cleaved peptide [7].

There are three natriuretic peptide receptors (NPR) A, B, and C with which BNP binds. NPR-A and -B are linked to guanylyl cyclase and also contribute to the biological effects of BNP, including diuresis, natriuresis, vasodilation, and reduced cardiovascular hypertrophy and fibrosis, while NPR-C internalizes and degrades BNP [11].

BNP has both active and passive clearance mechanisms, while NT-proBNP neither binds NPR nor is degraded by neprilysin and is cleared passively; the former peptide has a considerably shorter half-life [12].

14.3 Edema of One Leg

Deep vein thrombosis (DVT) is a multifactorial disease caused due to the interaction in between various acquired and genetic risk factors [13]. Acquired risk factors may be surgery, immobilization, cancer, trauma, antiphospholipid syndrome (APS), and pregnancy, whereas the inherited ones may be deficiency of anticoagulant proteins, mutations upregulating procoagulant pathway (factor V Leiden), or procoagulant proteins (fibrinogen, prothrombin, factor VII, factor VIII, factor IX, and factor XI) [14]. Single-nucleotide polymorphisms (SNPs), the common genetic variants, have modest effect on the risk of DVT [15]. Physiologically, DVT is a condition in which blood clots in the large veins in the thigh or calf, resulting in swelling of just one leg, but not so often, inferior vena cava that goes from the pelvis to the heart is blocked causing the swelling in both of the legs [1].

Apolipoprotein E (APOE) genotypes show modest association with DVT [16]. A polymorphic glycoprotein, ApoE, is a member of apolipoprotein family which has a role in lipoprotein metabolism as well as cell membrane maintenance. APOE gene is located on chromosome 19q13.32 and codes for 299-amino acid protein [17]. Two SNPs in exon 4 of APOE gene give rise to three haplotypes—e2, e3, and e4 resulting in six genotypes, e2/e2, e2/e3, e2/e4, e3/e3, e3/e4, and e4/e4 and eventually three different protein isoforms (ApoE2, ApoE3, ApoE4) [14]. Based on the presence or absence of several risk factors, association with APOE polymorphism revealed that the e2/e3 genotype was significantly more frequent in the pregnant females with DVT than those who were not pregnant and e3/e3 genotype was more frequent in females with DVT who suffered recurrent pregnancy loss than those who never suffered pregnancy loss [18]. This suggests DVT could be a predisposing factor for recurrent pregnancy loss.

The pathogenesis of APOE gene polymorphism in DVT was proposed by Ulrich et al. in 2014 [19]. Endothelial cells express the receptor for APOE (APOER2) which exhibits differential response to its three isoforms. The "wild"-type APOE3 stimulates endothelial nitric oxide synthase to produce nitric oxide, maintains single monolayer of endothelial cells by endothelial cell migration in response to injury at the time of repair, and reduces the leukocyte–endothelial adhesion and, hence, prevent thrombogenesis (Fig. 14.3). On the other hand, another isoform of APOE, APOE4, acts as a prothrombotic factor and is also an antagonist to APOE3. Antiphospholipid syndrome (APS)-related antibodies attenuate the downstream action of APOER2, which suggests that the combination of e4 allele and APS-related antibodies can predispose to DVT [16].

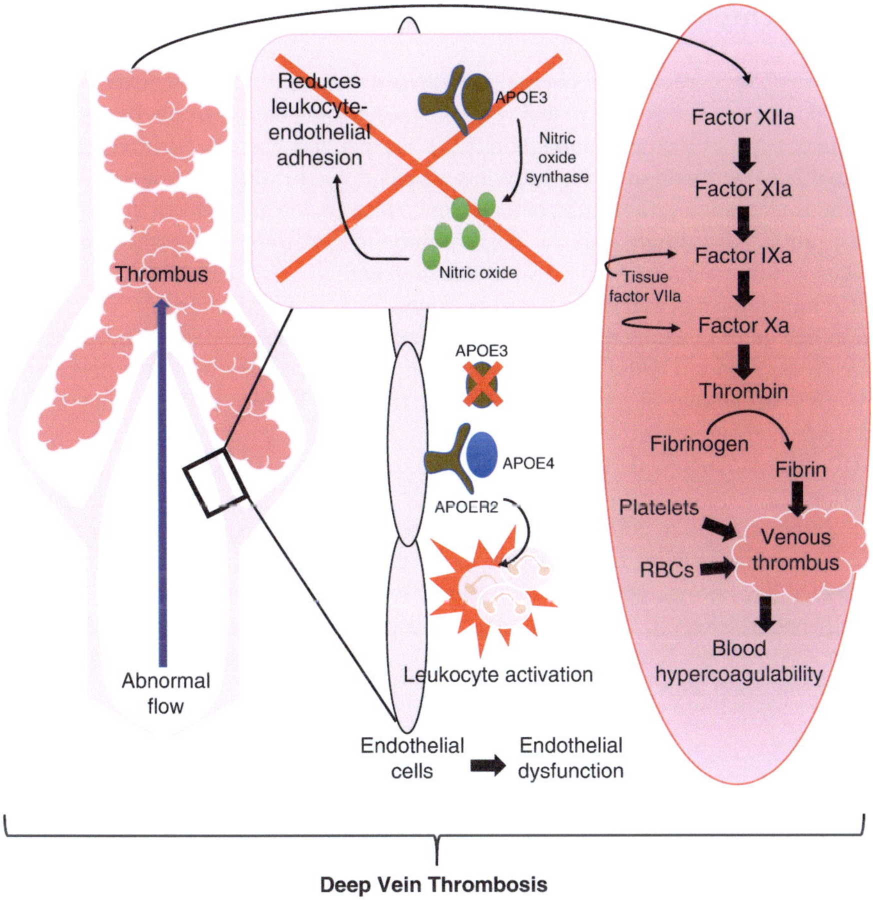

Fig. 14.3 Mechanism and genetic implication and development of deep vein thrombosis

14.4 Edema of One or Both Legs

A number of vascular disorders cause the swelling of one or both the legs. Veins help in the prevention of backward flow of blood, but when veins become enlarged, valves cannot close properly leading to backward flow of blood in the leg. This causes high pressure in the veins which leaks out into the tissue. These chronic vein troubles may lead to venous hypertension or chronic venous insufficiency (CVI) [20]. Patient earlier having DVT can also suffer from venous hypertension. Post-thrombotic syndrome (PTS) may also arise because of the damaged or blocked valves which causes backward flow of blood toward the heart [21]. Lymphedema is another vascular cause of swelling that can affect one or both legs.

14.4.1 Chronic Venous Insufficiency

CVI involves a spectrum of overlapping diseases or a multifactorial disease, usually caused due to damaged valve and venous hypertension, but precisely the underlying pathogenesis still remains ambiguous [22]. The patients with CVI exhibit symptoms like edema and pain in lower extremity, change in skin, varicose veins (VVs), and venous ulceration [20]. It may happen due to defects in vein walls or valves reflecting primary condition, and the post-thrombotic syndrome is the secondary one. Many studies suggested the possible role of genetics in CVI. Serra et al. [23] evaluated nine family genealogical trees and found obvious segregation of CVI in all the families in an autosomal dominant manner with incomplete penetrance [23]. The candidate marker D16S520 on chromosome 16q24 was linked with the occurrence of VVs, which may account for the linkage to FOXC2 which indicates that there is a functional variant within, or in the vicinity of, which predisposes to varicose veins. Affected patients with the D16S520 marker suggests saphenofemoral junction reflux [23].

Zamboni et al. in 2005 studied the association of hemochromatosis gene (HFE) C282Y mutation with venous leg ulcer on the basis of the information that in the affected leg, chronic venous disease causes localization of excessive iron [24]. The study cohort involved 238 patients which were divided into groups with and without skin lesions. They found that C282Y mutation was significantly associated with the ulcer subgroup within the CVD population [24].

14.4.2 Varicose Veins

Varicose veins (VVs) serve as the indication for CVI and are a type of chronic venous disease which is caused due to venous hypertension and loss of vessel wall homeostasis [25]. VVs of lower limbs are multifactorial vascular disease and are caused by extensive extracellular matrix remodeling, leading to weak vein wall or its dysfunction [26]. Vein dilation, distortion, leakage, and inflammation, wall disease, and reflux are the result of venous hypertension [25]. These are also found to be hereditary in nature, but still genetic factors are mostly not known. Shadrina et al. (2019) identified 12 associated loci that elucidate 13.4% of the SNP-based heritability and selected CASZ1, PIEZO1, PPP3R1, EBF1, STIM2, HFE, GATA2, NFATC2, and SOX9 genes as the underlying cause [27]. Within these loci, VVs-associated variants showed pleiotropic effects on some phenotypes comprising blood pressure/hypertension and blood cell traits. When genetic correlation analysis was done, it established epidemiological associations between VVs and DVT, weight, rough labor, and standing job, and came across a genetic overlap with multiple traits. Approximately, 27% of the variance supported by 12 SNPs ascribe to the polymorphism in the CASZ1 gene which is implicated in blood vessel development. A pressure-activated ion channel which senses shear stress and controls vascular architecture is encoded by PIEZO1 [28]. Taking this into account, the fact that mice embryos that are devoid of functional Piezo1 die at mid-gestation might be because of defects in vascular remodeling [29]. Region near rs3101725 contains two genes, *SLC12A2* and *FBN2*, which are possibly involved in varicose transformation. Potassium voltage-gated channels, which are encoded by KCNJ16 and KCNJ2 genes tagged by rs236530, also may have a role in vascular biology which is largely unknown. COL2A1 gene is under direct control of the *SOX9* gene product and encodes an extracellular matrix component whose transcription is regulated by RAPGEF3 gene in the rs73107980 locus. RAPGEF3 gene also regulates vascular permeability and further promotes vascular smooth muscle cell migration (Fig. 14.4) [27]. Finan et al. [30] placed SLC12A2, FBN2, STIM2, HFE, KCNJ16, KCNJ2, and COL2A1 genes in the category of druggable gene set, whereas PIEZO1 and the KCNJ2 gene products into the "potential drug target" class as according to the Human Protein Atlas (https://www.proteinatlas.org/) [30, 31]. The underlying effect of the plasma level of MHC class I polypeptide-related sequence B protein (MICB) and CD209 antigen was assessed by Mendelian randomization analysis. MICB, a ligand for activation of NKG2D receptor present on natural killer and other immune-related cells and CD209 (DC-SIGN), is a C-type lectin receptor expressed on dendritic cells and macrophages. Hence, both of them are implicated in innate and adaptive immune response. VVs is associated with ABO gene polymorphism as well as blood group A which is facilitated by CD209 protein [27].

The first gene that was found to be associated with primary venous valve failure in both the superficial and deep veins of the lower limbs was FOXC2 [32]. Lymphedema distichiasis is a rare inherited condition of which VVs are a common attribute and is caused due to mutation in single FOXC2 gene [33]. Mellor et al. [32] found venous reflux in the participant with the FOXC2 mutation when compared with the control. Due to this FOXC2 mutation, the superficial veins valves were always affected [32]. This is an instance where a rare monogenic trait is playing an important role in the disease pathogenesis.

Another candidate gene for VVs is thrombomodulin which is an endothelial cell surface glycoprotein receptor to which thrombin binds [34]. Subjects having venous thrombosis were studied for the candidate polymorphisms in the promoter region of the thrombomodulin gene, and it was found that 19% of venous thrombosis patients had VVs [35]. Venous thrombosis patients having del TT allele were having more chance of having VVs than the patients with the wild-type allele.

The C677T methylenetetrahydrofolate reductase (MTHFR) functional polymorphism was found to be associated with the development of VVs which was earlier known to be constantly associated with arterial disease. Sverdlova et al. [36] found that the subjects with VVs had higher frequency of at least one C677T MTHFR allele than the control group [36]. Hence, they reported the association of the C677T MTHFR functional polymorphism with the risk of developing VVs [36].

Patients with varicose veins without ulcer disease had not any changed C282Y allele frequency. Moreover, the frequency of this allele in the patients was found to be lower than the control suggesting the significance of C282Y variant with the ulcer biology than to the development of varicose veins [24]. When the factor XIII V34L gene polymorphism was analyzed, low-factor XIII activity was found in the blood of patients suffering with venous ulceration [37]. A group of 91 patients with

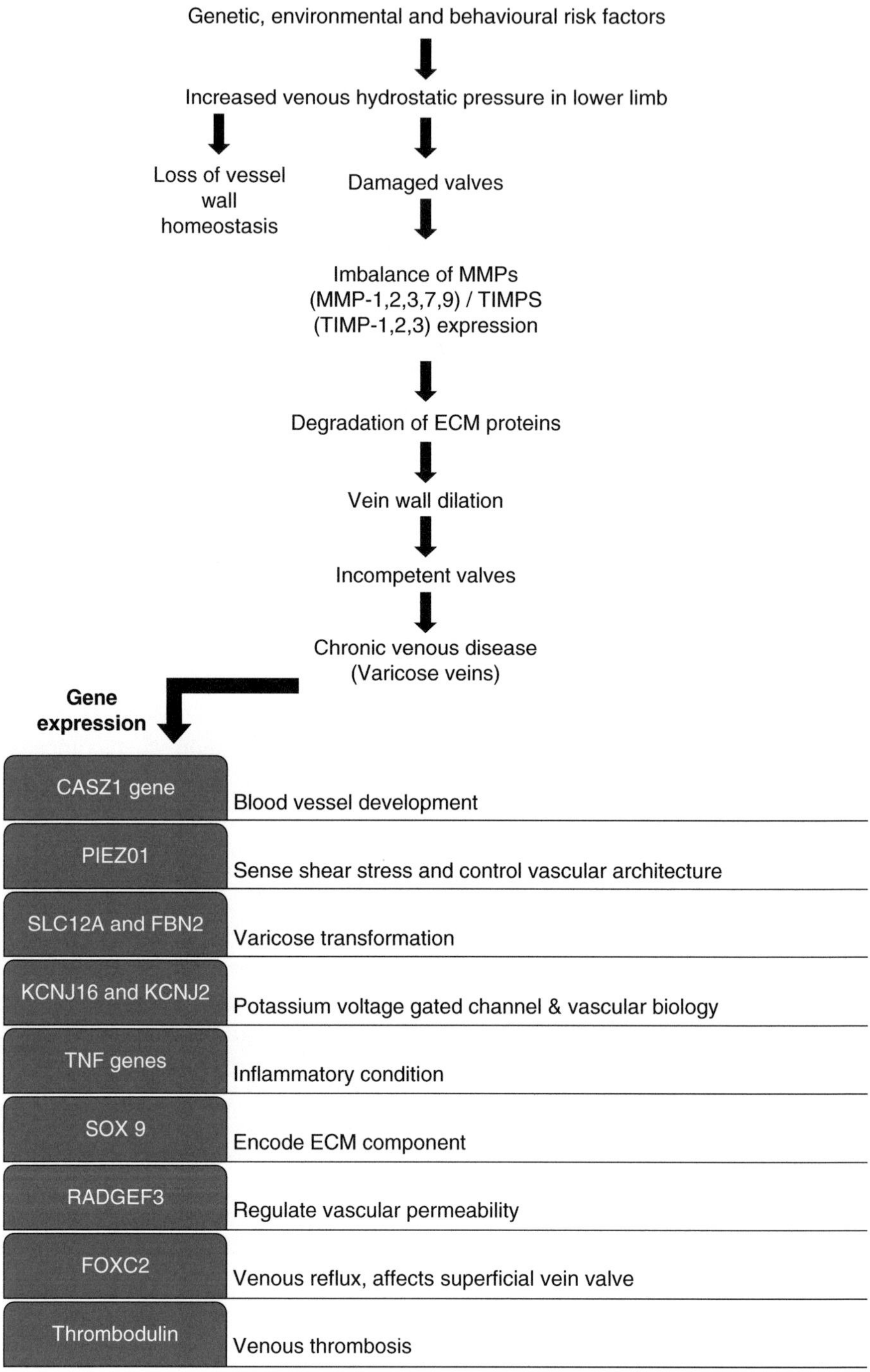

Fig. 14.4 Varicose veins of lower limbs are multifactorial vascular disease in which genetic overlap also play an important role

primary venous ulceration and post-thrombotic and mixed etiology was studied, but no significant difference was found in the factor XIII genotype frequencies when compared with 195 control donors but the association of ulcer size was found [38]. Patients excluding those with PTS revealed that the factor XIII-34 L variant was significantly associated with shorter healing time after superficial venous surgery that indicated function in the healing and tissue regeneration stages [39].

Venous ulcer is also associated with polymorphic variants of the estrogen and tumor necrosis factor (TNF) genes. Estrogen helps in the improvement of the rate of wound healing process and TNF-A polymorphism is associated with inflammatory conditions [40]. Genetic polymorphic variation in the promoter region of estrogen receptor-B (ERB) was studied in 125 venous ulcer cases, with venous insufficiency showing change in the frequencies of polymorphism flanking 5′ regulatory elements, which suggests that ERB acts as a regulator in both inflammatory and repair processes. When the healing starts in the leg ulcer wound, the fluid levels of TNF-A decrease. The promoter of the TNF-A gene polymorphisms frequency in 181 venous ulcer patients was compared with 181 controls and found the risk of ulceration in carriers of the TNFA 308A allele increased two fold [41].

All these findings associated with HFE C282Y, factor XIII V34L, ERB, or TNFA-308A support the fact that the genetic markers are associated with the CVI severity progression but not necessarily with primary varicose vein susceptibility suggestive of precision in disease phenotype selection, association studies designing, and meta-analysis. Studies also revealed that the patients with venous ulceration have an increased prevalence of genetic thrombophilia, similar to that observed in patients with deep vein thrombosis [42]. It was also found that the patients with varicose veins and chronic ulcer group had higher incidence of thrombophilia than the controls [43].

14.4.3 Post-Thrombotic Syndrome (PTS)

CVI includes a spectrum of chronic venous disease symptoms like VVs, venous ulceration, lipodermatosclerosis, and PTS [20]. Damaged valves, constant blockage of blood flow toward the heart, or a blood clot in leg veins causes condition [44]. Achy, painful, numbness/tingling, restless legs, and the muscle cramps due to prolonged sitting or standing are the symptoms in case of both VVs and PTS. Risk factors include incomplete DVT symptom resolution, proximal or previous ipsilateral DVT, obesity, and increased age. Treatment involves symptomatic relief using graduated elastic compression stockings or compression devices, leg elevation, or a trial of horse chestnut seed extract as a last resort [45].

Patients ae frequently diagnosed with PTS, but still it is poorly understood complication of DVT. Polymorphisms in the genes associated with CVI were also investigated to address the concern of involvement of those genes in increased risk of PTS. Extensively studied genes are the matrix metalloproteinases (MMPs) and tissue inhibitors of metalloproteinases (TIMPs) in venous diseases. MMP-1, 2, 3, 7, 9 and TIMP-1, 3 were highly expressed in VVs [46]. Raffetto and Khalil (2008) stated that MMPs are highly implicated in the pathogenesis of CVD; they cause degradation of extracellular membrane leading to venous remodeling, structural wall change, and subsequently venous dilation and valve dysfunction (Fig. 14.5) [47]. MMPs regulate or degrade the extracellular membrane through hydrolysis, and TIMPs are the tissue inhibitors of MMPs that have an effect on vascular remodeling. Therefore, the balance between two may cause vessel wall anomalies, eventually vascular disease such as varicosity and ulceration [48]. The dysregulation of MMP and TIMP activity causes impaired ulcer healing. According to Saito et al. [49], pro-ulcer condition is caused due to elevated MMP-2 level which affects tissue remodeling [49]. In fact, Herouy et al. (2001) found increased MMP-1, -22, and -213 and decreased TIMP-1, -22 in skin lesions while observing stasis dermatitis which is the result of impaired venous drainage described by dermal neovascularization [50]. Subsequently, Xu et al. [48], demonstrated that MMP-9 and TIMP2 gene polymorphisms impose higher risk to the patients for developing VVs [48]. Deatrick et al. (2011) found that after 6 months of vein remodeling an acute DVT was associated with MMP-9, which is precisely associated with resolution and prediction of PTS [51]. In acute DVT, there was increased MMP-9 and decreased Toll-like receptor 9 expression. Deatrick et al. [52] studied mouse model and found that MMP-9 modulates collagen content in the vein wall which also promotes inflammation and fibrosis, thus marking it as a potent target to decrease the fibrotic complications of PTS [52]. In addition, Beidler et al. [53] demonstrated that all the MMPs (except MMP-7), mainly MMP-8 and MMP-9, were highly expressed in venous leg ulcers [53]. In fact, Singh et al. in 2010 identified MMP-12 gene polymorphisms among numbers of SNPs associated with venous leg ulcers to have function in development

Fig. 14.5 The pathway leading to post thrombotic syndrome

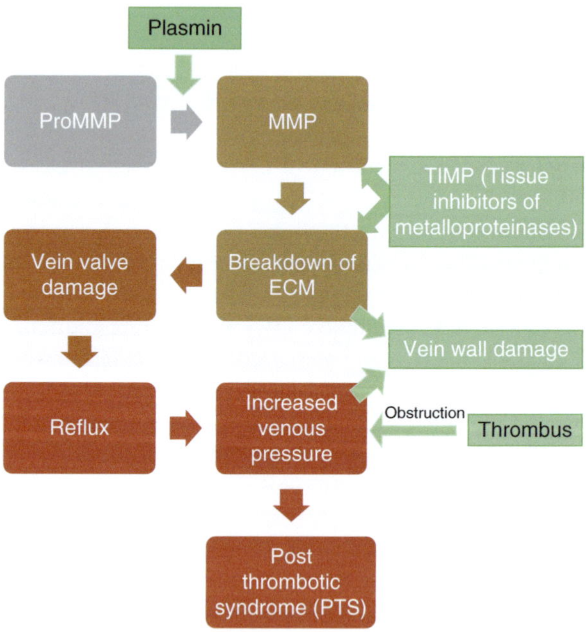

of ulcer [54]. Wojcik et al. [55] correlated IL-6 with decreased monocyte recruitment which causes reduced vein wall thickness and fibrosis, in a mouse model [55]. As it is known that extensive perivenous and mural fibrosis is implicated in PTS, IL-6 may play an important role as a therapeutic target to avert fibrotic complications.

14.4.4 Lymphedema

Lymphedema, or lymphatic obstruction, is a long-term condition in which there is accumulation of excess fluid in the tissues causing swelling or edema that can affect one or both legs [1]. It can be primary, also called congenital lymphedema, which occurs at birth or shortly after puberty, whereas secondary lymphedema is a consequence of infection, injury, trauma, or cancer that affects the lymphatic system. Hereditary lymphedema type IA or often called Milroy's disease is described by edema that occurs soon after the birth, but in rare cases it may also develop later in one's life and legs are mostly affected. Hereditary lymphedema type II, Meige disease, or also known as lymphedema praecox develops around puberty or after some time in most of the affected patients, being the most common kind of primary lymphedema (Fig. 14.6). The legs and also other body parts like the arms, face, and larynx are affected.

14.4.5 Milroy's Primary Congenital Lymphedema

Nonne-Milroy lymphedema or Milroy's primary congenital lymphedema (hereditary lymphedema I, and Milroy disease, OMIM 153100) is an autosomal dominant lymphatic disease with penetrance of 80–90% [56, 57]. This developmental disorder was mapped to the telomeric part of chromosome 5q (5q34-q35) in numerous families [58]; however, in a single inbred Pakistani family, a second locus was mapped to chromosome 6q (6q16.2-q22.1) [59]. This primary congenital lymphedema is caused due to autosomal dominant c.3109G>C mutations in the FLT4 (or vascular endothelial growth factor receptor 3 (VEGFR3)) gene. This is a missense mutation in which an aspartic acid is substituted with a histidine on amino acid position 1037 (p.D1037H) of the protein [60]. The probability of finding FLT4 mutations is very less, that is less than 5% in the patients who do not have typical symptoms of Milroy's disease. Though FLT4 mutations are autosomal dominant in nature, but still a single homozygous hypomorphic mutation was observed in an autosomal recessive form of non-syndromic primary congenital lymphedema [61]. The FLT4 gene encodes Fms-like tyrosine kinase 4 or VEGFR3 which is a receptor tyrosine kinase [62]. VEGFR3 is activated by VEGF-C and VEGF-D which is also required at the time of embryogenesis for lymphatic development [58]. All the mutations were detected in either of the two intracellular kinase domains and are supposed to interfere with tyrosine kinase activation [62]. FLT4/VEGFR3 happens to be the most essential receptors involved in lymphatic development [63]. FLT4

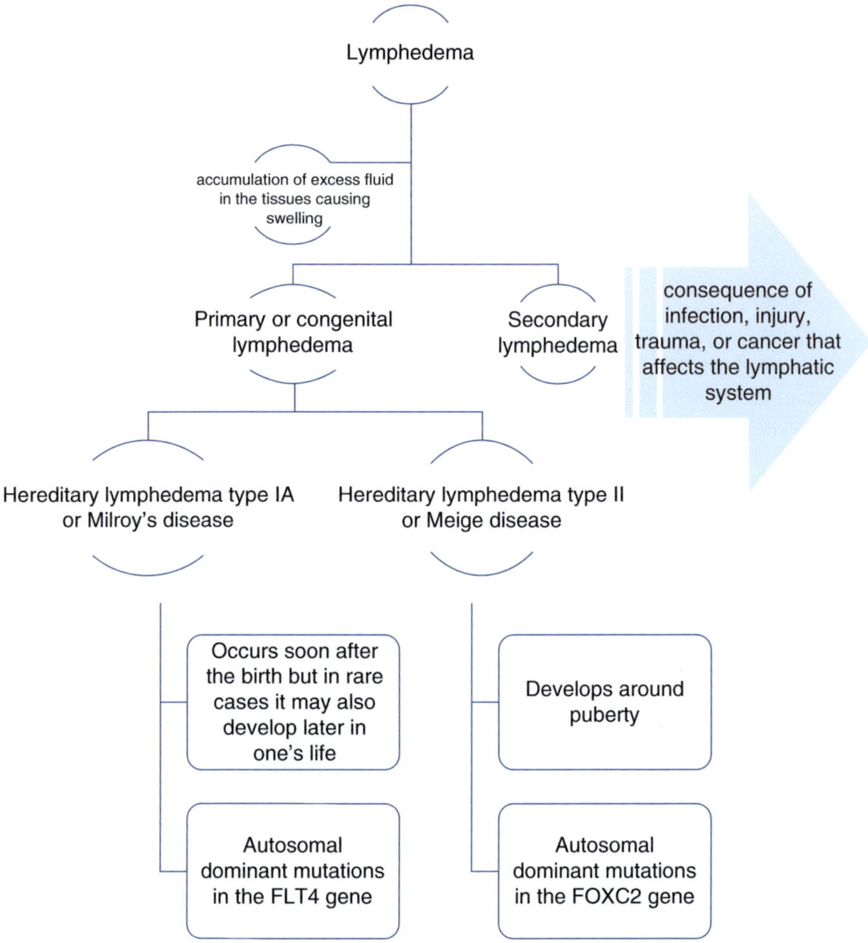

Fig. 14.6 Lymphedema may be inherited (primary) or caused by injury to the lymphatic vessels (secondary). Genetic mutations are implicated in the primary lymphedema (Milroy's disease and Meige disease)

gene is a member of the platelet-derived growth factor receptor subfamily of class III receptor tyrosine kinases and comprises 31 exons which are transcribed as two alternatively spliced transcripts which encode proteins with 7 immunoglobulins like repeat domains and 2 tyrosine kinase domains [64]. VEGFR genes contribute to angiogenesis and lymphangiogenesis process, including endothelial cell migration, proliferation, and survival [62].

14.4.6 Meige Disease

Meige syndrome or hereditary lymphedema type II (OMIM 153200), as well as nail syndrome, distichiasis-lymphedema syndrome, and lymphedema-ptosis syndrome, happens due to different mutations in the FOXC2 gene and inherited as an autosomal dominant trait. So far only FOXC2 transcription factor has been found to be implicated in the pathogenesis where mutations are known to produce lymphedema with distichiasis and in very rare condition SOX18 has been found to be associated with hypotrichosis-lymphoedema-telangiectasia. Rezaie et al. (2008) studied 23 affected individuals with Meige disease by analyzing FOXC2 gene sequence and identified a c.563-584del mutation, a novel truncating mutation in a family which was segregating with the disease in eight affected relatives over three generations [65]. This deletion truncates the normal protein by 38% by causing a frameshift mutation by causing a premature stop at nucleotide 599. The affected patient had lymphedema without distichiasis, but one of his affected relatives carried the FOXC2 mutation with accessory eyelashes (distichiasis-lymphedema) originating from their meibomian glands which further confirmed that distichiasis is caused by FOXC2 mutations [65].

14.4.7 Hereditary Angioedema (HAE)

HAE is an autosomal dominant disorder characterized by recurrent episodic swelling of the face, upper airway, oropharynx, extremitics, genitalia, and gastrointestinal tract, mostly limbs. Mostly HAE is caused due to mutation in serine protease inhibitor family G member 1 (SERPING1) gene which leads to functional plasma C1 esterase inhibitor (C1EI or C1INH) deficiency [66]. C1EI is the largest member of a serine protease inhibitor (SERPIN) superfamily that in general is a protease inhibitor of the complement and fibrinolytic systems [67]. C1EI inhibits C1r, C1s, mannose binding lectin-associated serine protease MASP-1, MASP-2, factor XII and kallikrein in the contact system, factor XI and thrombin in the coagulation system, and tissue plasminogen-activator (tPA) and plasmin in the fibrinolytic system and is largely produced by the liver and is secreted in blood [67]. Reduced C1EI functional activity causes increased C1 and decreased C2 and C4 activity leading to increased kallikrein formation and consequential bradykinin accumulation which elicits episodes of increased vascular permeability secreted in blood [68]. Globally more than 200 different mutations have been reported in the SERPING1 gene (http://hae.enzim.hu/) [69].

HAE is characterized into three different types (type I, II, and III) depending upon their underlying causes and C1 inhibitor protein level in the blood, though having similar signs and symptoms [70]. In 85% of cases type I mutation may cause synthesis of truncated or a misfolded protein that cannot be secreted [68]. And in HAE type II, 15% of cases are the result of mutations in the active site of protein or any adjacent amino acids leading to inactive enzyme [71]. C1 inhibitor protein inhibits the activity of certain proteins that induce inflammation; hence, the inflammation is regulated by C1 inhibitor protein whose synthesis is directed by SERPING1 gene [72]. HAE type I and type II are caused due to SERPING1 gene mutation [73]. In type I the C1 inhibitor level is decreased in the blood, whereas in type II, the function of C1 inhibitor is aberrant [74]. Abnormal level of functional C1 inhibitor causes too much increase in bradykinin production. Bradykinin increases the fluid leakage through the blood vessel walls into the tissues leading to increased inflammation. And this excessive accumulation consequently leads to the episodes of swelling in the patients with type I and type II HAE [75]. HAE type III is caused due to mutation in the F12 gene which directs the coagulation factor XII protein synthesis [76]. Factor XII is a blood clotting factor and also produces bradykinin which promotes inflammation. Mutation in F12 gene causes increased factor XII as well as increased bradykinin production leading to increased fluid leakage from the wall of blood vessels which contributes to episodes of swelling type III HAE patients [77].

14.4.8 Erythromelalgia

Erythromelalgia is a neurovascular disorder in which patient suffers from pain, swelling, erythema, and warmth of the distal extremities [78]. It is of two types - primary erythromelalgia and secondary erythromelalgia. Yang in 2004 reported for the first time that primary erythromelalgia is caused due to an autosomal dominant mutation in the SCN9A gene which is localized at the 7.94 cM region on chromosome 2q [79]. SCN9A gene encodes the α-subunit of the NaV 1.7 voltage-gated sodium channel which is expressed in sympathetic and sensory neurons [80]. These voltage-gated sodium channels have an important role in pain perception and the mutation causes the change in their biophysical properties [81], whereas secondary erythromelalgia is a multifactorial condition having a number of underlying etiologies, including drug and toxin exposures [82]. Under the influence of hematological conditions, the pathogenesis is associated with the changes in arterioles due to platelet activation. The symptoms of the distal extremities are caused as a result of the proliferation of intimal cells and smooth muscle cells along with thrombotic occlusions ensuing platelet aggregation. These activation pathways ultimately cause inflammation because of increased prostaglandin production leading to initiation of coagulation pathways [83].

14.5 Conclusion

With the many ambiguities associated with the pathophysiology of leg edema or swelling, the approach of reverse genetics may serve as one possible research path. Knowledge about the genetic association and family studies using genetic linkage analysis would facilitate understanding of the underlying genetic causes responsible for the disease. This will also help the researchers to conduct genotype-phenotype analysis when one or more genetic mutations are found to be involved (Fig. 14.7). Another promising benefit would be the identification of new drug target treatments and possibly considerations for gene therapy. Essentially, huge global burden of the disease and the scarcity of treatment options currently available warrant rigorous study of genes associated with disease and the involved polymorphisms which may help better identification of patients at higher risk of development of edema.

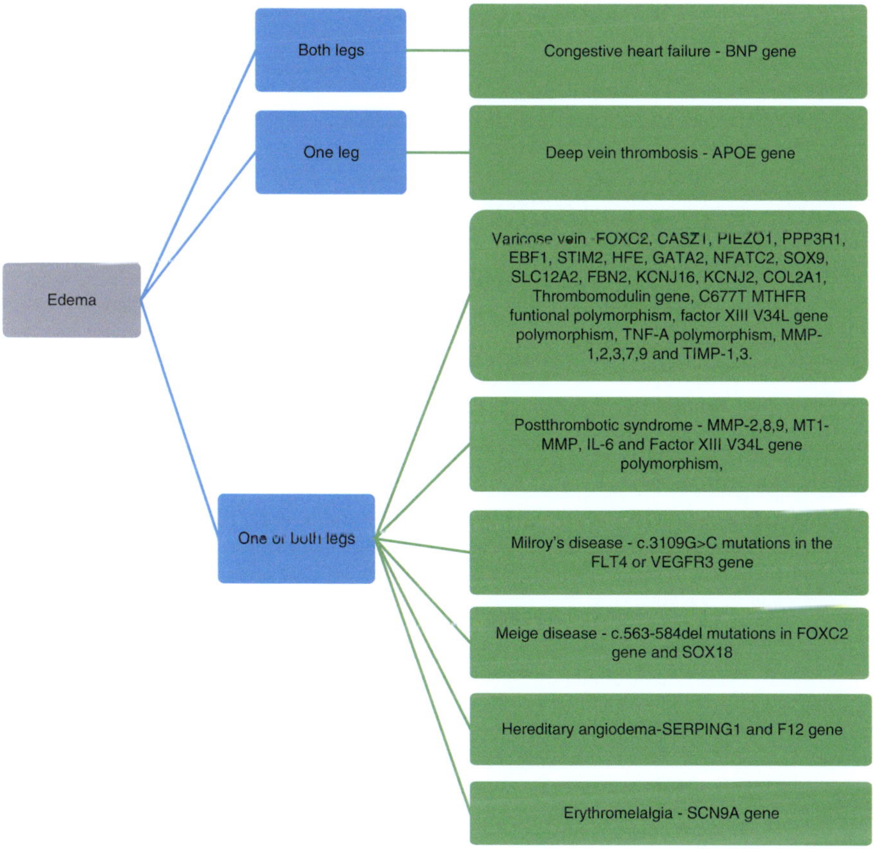

Fig. 14.7 Leg edema is caused due to various underlying genetic causes which can be categorized on the basis of the swelling in—one leg versus both the legs, and others involving one or both the legs. There are a number of genes and proteins associated with the different cases of leg swelling

References

1. Evans NS, Ratchford EV. The swollen leg. Vasc Med. 2016;21(6):562–4.
2. Garza R, Skoracki R, Hock K, Povoski SP. A comprehensive overview on the surgical management of secondary lymphedema of the upper and lower extremities related to prior oncologic therapies. BMC Cancer. 2017;17(1):468.
3. Mortimer PS. Disorders of lymphatic vessels. Rook's textbook of. Dermatology. 2010:1–31.
4. Navas JP, Martinez-Maldonado M. Pathophysiology of edema in congestive heart failure. Heart Dis Stroke. 1993;2(4):325–9.
5. Yeboah J, Bertoni A, Qureshi W, Aggarwal S, Lima JAC, Kawel-Boehm N, et al. Pedal Edema as an indicator of early heart failure in the community. Circ Heart Fail. 2016;9(12):e003415.
6. Cao Z, Jia Y, Zhu B. BNP and NT-proBNP as diagnostic biomarkers for cardiac dysfunction in both clinical and forensic medicine. Int J Mol Sci. 2019;20(8)

7. Weber M. Role of B-type natriuretic peptide (BNP) and NT-proBNP in clinical routine. Heart. 2005;92(6):843–9.
8. Jacob J, Chopra S, Cherian D, Verghese P. Physiology and clinical significance of natriuretic hormones. Indian J Endocrinol Metab. 2013;17(1)
9. Ichiki T, Huntley BK, Burnett JC. BNP molecular forms and processing by the cardiac serine protease Corin. Adv Clin Chem. 2013:1–31.
10. Parcha V, Arora P. Glycosylation of natriuretic peptides in obese heart failure: mechanistic insights. Ann Transl Med. 2019;7(22):611.
11. Potter LR, Yoder AR, Flora DR, Antos LK, Dickey DM. Natriuretic peptides: their structures, receptors, physiologic functions and therapeutic applications. cGMP: generators, effectors and therapeutic implications. Handb Exp Pharmacol. 2009:341–66.
12. Potter LR. Natriuretic peptide metabolism, clearance and degradation. FEBS J. 2011;278(11):1808–17.
13. Franco RF, Reitsma PH. Genetic risk factors of venous thrombosis. Hum Genet. 2001;109(4):369–84.
14. Diz-Kucukkaya R, Hancer VS, Artim-Esen B, Pekcelen Y, Inanc M. The prevalence and clinical significance of inherited thrombophilic risk factors in patients with antiphospholipid syndrome. J Thromb Thrombolysis. 2009;29(3):303–9.
15. Bezemer ID. Gene variants associated with deep vein thrombosis. JAMA. 2008;299(11)
16. Rastogi P, Kumar N, Ahluwalia J, Das R, Varma N, Suri V, et al. Thrombophilic risk factors are laterally associated with apolipoprotein E gene polymorphisms in deep vein thrombosis patients: an Indian study. Phlebol J Venous Dis. 2018;34(5):324–35.
17. Van Giau V, Bagyinszky E, An SS, Kim S. Role of apolipoprotein E in neurodegenerative diseases. Neuropsychiatr Dis Treat. 2015;
18. Zhu S, Wang Z, Wu X, Shu Y, Lu D. Apolipoprotein E polymorphism is associated with lower extremity deep venous thrombosis: color-flow Doppler ultrasound evaluation. Lipids Health Dis. 2014;13(1)
19. Ulrich V, Konaniah ES, Herz J, Gerard RD, Jung E, Yuhanna IS, et al. Genetic variants of ApoE and ApoER2 differentially modulate endothelial function. Proc Natl Acad Sci. 2014;111(37):13493–8.
20. Youn YJ, Lee J. Chronic venous insufficiency and varicose veins of the lower extremities. Korean J Intern Med. 2019;34(2):269–83.
21. Schleimer K, Barbati ME, Gombert A, Wienert V, Grommes J, Jalaie H. The treatment of post-thrombotic syndrome. DeutschesAerzteblatt Online. 2016.
22. Spiridon M, Corduneanu D. Chronic venous insufficiency: a frequently underdiagnosed and undertreated pathology. Maedica (Bucur). 2017;12(1):59–61.
23. Serra R, Buffone G, de Franciscis A, Mastrangelo D, Molinari V, Montemurro R, et al. A genetic study of chronic venous insufficiency. Ann Vasc Surg. 2012;26(5):636–42.
24. Zamboni P, Tognazzo S, Izzo M, Pancaldi F, Scapoli GL, Liboni A, et al. Hemochromatosis C282Y gene mutation increases the risk of venous leg ulceration. J Vasc Surg. 2005;42(2):309–14.
25. Mansilha A, Sousa J. Pathophysiological mechanisms of chronic venous disease and implications for venoactive drug therapy. Int J Mol Sci. 2018;19(6)
26. Kucukguven A, Khalil RA. Matrix metalloproteinases as potential targets in the venous dilation associated with varicose veins. Curr Drug Targets. 2013;14(3):287–324.
27. Cordell HJ, Shadrina AS, Sharapov SZ, Shashkova TI, Tsepilov YA. Varicose veins of lower extremities: insights from the first large-scale genetic study. PLOS. Genetics. 2019;15(4)
28. Li J, Hou B, Tumova S, Muraki K, Bruns A, Ludlow MJ, et al. Piezo1 integration of vascular architecture with physiological force. Nature. 2014;515(7526):279–82.
29. Ranade SS, Qiu Z, Woo SH, Hur SS, Murthy SE, Cahalan SM, et al. Piezo1, a mechanically activated ion channel, is required for vascular development in mice. Proc Natl Acad Sci. 2014;111(28):10347–52.

30. Finan C, Gaulton A, Kruger FA, Lumbers RT, Shah T, Engmann J, et al. The druggable genome and support for target identification and validation in drug development. Sci Transl Med. 2017;9(383)
31. The Human Protein Atlas. 2005. http://www.proteinatlas.org
32. Mellor RH, Brice G, Stanton AWB, French J, Smith A, Jeffery S, et al. Mutations in FOXC2 are strongly associated with primary valve failure in veins of the lower limb. Circulation. 2007;115(14):1912–20.
33. Brice G. Analysis of the phenotypic abnormalities in lymphoedema-distichiasis syndrome in 74 patients with FOXC2 mutations or linkage to 16q24. J Med Genet. 2002;39(7):478–83.
34. Le Flem L, Mennen L, Aubry ML, Aiach M, Scarabin PY, Emmerich J, et al. Thrombomodulin promoter mutations, venous thrombosis, and varicose veins. Arterioscler Thromb Vasc Biol. 2001;21(3):445–51.
35. LeFlem LN, Picard VR, Emmerich J, Gandrille S, Fiessinger J-NL, Aiach M, et al. Mutations in promoter region of Thrombomodulin and venous thromboembolic disease. Arterioscler Thromb Vasc Biol. 1999;19(4):1098–104.
36. Sverdlova AM, Bubnova NA, Baranovskaya SS, Vasina VI, Avitisjan AO, Schwartz EI. Prevalence of the methylenetetrahydrofolate reductase (MTHFR) C677T mutation in patients with varicose veins of lower limbs. Mol Genet Metab. 1998;63(1):35–6.
37. Wozniak G, Dapper F, Alemany J. Factor XIII in ulcerative leg disease: background and preliminary clinical results. Semin Thrombosis Haemostasis. 2008;22(05):445–50.
38. Gemmate D, Tognazzi S, Sereno ML, Fugato L, Car Andina S, De Palma M, et al. Factor XIII V34L polymorphism modulates the risk of chronic venous leg ulcer progression and extension. Wound Repair Regen. 2004;12(5):512–7.
39. Gemmate D, Tognazzi S, Catozzi L, Federici F, De Palma M, Guanosine S, et al. Influence of gene polymorphisms in ulcer healing process after superficial venous surgery. J Vasc Surg. 2006;44(3):554–62.
40. Ashcroft GS, Dodsworth J, Boatel EV, Tarnisher RW, Horan MA, Schultz GS, et al. Strogen accelerates cutaneous wound healing associated with an increase in TGF-β1 levels. Nat Med. 1997;3(11):1209–15.
41. Ashworth JJ, Smyth JV, Pendleton N, Horan M, Payton A, Worthington J, et al. Polymorphisms spanning the 0N exon and promoter of the estrogenic receptor-beta (ERβ) gene ESR2 are associated with venous ulceration. Clin Genet. 2007;73(1):55–61.
42. Sam RC, Burns PJ, Hobbs SD, Marshall T, Wilkin ABM, Silverman SH, et al. The prevalence of Wilkin, methylene tetrahydrofolate reductase C677T mutation, and vitamin B12 and folate deficiency in patients with chronic venous insufficiency. J Vasc Surg. 2003;38(5):904–8.
43. Darnall KAL, Sam RC, Adam DJ, Silverman SH, Fegan CD, Bradbury AW. Higher prevalence of thrombophilia in patients with varicose veins and venous ulcers than controls. J Vasc Surg. 2009;49(5):1235–41.
44. Beckman JA. Diseases of the veins. Circulation. 2002;106(17):2170–2.
45. Kahn SR. The post-thrombotic syndrome. Haematology. 2010;2010(1):216–20.
46. Lim CS, Davies AH. Pathogenesis of primary varicose veins. Br J Surg. 2009;96(11):1231–42.
47. Raffetto J, Khalil R. Matrix metalloproteinases in venous tissue remodelling and varicose vein formation. Curr Vasc Pharmacol. 2008;6(3):158–72.
48. Xu H-m, Zhao Y, Zhang X-m, Zhu T, Fu W-g. Polymorphisms in MMP-9 and TIMP-2 in Chinese patients with varicose veins. J Surg Res. 2011;168(1):e143–e8.
49. Saito S, Trovato MJ, You R, Lal BK, Fushun F, Patberg FT, et al. Role of matrix metalloproteinases 1, 2, and 9 and tissue inhibitor of matrix metalloproteinase-1 in chronic venous insufficiency. J Vasc Surg. 2001;34(5):930–8.
50. Haroun Y, Melius P, Bandemir E, Wichmann S, Nowakowski P, Schimpf E, et al. Inflammation in stasis dermatitis upregulates MMP-1, MMP-2 and MMP-13 expression. J Dermatol Sci. 2001;25(3):198–205.
51. Deitrick KD, Elfline M, Baker N, Luke CE, Blackburn S, Stabler C, et al. Post thrombotic vein wall remodelling: preliminary observations. J Vasc Surg. 2011;53(1):139–46.

52. Deatrick KB, Obi A, Luke CE, Elfline MA, Stood V, Upchurch GR, et al. Matrix metalloproteinase-9 deletion is associated with decreased mid-term vein wall fibrosis in experimental stasis DVT. Thromb Res. 2013;132(3):360–6.
53. Beidler SK, Douillet CD, Berndt DF, Keagy BA, Rich PB, Marston WA. Multiplexed analysis of matrix metalloproteinases in leg ulcer tissue of patients with chronic venous insufficiency before and after compression therapy. Wound Repair Regen. 2008;16(5):642–8.
54. Singh AV, Subhashree L, Milani P, Gemmate D, Zamboni P. Review: interplay of iron malariology, metalloproteinases, and FXIII, and role of their gene variants in venous leg ulcer. Int J Low Extrem Wounds. 2010;9(4):166–79.
55. Wojcik BM, Wrobleski SK, Hawley AE, Wakefield TW, Myers DD, Diaz JA. Interleukin-6: a potential target for post-thrombotic syndrome. Ann Vasc Surg. 2011;25(2):229–39.
56. Ferrell R. Hereditary lymphedema: evidence for linkage and genetic heterogeneity. Hum Mol Genet. 1998;7(13):2073–8.
57. Brice G. Milroy disease and the VEGFR-3 mutation phenotype. J Med Genet. 2005;42(2):98–102.
58. Arthur A, Markkanen MJ, Defriend K, Alitalia K, Vakala M. Congenital hereditary lymphedema caused by a mutation that inactivates VEGFR3 tyrosine kinase. Am J Hum Genet. 2000;67(2):295–301.
59. Malik S, Gresik K-H. Congenital, low penetrance lymphedema of lower limbs maps to chromosome 6q16.2–q22.1 in an inbred Pakistani family. Hum Genet. 2008;123(2):197–205.
60. Gresik S, Vrettos C, Laze E, Marathonists P, Kananaskis E, Willems P. Milroy's primary congenital lymphedema in a male infant and review of the literature. In Vivo. 2010;24(3):309–14.
61. Kananaskis A, Debauched C, Hana E, Van Reredorter N, Sinauer Y, Thomas D, et al. Sporadic in utero generalized enema caused by mutations in the Lymphangiogenic genes VEGFR3 and FOXC2. J Paediat. 2009;155(1):90–3.
62. Markkanen MJ, Haiku P, Sainio K, Partanen J, Taipale J, Petrova TV, et al. Vascular endothelial growth factor C is required for sprouting of the first lymphatic vessels from embryonic veins. Nat Immunol. 2003;5(1):74–80.
63. Ferrell RE and Finegold D. Research perspectives in inherited lymphatic disease. Ann N Y Acad Sci 2008;1131(1):134–139.
64. Butler MG, Dagenais SL, Rockson SG, Glover TW. A novelVEGFR3 mutation causes Milroy disease. Am J Med Genet A. 2007;143A(11):1212–7.
65. Rezaei T, Homochain R, Bell R, Brice G, Hasan A, Burnand K, et al. Primary non-syndromic lymphoedema (Miege disease) is not caused by mutations in FOXC2. Eur J Hum Genet. 2008;16(3):300–4.
66. Cugno M, Zanichelli A, Foieni F, Caccia S, Ciardi M. C1-inhibitor deficiency and angioedema: molecular mechanisms and clinical progress. Trends Mol Med. 2009;15(2):69–78.
67. Zuraw BL, Christiansen SC. HAE pathophysiology and underlying mechanisms. Clin Rev Allergy Immunol. 2016;51(2):216–29.
68. Zuraw BL. The pathophysiology of hereditary angioedema. World Allergy Org J. 2010;3(Supplement):S25–S8.
69. C1 inhibitor gene mutation database. 2018. http://hae.enzim.hu/
70. Bork K. Diagnosis and treatment of hereditary angioedema with normal C1 inhibitor. Allergy, Asthma Clin Immunol. 2010;6(1)
71. Kaplan AP. Angioedema. World Allergy Org J. 2008;1(6):103–13.
72. Haslund D, Rye LB, Rye S, Rose I, Skipper KA, Fryland T, et al. Dominant-negative SERPING1 variants cause intracellular retention of C1 inhibitor in hereditary angioedema. J Clin Investig. 2018;129(1):388–405.
73. Steiner UC, Keller M, Schmid P, Chicon S, Guillemin WA. Mutational spectrum of the SERPING1 gene in Swiss patients with hereditary angioedema. Clin Exp Immunol. 2017;188(3):430–6.
74. Gower RG, Buses PJ, Buses E, Barakat AJ, Caballero T, Davis-Lorton M, et al. Hereditary angioedema caused by C1-esterase inhibitor deficiency: a literature-based analysis and clinical commentary on prophylaxis treatment strategies. World Allergy Org J. 2011;4(2):S9–S21.

75. Sala-Cunill A, Jerkiest J, René T. Hereditary angioedema: a bradykinin-mediated swelling disorder. Thromb Haemost. 2017;109(03):368–74.
76. Björkqvist J, de Maat S, Lewandowski U, Di Gennaro A, Schatz C, Schurig K, et al. Defective glycosylation of coagulation factor XII underlies hereditary angioedema type III. J Clin Investig. 2015;125(8):3132–46.
77. Cichon S, Martin L, Hennies HC, Müller F, Van Driesch K, Kampuchea A, et al. Increased activity of coagulation factor XII (Hageman factor) causes hereditary angioedema type III. Am J Hum Genet. 2006;79(6):1098–104.
78. Kang BC, Nam DJ, Ahn EK, Yoon DM, Cho JG. Secondary Erythromelalgia - a case report. Korean J Pain. 2013;26(3):299–302.
79. Yang Y. Mutations in SCN9A, encoding a sodium channel alpha subunit, in patients with primary arthralgia. J Med Genet. 2004;41(3):171–4.
80. Waxman SG, Dib-Hajj SD. Erythromelalgia: a hereditary pain syndrome enters the molecular era. Ann Neurol. 2005;57(6):785–8.
81. Mann N, King T, Murphy R. Review of primary and secondary erythromelalgia. Clin Exp Dermatol. 2019;44(5):477–82.
82. Bibb LA, Winter RP, Leicht SS. Cyclosporine-induced Erythromelalgia. Cureus. 2018.
83. Michiels JJ, van Joost T. Erythromelalgia and thrombocythemia: a causal relation. J Am Acad Dermatol. 1990;22(1):107–11.

Vascular Malformations and Edema

15

Raul Mattassi and Valter Pozzoli

15.1 Introduction

Congenital vascular malformations (CVM) are errors in the morphogenetic process that regulates vascular development [1]. According to the type of vessel involved, there may be arterial, venous, arteriovenous, lymphatic, and combined defects. Venous malformations (VM) are by far the most frequent anomaly, with an incidence of over 60%. Modern classification distinguishes two groups, according to the type of vessels:

- Defects of the main vessels or "truncular" anomalies. These are anomalies of the main vessels, like aplasia, hypoplasia, or dilatation (congenital aneurysms)
- Areas of dysplastic more or less smaller vessels, located in the normal tissues. These defects, the most common (over 70% of cases) [2], are called "extratruncular" or "simple" vascular dysplasias [3, 4]

Frequency of the Different Type of Vascular Malformations
(Castellanza, 1497 cases, 2011–2017)

- Venous defects 918 (61%)
- Arteriovenous defects 271 (18%)
- Lymphatic defects.................... 164 (11%)
- Capillary defects 111 (7.5%)
- Combined forms 26 (2%)
- Arterial defects 7 (0.5%)

R. Mattassi (✉) · V. Pozzoli
Center for Vascular Malformations "Stefan Belov", Clinical Institute Humanitas "Mater Domini", Castellanza (Varese), Italy

S. K. Tiwary (ed.), *Approach to Lower Limb Oedema*,
https://doi.org/10.1007/978-981-16-6206-5_15

Vascular malformations may be sited in almost any part of the body. About 50% of cases have CVM on the lower limbs [5]; as this chapter is dedicated to edema, it will be focused on lower limbs.

15.2 Type of Defects

15.2.1 Venous Defects (VM)

Venous malformations of the lower limbs may be of different types:

- Aplasia or hypoplasia of the main deep veins
- Persistence of marginal vein
- Venous aneurysms
- Dysplastic superficial veins
- Dysplastic venous areas infiltrating tissues

15.2.2 Arteriovenous Malformations (AVM)

Two types of anomalies are possible:

(1) Direct communication between two main vessels (truncular forms)
(2) More or less small fistulous vessels infiltrating tissues

15.2.3 Lymphatic Malformations (LM)

(1) Defects of the main lymphatics (aplasia or hypoplasia) and lymph nodes
(2) Areas of dysplastic small lymphatics infiltrating tissues

15.3 Pathology and Clinical Picture

Aplasia or hypoplasia of main deep veins is an uncommon anomaly. Main vein tracts involved in the lower limbs are superficial femoral, popliteal, and common femoral vein [6]. Iliac veins and even inferior cava vein aplasia are also possible (Fig. 15.1). As these anomalies appear during intrauterine life, collateral venous circulation develops. This patient shows superficial dilated veins, more or less extended, with atypical varicose, located mainly on the lateral part of the limb (Fig. 15.2). In case of iliac aplasia, abdominal subcutaneous collateral circulation may be visible which bypasses the obstructed venous tract connecting with superficial thoracic veins, draining in the superior cava territory (cava–cava bypass).

Marginal vein, is an abnormal, valveless, more or less dilated vein, located on the lateral edge of the lower limb. This vein is a remnant of an embryonic vessel that

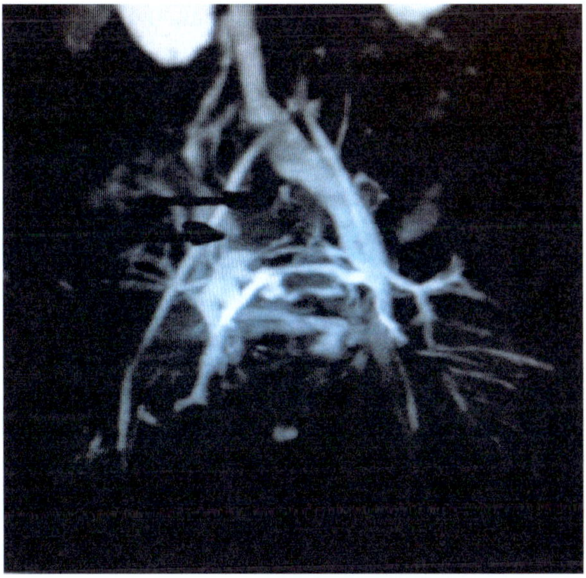

Fig. 15.1 MR demonstrating an aplasia of the right iliac vein (arrows)

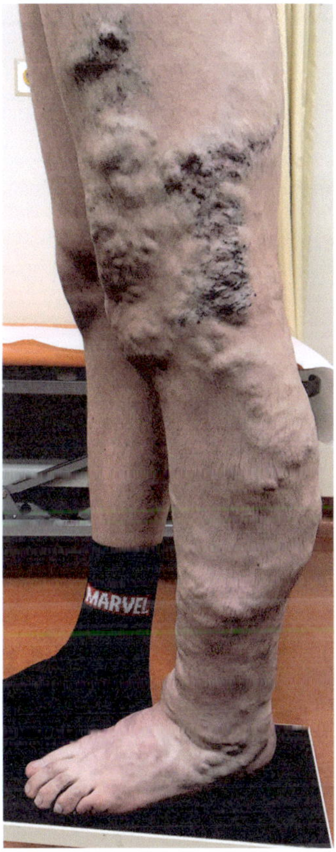

Fig. 15.2 Dysplastic superficial veins on the lateral side of the limb

normally disappears before birth. Marginal vein may have different extension, ending through abnormal lateral perforators or through gluteal perforators in the deep venous system [7] (Fig. 15.3).

Marginal vein may be of different caliber: sometimes not larger than a normal saphena, but in other cases the vessel can be extremely large and connected to the deep system through huge perforators. Clinically, the abnormal vein may be visible on the lateral side of the limb. However, sometimes the vein may be not visible because of smaller caliber and subcutaneous fat. Other dilated veins, extended until the dorsum of the foot, can be seen (Fig. 15.4)

Venous aneurysms may be located in different parts of the body. The most frequent site is in the lower limbs, like popliteal vein, superficial femoral, and common femoral vein [8]. Clinically, they are rarely visible because of the deep location, except in the inguinal region.

Dysplastic superficial veins are anomalous subcutaneous veins located often in atypical sites, like the lateral edge of a limb. They are incontinent and with reflux [9] (Fig. 15.5).

Infiltrating extratruncular venous malformations of the lower limb are a mass of dysplastic venous structures which infiltrate tissues, mainly muscles. These defects may manifest clinically by an enlargement of the interested area, like in the thigh or in the calf (Figs. 15.6 and 15.7).

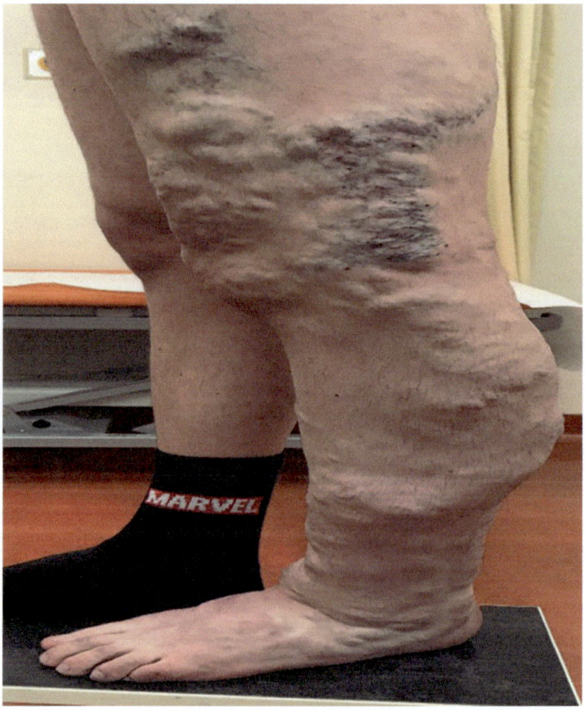

Fig. 15.3 Marginal vein (arrows). A huge perforator on the proximal lateral side of the thigh is the upper connection with the deep venous system

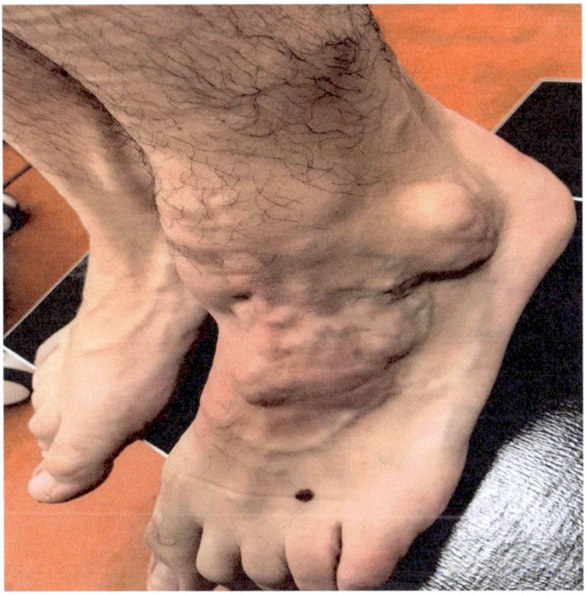

Fig. 15.4 Dilated dysplastic veins on external ankle and dorsum of the foot

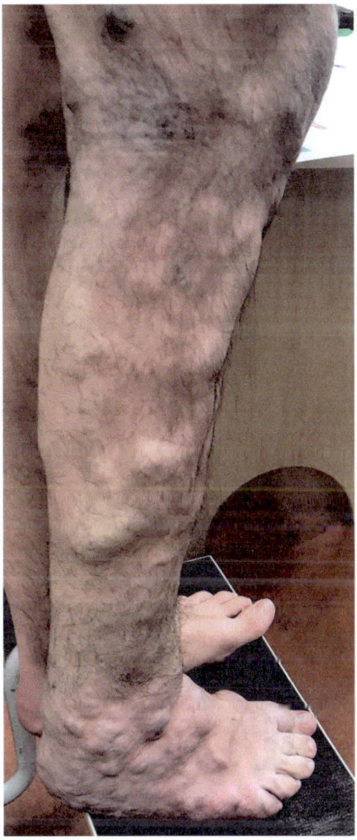

Fig. 15.5 Superficial dysplastic veins extended to the dorsum of the foot. Right foot is hypoplastic due to compression of the hypertonic veins on bones

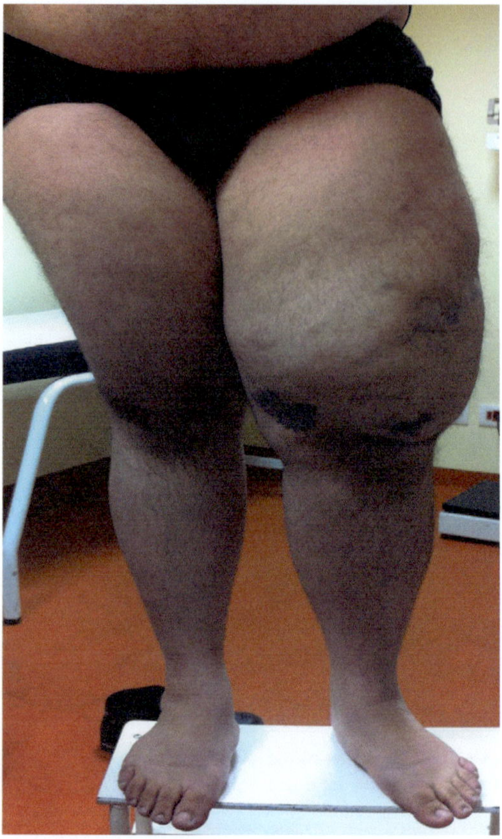

Fig. 15.6 Remarkable swelling of left thigh due to area of dysplastic veins. Notice edema of the calf

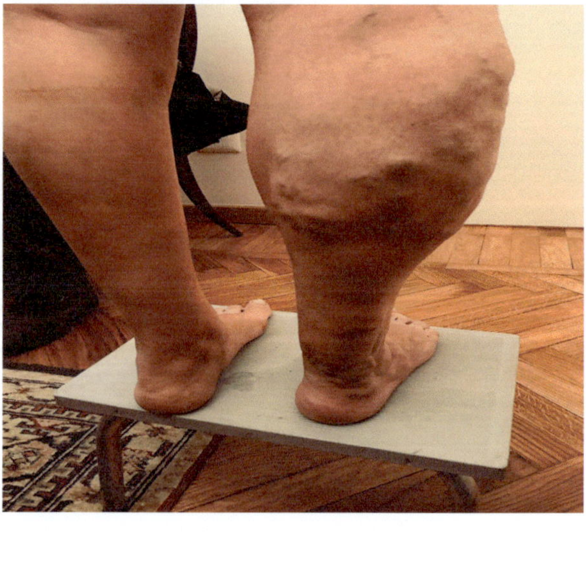

Fig. 15.7 Swelling of the calf because of dysplastic veins

Direct arteriovenous malformations are direct connections between a main artery and a vein. This type of anomaly, fortunately uncommon (3% in a series of 261 cases: [10]), may create a high overloading of the circulation and of the heart. As located on main vessels, they are usually deep sited and not visible; sometimes they manifest with visible dilated superficial veins.

Infiltrating or peripheral AVM: this type of defect may be limited or infiltrating and diffuse; it may be sited more or less superficially or deep inside the tissues. It may manifest as a mass more or less pulsating, sometimes with visible superficial veins or as a swelling of the whole limb (Figs. 15.8 and 15.9).

Truncular lymphatic defects are mainly an aplasia or hypoplasia of the main lymphatic draining trunks and/or lymph nodes [11]. Lower limbs are the most common site of that defect. Main lymphatic trunks of this area are the deep and the superficial system, the deep one following main artery and the superficial one following the great saphenous vein. Absence of a segment or of the whole lymphatic trunk is the most common defect; aplasia of both systems is rare, but possible. Lymph nodes may lose their function and become a blockade of lymph outflow. The deep lymphatic trunk is the most common site of a defect; very often the superficial system is able to compensate even completely so that there may be a clinically

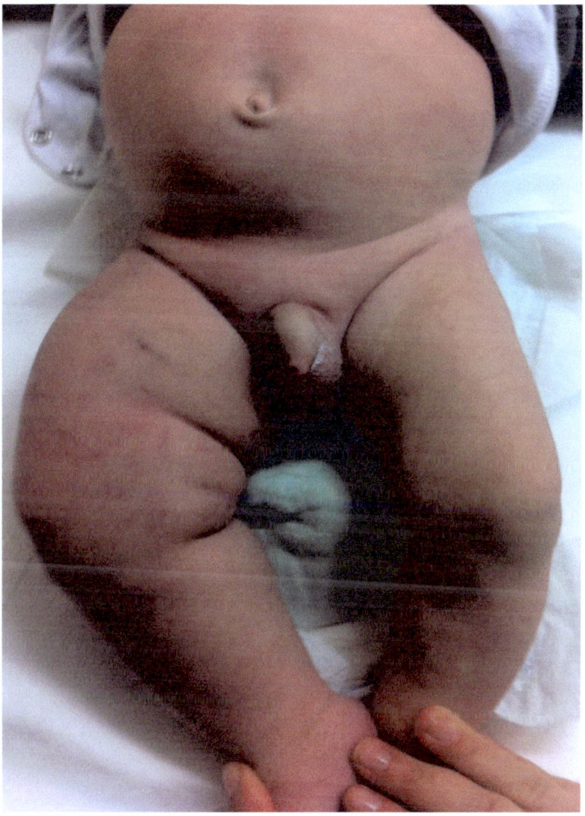

Fig. 15.8 Diffuse swelling of the right lower limb in a 6-month-old child due to extensive AVM on the thigh. Duplex scan recognizes a hypoplasia of the superficial femoral vein. Two years later, femoral vein dilates spontaneously and fistulas disappear

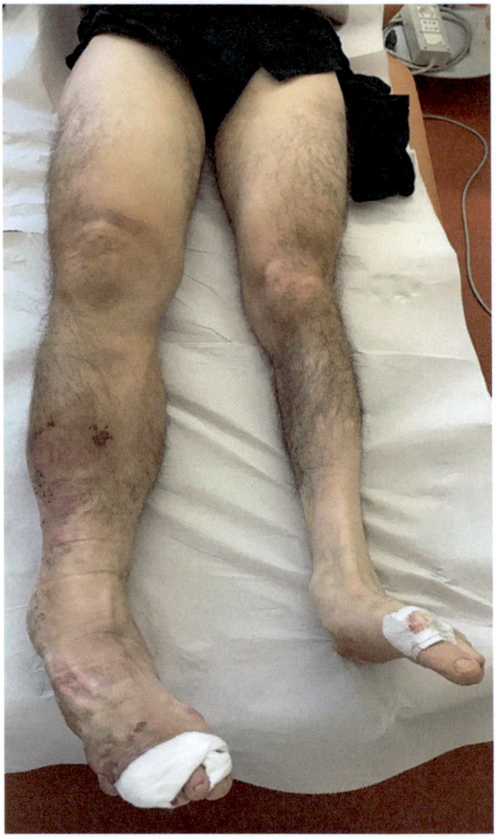

Fig. 15.9 Diffuse swelling of the right limb because of an infiltrating AVM on the ankle and foot. Medications are due to ulcers on fingers

normal picture and the defect is discovered only after a specific test, like lymphoscintigraphy. Foot or calf and, sometimes the whole limb, may be increased in volume (Fig. 15.10).

Extratruncular lymphatic malformations are areas of dysplastic lymphatics infiltrating tissues. They are composed by lymphatic cysts of different size: microcystic, in case of small cysts, or macrocystic, in case of larger size of cysts. They manifest as swollen, limited area, non-compressible (Fig. 15.11).

All these malformations may show a cutaneous nevus, more or less extended (Fig. 15.12).

15.4 Hemodynamics of Vascular Malformations of the Lower Limbs

There are three mechanisms that cause edema in CVM:

- Venous reflux and venostasis in venous malformations
- Venous hypertension in arteriovenous malformations
- Lymphatic stasis in defects of the main draining trunks

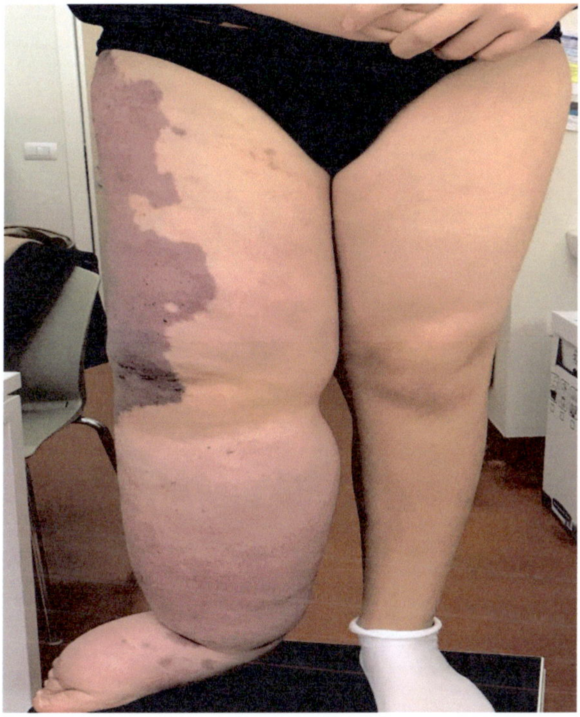

Fig. 15.10 Diffuse edema of the whole right limb due to a truncular lymphatic dysplasia. Extratruncular lymphatic malformations are also present on the foot and calf

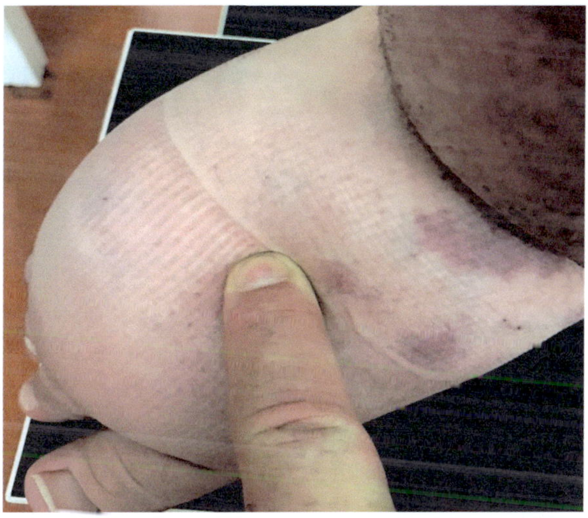

Fig. 15.11 Swelling of the dorsum of the foot due to extratruncular lymphatic malformation. The area is compact and not compressible

(1) Venous reflux exists in abnormal insufficient veins, like marginal vein, superficial dysplastic veins, and deep insufficient main veins. In a study with color doppler about hemodynamic defects in 52 cases of complex venous dysplasia of the lower limbs, reflux was recorded in all dysplastic superficial veins and marginal veins; in 22 of 52 cases (42%) a reflux in the deep venous system was

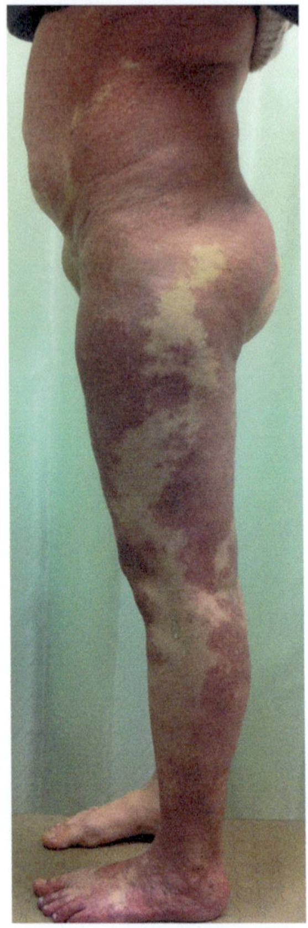

Fig. 15.12 Diffuse cutaneous nevus in venous malformation

noticed. A venous stasis without reflux was recorded in extratruncular infiltrating malformations, mainly intramuscular, and also in 8 cases (16%) of abnormal dilatation of calf veins [9].

(2) Venous hypertension in AVM is due to an increased inflow of blood in the venous system. The shunt between arterial and venous system is a low resistance condition in which more blood than normal enters the veins. Outflow veins dilate and pulsating venous flow may be sometimes recognized. Peripheral veins, located distally to the shunt, have stasis with hypertension [12].

(3) Lymphatic outflow defects, due to an obstruction of the main draining lymphatic trunks. As explained before, absence or stenosis of a main trunk may create distal lymph stasis. However, even in the absence of a main lymphatic, the phenomenon of dermal backflow is very rare in CVM [13].

15.5 Symptomatology

Aplasia or hypoplasia of main veins of the lower limb may even cause no symptoms, especially if larger veins are obstructed, like iliac or cava vein, because development of collateral circulation is possible. In more distal obstruction, like superficial or popliteal vein, main disturbances are due to venous stasis, in the normal main veins and in superficial dysplastic veins.

Extranuclear venous malformations my cause heaviness and edema, due to venous stasis. Pain, due to blood stasis, or even related to a localized thrombosis in the malformation may be claimed by the patient. If this type is sited on the foot, infiltrating the plantar muscles or extending subcutaneously, the clinical picture will be of a swollen foot. However, rather than due to edema, the swollen aspect is caused by the dysplastic vascular mass itself. In diffuse infiltration of the foot, this malformation may substitute main part of the muscles. By elevation of the limb, typically the outflow of the resting blood will be thinning out the foot (Figs. 15.13 and 15.14).

Arteriovenous malformations on the limbs may show a hyperemic area with swelling and abnormal pulsation (Fig. 15.15). Pain appears with worsening of the condition. If ulcers appear they may be complicated by sudden bleeding, which is a sign of progression of the disease. Heart decompensation is rare and is more common in direct AVM.

Lymphatic defects often manifest with edema by aplasia or malfunction of main lymphatic trunks. The deep lymphatic system is much more often involved. The defect exists since birth but, for unknown reasons, edema may appear late (Fig. 15.16).

In complex and extended venous malformations, there may coexist lymphatic dysplasia of the main trunks or even extratruncular lymphatic anomalies: this is the so-called Klippel-Trenaunay syndrome [14, 15] (Fig. 15.17).

Extratruncular lymphatic malformations are less common on the lower limbs. They manifest as lymphatic masses infiltrating muscles. The microcystic form is much more common in lower limbs. These defects, if truncular lymphatic malformations do not coexist, rarely originate edema (Fig. 15.18).

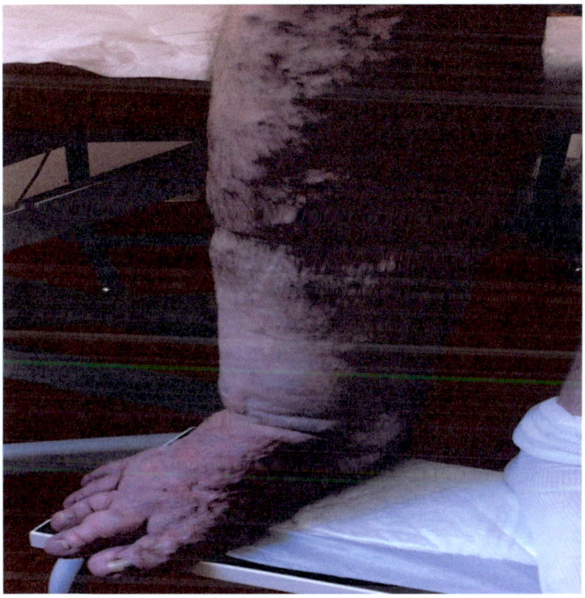

Fig. 15.13 Diffuse infiltrating extratruncular venous malformations of the calf and foot. The malformation also infiltrates extensively muscles of calf and also planta pedis. Patient complains swelling of dysplastic veins by gravity in standing position

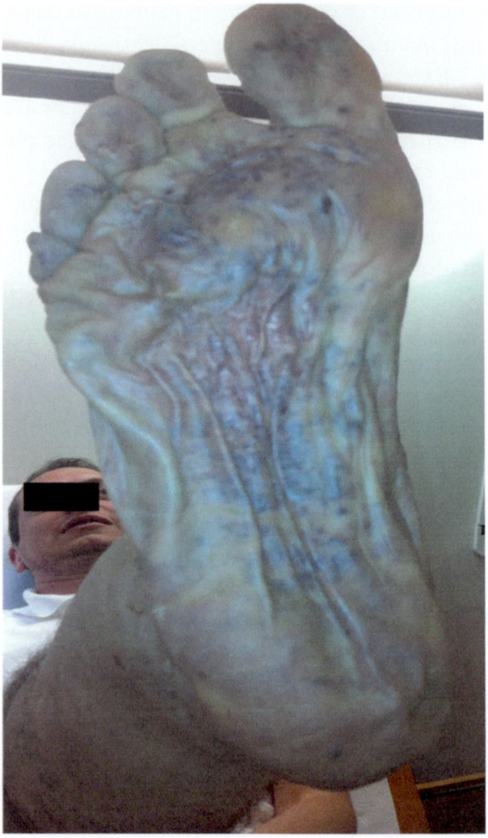

Fig. 15.14 Same patient of Fig. 15.13: by limb lifting, blood flows out shrinking the foot and demonstrating the extension of the venous dysplastic mass

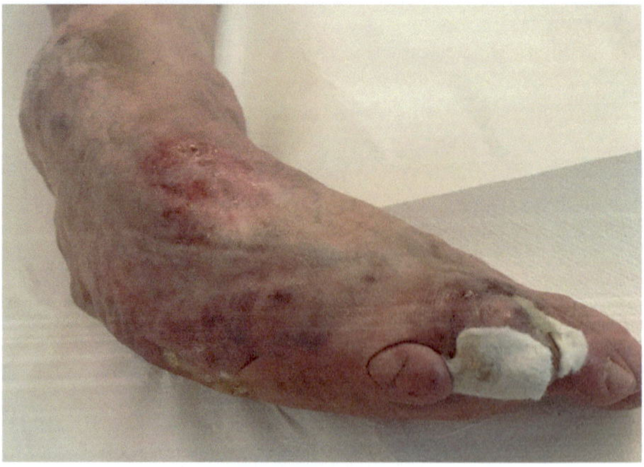

Fig. 15.15 Swelling of the lateral site of foot and ankle in a patient with AVM. Details of the same patient of Fig. 15.9

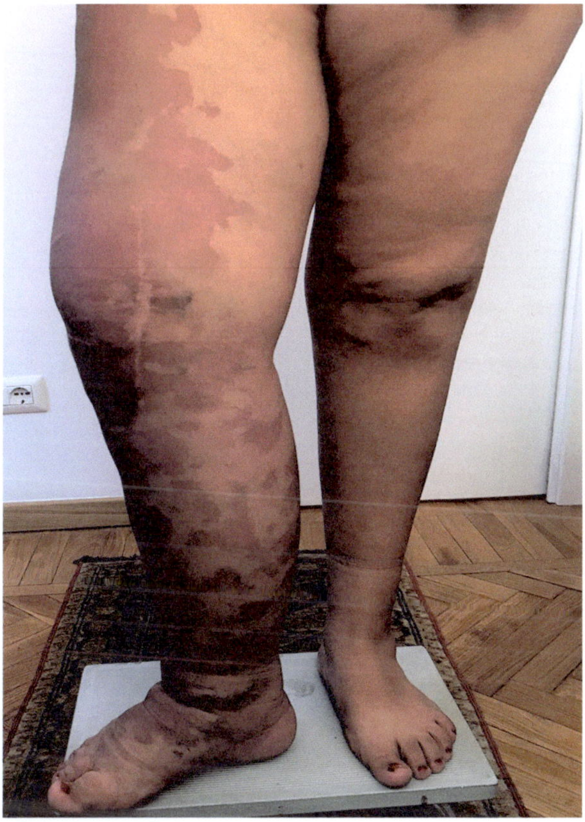

Fig. 15.16 Swelling of the limb in lymphatic truncular dysplasia

15.6 Clinical Picture of Edema in CVM

In venous malformations, swelling may have different aspects. The classical edema that involves foot, ankle, and sometimes also the calf is often visible. However, because of great variability in location of dysplastic tissue, sometimes swelling may be seen mainly in a part of the foot rather than in the whole distal extremity (Fig. 15.19).

Another cause of swollen appearance of a limb in CVM is a "false edema," not due to fluid stasis, but because of other causes:

- Subcutaneous fat overgrowth in the site of the malformation. This condition increases volume of the involved area but is not due to edema. New data demonstrate that it may be related to gene mutations, like PIK3Ca [16, 17] (Fig. 15.20).
- Intramuscular CVM with enlargement of the involved muscle. The most common cause is venous malformation; lymphatic and also AVM are possible. Intramuscular fibro-adipose vascular anomaly, called FAVA, a rare entity due to

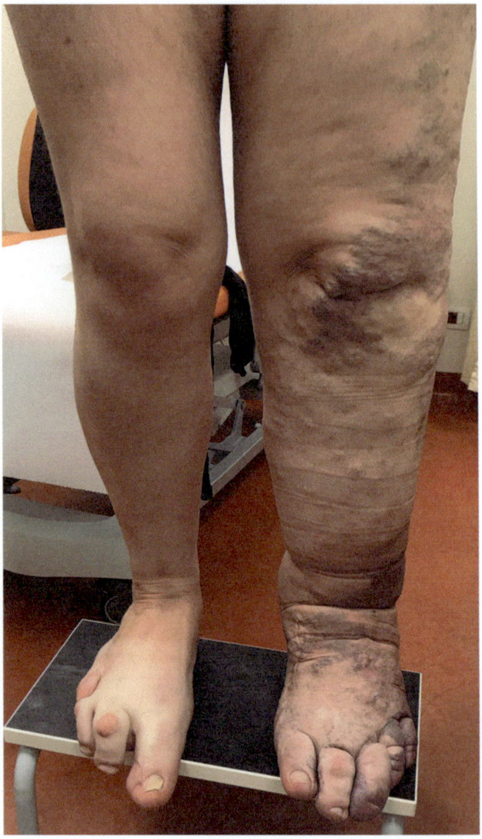

Fig. 15.17 Patient with a combined truncular lymphatic (absence of the deep lymphatics) and venous extratruncular malformations. Superficial nevus, dilated abnormal veins, and limb overgrowth. This case can be defined as "Klippel-Trenaunay syndrome" (KTS). Diagnosis of KTS is often not correct, as the syndrome requires a combination of malformations (venous and lymphatic) and not AVM. The term "Klippel-Trenaunay-Weber" is also incorrect because it is a mixture between KTS (without AVM) and Parkes Weber syndrome (with AVM). The incorrect terminology is often the cause of confusion

intramuscular infiltration of fibrofatty tissue, together with venous anomalies and muscle contraction may also create limb enlargement and simulate true edema [18] (Fig. 15.21).

15.7 Diagnosis

Clinical examination is the first step. Location of edema and extension on the foot and on the calf should be noticed. Effect of compression of the swollen part is helpful to distinguish true edema (compressible subcutaneous fluid) (Fig. 15.22), from limb enlargement due to subcutaneous dilated vessels (Fig. 15.23) (compressible but slowly filling again - venous; pulsating and quickly filling again - arteriovenous) or dysplastic masses. Lymphatic extratruncular malformations are normally not compressible (Fig. 15.11). Venous extratruncular malformations may be easily compressible and fill out slowly. Abnormal located superficial veins, cutaneous nevus, limb enlargement, and limb length discrepancy are all signs of vascular malformations. Abnormal superficial masses, pulsating or not, are also signs that should orient on a vascular defect.

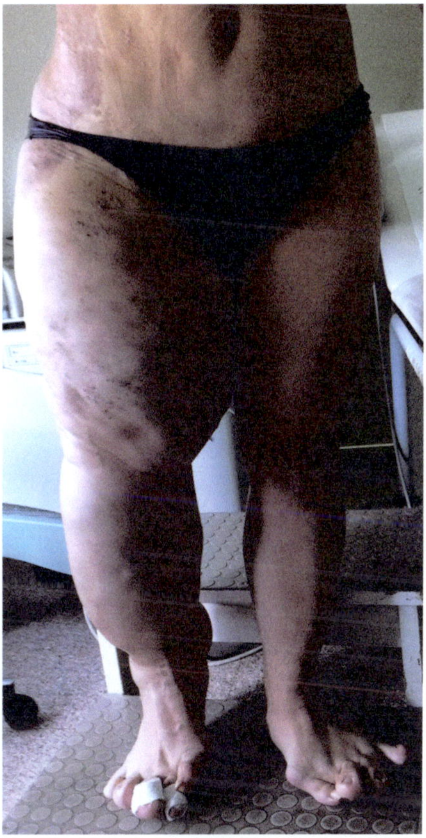

Fig. 15.18 Young girl with extensive extratruncular lymphatic malformation. Visible masses are firm and not compressible. This patient was treated by surgical removal, step by step, of the malformation with significant improvement

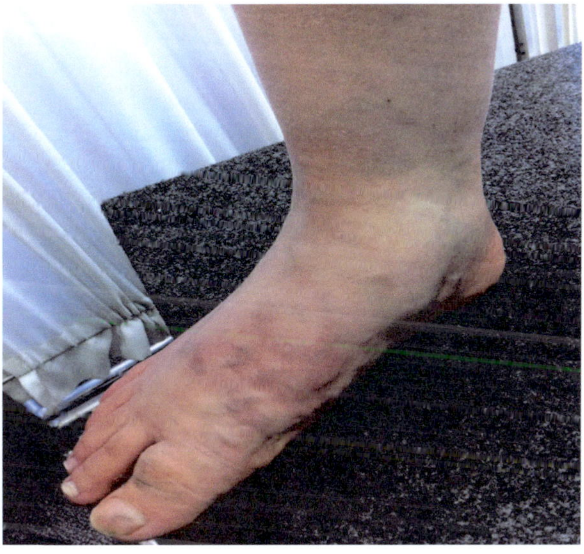

Fig. 15.19 Swelling of the medial part of the dorsum of the foot and of the first toe, due to a venous malformation. In this case, swollen aspect was increased by fat overgrowth (see text)

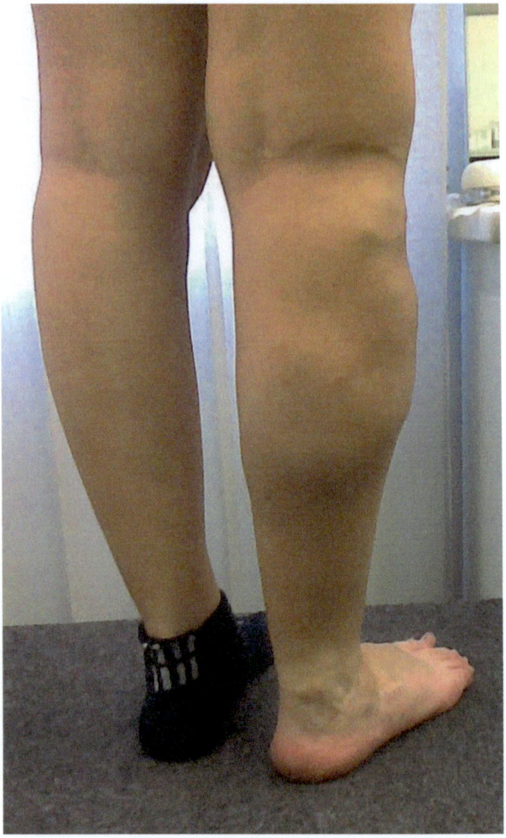

Fig. 15.20 Increase of volume of the calf due to small venous malformations surrounded by extensive fat overgrowth

The second step of diagnosis is color Doppler examination. This exam is as much effective as the examiner has experience in CVM and knows what can be found. A standard color Doppler investigation is currently an incomplete test. Deep and superficial veins, their caliber and flow, as well as arterial flow should be studied. Aplasia or hypoplasia should be investigated (Fig. 15.24). Existence of a marginal vein is a mandatory step in a case with a clinical picture that suggests a venous malformation. Search of intramuscular vascular masses is also necessary. The quantity of non-vascular tissue (relation tissue/vessels) is useful for the correct treatment: in case of a high non-vascular tissue component of a dysplastic mass, sclerotherapy is ineffective (Fig. 15.25). High flow areas (AVM) should be recognized as well as no flow vascular tissue (lymphatic).

The next step is to choose an imaging investigation and that should be guided by the result of the Duplex scan test. In case of low flow (venous) or no flow (lymphatic) data, MR is the best test (Fig. 15.26 a, b). Contrast media is not necessary in venous and lymphatic defects as a high-quality exam will demonstrate all necessary

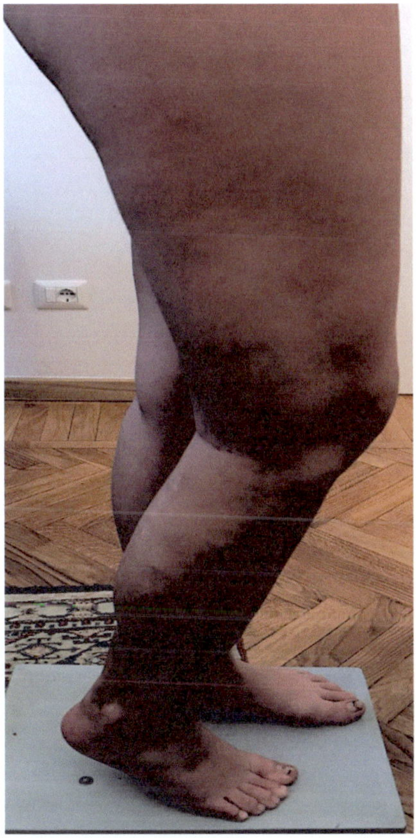

Fig. 15.21 Infiltrating venous malformation of the calf with muscle retraction and equinism, in a case of FAVA. Pain by walking and edema of the ankle and foot

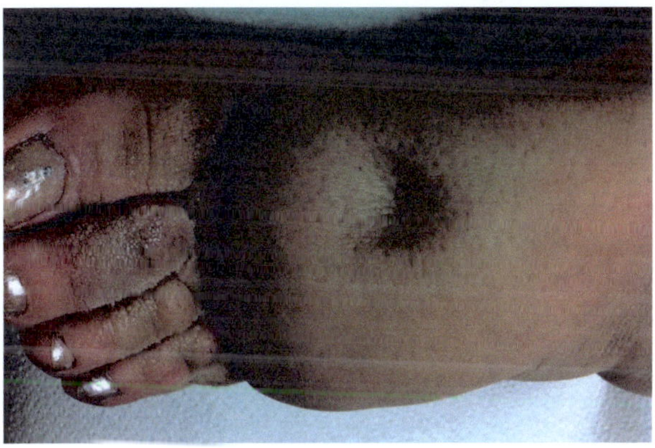

Fig. 15.22 Effect of digit pressure on true edema

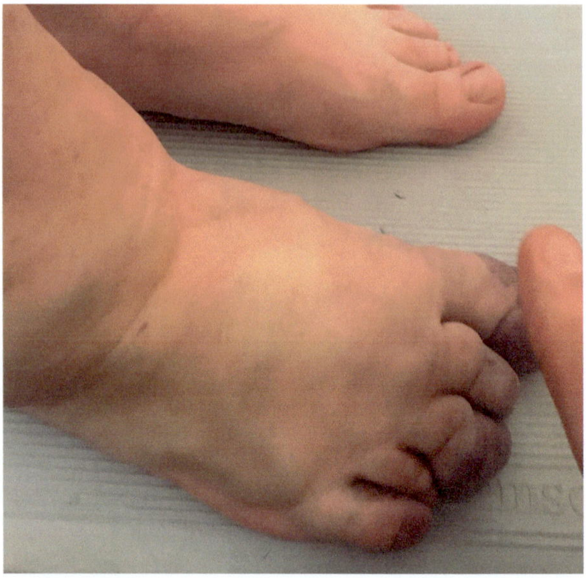

Fig. 15.23 Swelling of the foot due to infiltration of diffuse venous malformations. These masses are compressible and fill out again after release, slowly. In case of AVM, filling is quick and often pulsation is perceptible

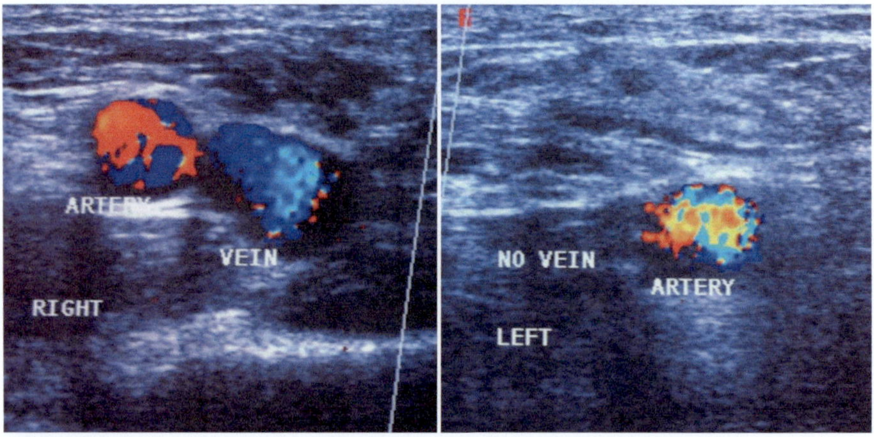

Fig. 15.24 Aplasia of left superficial femoral vein, demonstrated by echo Doppler

data about the location and extension of the malformation [19]. In case of high flow signal (AVM), MR with contrast media or also Angio-MR is the best test. Angio-CT with 3D images can also be useful (Figs. 15.27 and 15.28).

Angiography is no more a first option diagnostic test, as MR and CT offers excellent results. It should be reserved only to AVM in an intention to treat procedure, after diagnostic process has been completed [20]. There is no indication for angiography in venous and lymphatic malformations [2].

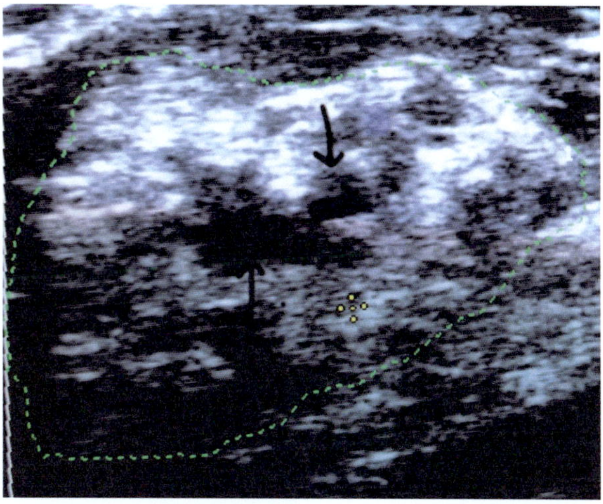

Fig. 15.25 Echo Doppler of a venous malformation (bounded area) with prevalent non-vascular component. Vessels are indicated by arrows; the other area is composed by compact tissue. That type of defect, if treated by sclerosis, will not disappear

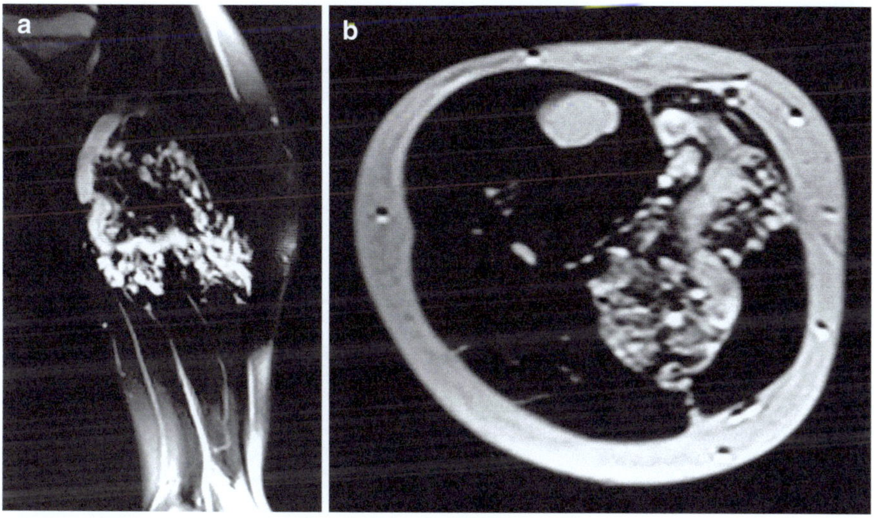

Fig. 15.26 (**a**) MR without contrast of a venous malformation of the calf. Frontal projection. The malformation is well demonstrated. Contrast media is not necessary for venous or lymphatic malformations. (**b**) MR without contrast of the same case in a transverse projection. The extension into the deep tissues is demonstrated. At least two projections are necessary to have a complete image of location, extension, and infiltration of tissues of the malformation

In case of whole swollen limb or in case of diffuse extended venous malformation, a lymphoscintigraphy should be performed. However, rather than a standard outflow test, a morphologic study of the main, superficial, and deep lymphatic trunks should be done. This test will demonstrate anomalies of the main lymphatic trunks or in lymph nodes [21] (Fig. 15.29 a, b).

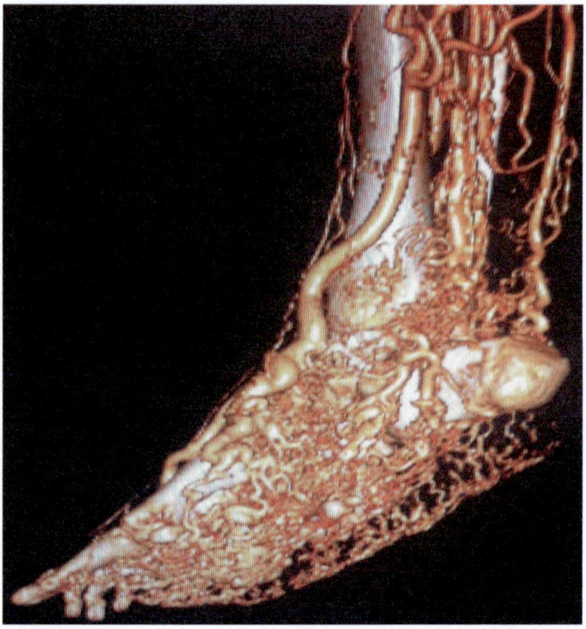

Fig. 15.27 Angio-CT with 3D elaboration of images in a case of AVM of the planta pedis. Anatomy of vessels and site of "nidus" of AVM are demonstrated. This report should be compared with echo Doppler in order to have complete data about site and hemodynamic of the malformation

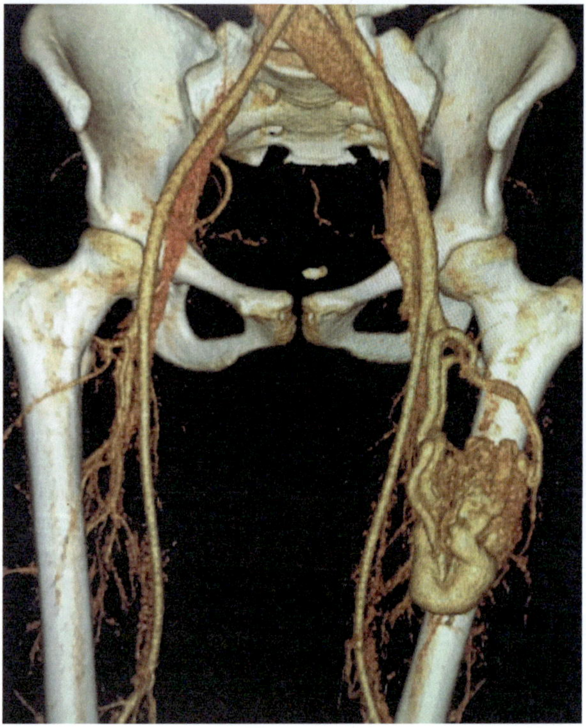

Fig. 15.28 Angio-CT with 3D elaboration of images in case of an intramuscular limited AVM of the thigh. Some feeders of the AVM mass are visible, as well as a large outflow vessel

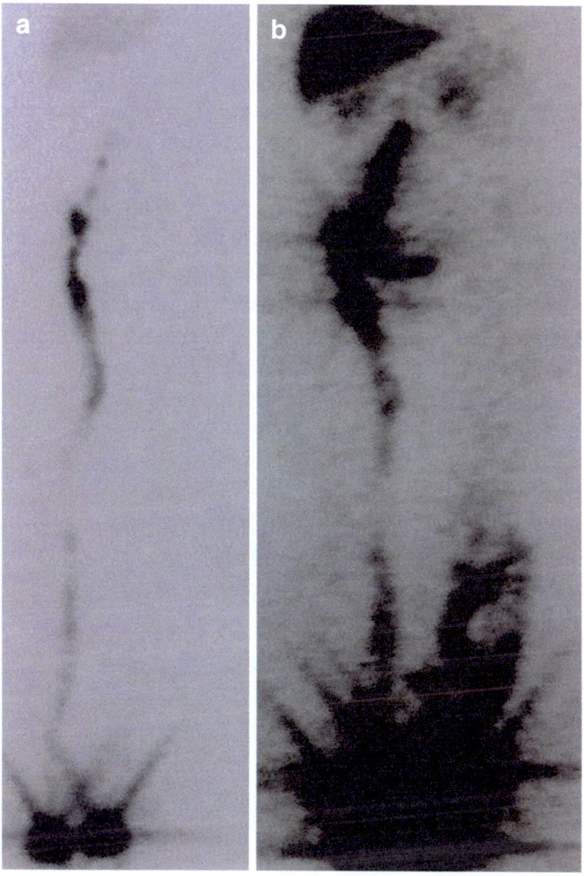

Fig. 15.29 (**a**) Lymphoscintigraphy for selective study of the deep lymphatic system by injection of the tracer on the planta pedis. Complete absence of the deep lymphatic trunk on the left lower limb; (**b**) Selective lymphoscintigraphy of the superficial lymphatic system by injection of the tracer in the interdigital spaces on the foot. On the left limb, some flow through abnormal and dilated lymphatics, which do not proceed beyond the knee. The right limb shows a single superficial outflow vessel. Popliteal lymph nodes are not visible. This patient has edema on the left limb but a clinically normal right one. The absence of edema in limbs with dysplastic lymphatics in CVM is not uncommon

15.8 Treatment

Vascular malformations are considered a difficult issue for treatment. However, often the difficulty is due to an incomplete or absent diagnostic procedure because of lack of knowledge and experience in the management of CVM. If the vascular defect has been correctly recognized, the choice of the best treatment will be much more easier [22]. Detailed discussion of the single technique is beyond the scope of this chapter; an overview of it will be given here.

Elastic compression can be the first choice in slight forms without symptoms. However, as the disease has the tendency to progress, regular controls should be performed [23].

Venous hypoplasia with superficial dilated veins can be treated successfully by surgery, as deep veins are able to dilate after removal of the superficial veins. That happens because superficial veins act as a functional bypass: if removed, blood flow is forced again to flow through deep veins which dilate spontaneously. This technique is called "derivation of venous flow" [24]. In case of aplasia (and not hypoplasia), this treatment is not possible because the superficial veins are the true outflow venous system. Dysplastic superficial veins, including marginal vein, can be removed by surgery [7] or treated by sclerosis, even if that last technique is not always effective in large dilated dysplastic veins. Laser or radiofrequency occlusion of marginal vein is also possible [2, 25, 26].

Extratruncular infiltrating venous malformations can be treated by surgical removal, by sclerotherapy, or by interstitial laser technique [27]. Sclerotherapy is an effective method for this type of VM. Different substances are available: polidocanol, alcohol, bleomycin, and others [26] (Figs. 15.30 and 15.31).

Treatment of AVM can be one of the most difficult problems, especially in infiltrating diffuse forms. According to location, extension, infiltration of tissues, and secondary effects, catheter embolization, surgery with "en bloc" removal, if possible, percutaneous alcohol occlusion, and interstitial laser are available (Fig. 15.32). Treatment strategy should be decided on a multidisciplinary basis, and in case of diffuse forms, step-by-step procedures should be planned [2, 20].

Truncular lymphatic malformations (primary lymphedema) are best treated conservatively and are explained in another chapter of this book. Extratruncular lymphatic malformations can be treated by surgical removal in limited cases. Macrocystic

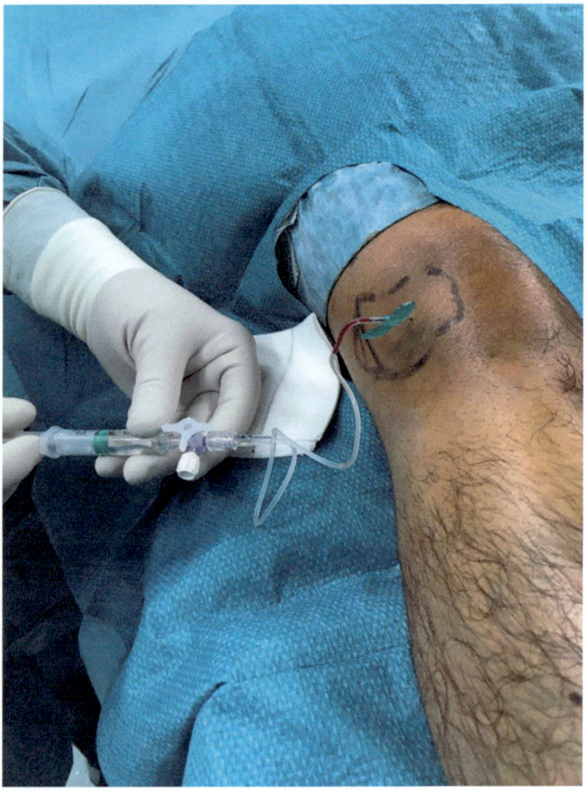

Fig. 15.30 Alcohol sclerosis of a superficial extratruncular venous malformation. The procedure requires a radioscopic control: after direct puncture of the malformation and blood backflow, contrast media is injected in order to find out the correct position of the needle. Only after that control, alcohol is injected (no more than 5 cc for each injection) and is immediately taken out by syringe aspiration. Alcohol is the most active sclerosing agent for VM, by far stronger than all other sclerosing liquids

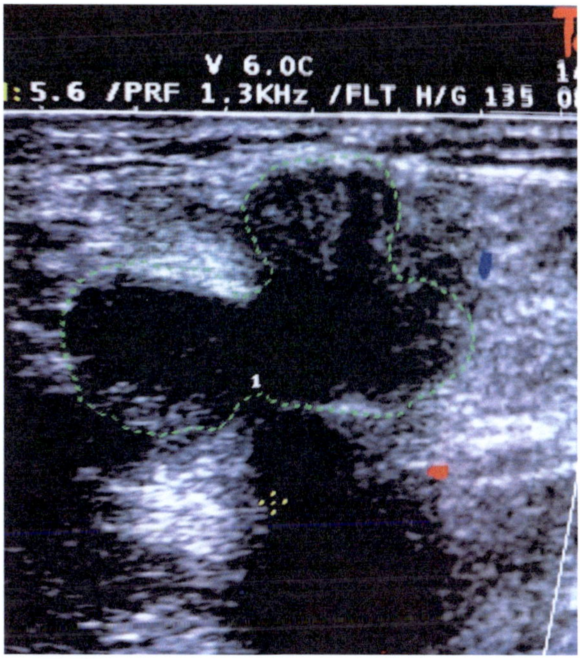

Fig. 15.31 Color doppler control after alcohol sclerosing session: complete occlusion of the malformation: color mode does not show any flow in the central dark area, which demonstrates the treated vessels

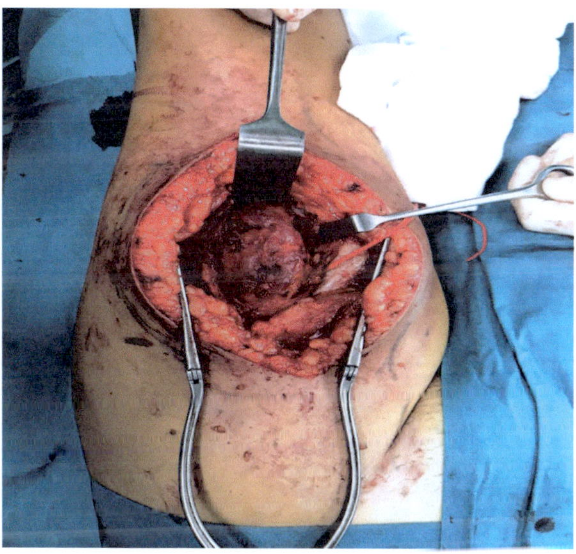

Fig. 15.32 Surgical resection of an intramuscular limited AVM area at the thigh. Same case of the MR shown in picture 28. This patient was completely healed after surgery. In limited easily accessible cases, surgery is often more effective than embolization because a complete removal of the malformation and definitive healing is possible, while embolization may have a higher chance of recurrence. This is a typical case in which a multidisciplinary approach should be done. However, if treatment decision depends only on which specialist the patient gets (radiologist or surgeon), the treatment may be not optimal. Angio-CT with 3D elaboration of images in a case of AVM

forms are successfully treated by percutaneous alcohol injections; however, macrocystic form is rare in lower limbs. Interstitial laser can be used in infiltrating, non-resectable forms, which have lymph leak and recurrent infections [5].

Medical therapy has been investigated in the last few years, especially after progress in genetics of CVM, showing different possibilities [28]. Several substances are under investigation; the best known is sirolimus, which seems to be effective, especially in extratruncular lymphatic malformations [29, 30]. However, more investigation is necessary.

15.9 Conclusion

Edema is a common symptom in CVM. However, it may manifest in different forms, due to the great variability of CVM. The aim of the diagnosis is to recognize the type of defect and the hemodynamics of it. After clinical examination, a correct instrumental diagnosis with duplex scan, followed by imaging (MR or CT), is required before deciding a treatment. Different types of treatments are available, even in combination. Choosing the best strategy of approach should be based on a multidisciplinary consultation, especially in complex cases.

References

1. Adams RH, Alitalo K. Molecular regulation of angiogenesis and lymphangiogenesis. Nat Rev Mol Cell Biol. 2007;8:464–9.
2. Lee BB, Baumgartner I, Berlien HP, et al. International Union of angiology. Consensus document of the international union of angiology (IUA) – 2013. Current concept on the management of arteriovenous malformations. Int Angiol. 2013;32(1):9–36.
3. Belov S. Surgical treatment of congenital vascular defects. Int Angio. 1990;9(3):175–82.
4. Wassef M, Blei F, Adams D, et al. and ISSVA Board and Scientific Committee. Pediatrics. 2015;136(1):e203–14. https://doi.org/10.1542/peds.2014-3673. Epub 2015 Jun 8
5. Lee BB, Laredo J, Neville RF. Lymphatic vascular malformations of the lower limbs: treatment of extratruncular malformations. In: Mattassi R, Loose DA, Vaghi M, editors. Hemangiomas and vascular malformations: an atlas of diagnosis and treatment. Milan: Springer; 2015. p. 431–44.
6. Eifert S, Villavicencio L, Kao T, et al. Prevalence of deep venous anomalies in congenital vascular malformations of venous predominance. J Vasc Surg. 2000;31(3):462–71.
7. Mattassi R, Vaghi M. Management of marginal vein: current issues. Phlebology. 2007;22:283–6.
8. Teter KA, Maldonado TH, Adelman MA. A systematic review of venous aneurysms by anatomic location. J Vasc Surg Venous Lymphat Disord. 2018;6(3):408–13.
9. Mattassi R, Pozzoli W. Hemodynamics in Klippel-Trenaunay syndrome. J Theoret Pract Vasc Res. 2018; https://doi.org/10.24019/jtavr.48.
10. Mattassi R, Di Giuseppe P, Grappolini S et al. Multidisciplinary, single center approach to 261 cases of peripheral arteriovenous malformations: a retrospective analysis. It J Vasc Endovasc Surg. 2020; (in publication).
11. Lee BB, Laredo J, Neville RF. Primary lymphedema as a truncular lymphatic malformation. In: Lee BB, Bergan J, Rockson SG, editors. Lymphedema. A concise compendium of theory and practice. London: Springer; 2011. p. 419–26.

12. Strandness DE, Sumner DS. Arteriovenous fistula. In: Hemodynamics for surgeons. New York: Grune & Stratton; 1975. p. 621.
13. Lee BB, Laredo J, Lee TS, et al. Terminology and classification of congenital vascular malformations. Phlebology. 2007;22(6):249–51.
14. Liu NF, Qing L, Zhi-Xin Y. Lymphatic malformation is a common component of Klippel-Trenaunay syndrome. J Vasc Surg. 2010;52(6):1557–63.
15. Mattassi R. Management of combined venous and lymphatic malformations. Phlebolymphology. 2016;23(2):112–9.
16. Lindhurst MJ, et al. Mosaic overgrowth with fibroadipose hyperplasia is caused by somatic activating mutations in PIK3CA. Nat Genet. 2012;44:928–33.
17. Keppler-Noreuil KM, Sapp JC, Lindhurst MJ, e al. Clinical delineation and natural history of the PIK3CA-relaes overgrowth spectrum. Am J Med Genet A. 2014;164(7):1713–33.
18. Alomari I, Spencer SA, Arnold RW, et al. Fibro-adipose vascular anomaly. Clinical-radiologic-pathologic features of a newly delineated disorder of the extremity. J Pediatr Orthop. 2014;34(1):109–17. https://doi.org/10.1097/BPO.0b013e3182a1f0b8.
19. Fayad L, Hazirolan T, Bluemke D, Mitchell S. Vascular malformations in the extremities: emphasis of MR imaging features that guide treatment options. Skeletal Radiol. 2006;35(3):127–37.
20. Mattassi R, Gandolfo C, Moneghini L, et al. Guidelines for vascular anomalies: arteriovenous malformations. Int Angiol. 2015;31(suppl 1):36–9.
21. Dentici R, Mattassi R, Nuclear Medicine Diagnostics. In: Mattassi R, Loose DA, Vaghi M, editors. Hemangiomas and vascular malformations: an altas of diagnosis and treatment. Milan: Springer; 2015. p. 223–36.
22. Madani H, Farrant J, Chhaya N, et al. Peripheral limb vascular malformations: an update of appropriate imaging and treatment options of a challenging condition. Br J Radiol. 2015;88:20140406.
23. Stout N, Partsch H, Szolnoky G, et al. Chronic edema of the lower extremities: international consensus recommendations for compression therapy clinical research trials. Int Angiol. 2012;31(4):316–29.
24. Belov S. Classification of congenital vascular defects. Int Angiol. 1990;9(3):141–6.
25. Greene AK, Alomari A. Management of venous malformations. Clin Plast Surg. 2011;38(1):83–93.
26. Hage AN, Cick JFB, Srinivasa RN, et al. Treatment of venous malformations: the data. Where we are and how it is done. Tech Vasc Interv Radiol. 2018;21(2):45–54.
27. Leghien GM. Sclerotherapy with adjunctive stasis of efflux (STASE) in venous malformations: techniques and strategies. Tech Vasc Interv Radiol. 2019;22(4):100630.
28. Paolacci S, Zulian A, Bruson A, et al. Vascular anomalies: molecular bases, genetic testing and therapeutic approaches. Int Angiol. 2019;38(2):157–70.
29. Freixo C, Ferreira V, Martins J, et al. Efficacy and safety of sirolimus in the treatment of vascular anomalies: a systematic review. J Vasc Surg. 2020;71:318–27.
30. Adams DM, Trenor CC 3rd, Hammill AM, et al. Efficacy and safety of sirolimus in the treatment of complicated vascular anomalies. Pediatrics. 2016;137(2):e20153257.

Infection Control in Lower Limb Oedema 16

Tuhina Banerjee, Rahul Garg, and Aradhana Singh

16.1 Introduction

Infection in lower limb oedema is a common entity. While an often unnoticed cutaneous barrier disruption in an oedematous limb is the initiation point of entry for pathogens causing infections, uncontrolled infections can result in limb loss and morbidity. In this chapter, we briefly summarize the recent insights into the microbiological aspects of infection, the diagnostic strategies, choices of antibiotics for early management and treatment and preventive approaches in form of non-pharmacological measures. Finally, we also discuss the challenges in management of such infections from the perspectives of developing countries.

16.2 Mechanisms of Infection in Lower Limb Oedema

In all tissues, passive fluid exchange between capillary microcirculation and the interstitial fluid is governed by Starling's principle of fluid exchange [1]. The 4 Starling forces namely Capillary hydrostatic pressure (Pc), Interstitial hydrostatic pressure (Pi), Capillary oncotic pressure (Πc) and Interstitial oncotic pressure (Πi) maintain a perfect balance in fluid exchange thus protecting against oedema formation. Any oedema, whatever might be the aetiology, is caused due to overwhelming capillary filtration in comparison to lymphatic drainage over a sufficient period of time. The physiological mechanism has been shown in Fig. 16.1.

T. Banerjee (✉) · R. Garg · A. Singh
Department of Microbiology, Institute of Medical Sciences, Banaras Hindu University, Varanasi, Uttar Pradesh, India
e-mail: drtuhina105@bhu.ac.in

S. K. Tiwary (ed.), *Approach to Lower Limb Oedema*,
https://doi.org/10.1007/978-981-16-6206-5_16

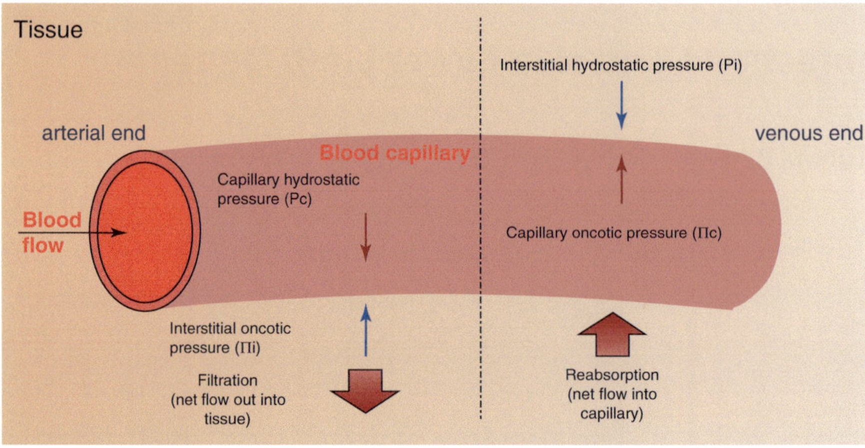

Fig. 16.1 Physiology of fluid exchange across capillary walls

The most commonly encountered types of leg oedema are venous oedema and lymphoedema [2]. While venous oedema due to venous insufficiency consists of low viscosity interstitial fluid which is poor in proteins ultimately leading to increased capillary filtration beyond the capacity of lymphatic drainage, lymphoedema on the other hand consists of protein-rich interstitial fluid [2]. This protein-rich or depleted stagnant fluid along with a state of local immune deficiency provides an excellent media for growth of microorganisms [3]. Additionally, lymphoedema in infected areas also impedes the action of antibiotics or action of phagocytes for the effective clearing of the pathogens [4].

The skin constitutes the first anatomical barrier that mechanically prevents entry of any microbes. There are several epidermal, dermal and subcutaneous protective factors in intact healthy skin. Among the prominent epidermal factors are also included the tightly linked corneocytes with a high rate of bacterial shedding and modulation of local immunity by the skin commensals [5]. Any breach in the skin due to underlying oedema can lead to dire consequences. These areas of broken skin are often the 'entry lesions' serving as potential sources of infection. Per se lower limb oedema does not itself cause infection but it probably facilitates its development by impairing local defence mechanisms.

16.3 Types of Infections and Microbiological Aspects

Along with the progression of oedema, changes in the overlying skin appear due to alterations in perfusion of the skin and in the levels of nutrients. The changes initially manifest as dry, flaky skin with a loss in elasticity. Hyperkeratosis and papilloma soon follow which later lead to blistering and 'weeping legs' [6]. Disruption of the cutaneous barrier results in acute bacterial cellulitis predominantly having a unilateral presentation. Cellulitis is an inflammatory condition of the skin and subcutaneous tissue, characterized by erythema, swelling, warmth and pain as hallmark presentations [7]. The aetiological agents are most often Gram-positive cocci namely *Streptococcus pyogenes* and *Staphylococcus aureus*, followed by non-group A β-haemolytic streptococci and Gram-negative bacilli. Among the Gram-negative bacilli, members of *Enterobacteriaceae* family along with *Pseudomonas* species often colonize infected areas thus causing delayed healing. In association with anaerobes, these organisms like *Escherichia coli, Klebsiella pneumoniae, Citrobacter*, are often present in wounds, especially associated with diabetes [8]. In cases of exposure to animal bites, rare organisms like *Pasteurella* and *Capnocytophaga* could be the probable cause, while infections following exposure of broken skin to brackish or fresh water are often associated with *Vibrio* species and *Aeromonas* species, respectively [5, 9]. Cellulitis is a known medical emergency, the severity of which differs from mild to severe infections with life-threatening consequences. Although dermatophytes do not cause cellulitis, they lead to scaling and fissure formation and by disruption of the skin provide a niche for bacteria facilitating their entry into the body. Tinea pedis often promotes the initiation of infection in an oedematous limb [10].

Erysipelas, a subtype of cellulitis with erythema is characterized by well-demarcated sharp palpable edges along with fever. Once thought to be only of streptococcal aetiology, there is growing evidence now that there is extensive overlap between these two entities. Consequently, these two conditions are preferably grouped together as skin and soft tissue infections (SSTIs) [5].

Cellulitis can progress as rapidly spreading erythema and severe sepsis along with excruciating pain, the condition known as necrotizing fasciitis [1]. This presentation commonly proceeds faster in the elderly and immunosuppressed patients with compromised skin elasticity and nutritional factors. Besides Group A streptococci which is often associated with the development of necrotizing fasciitis, a mixed group of organisms comprising Gram-negative bacilli and anaerobes are also involved [9]. Realizing the urgency to diagnose necrotizing fasciitis immediately in order to prevent devastating effects, one should be prompt in identifying the condition early. Some of the clinical features that hint towards the condition in comparison to simple cellulitis have been summarized in Table 16.1 [11]. Besides, a laboratory risk indicator for necrotizing fasciitis (LRINEC) is based on estimation of C-reactive protein (CRP), white blood cell counts (WBC), haemoglobin, sodium, creatinine and glucose. Magnetic resonance imaging (MRI) along with LRINEC have often been used to distinguish cellulitis from necrotizing fasciitis. However, clinical suspicion and prompt medication or surgical exploration is superior [5].

Table 16.1 Clinical features suggesting early suspicion of necrotizing fasciitis

Features	Findings
Symptoms	High fever, altered sensorium, lethargy, disproportionate pain
Signs	Hypotension, tachycardia, pallor
Limb examination	Watery discharge, crepitus, aggravated oedema, hypoesthesia of underlying skin, areas of normal skin surrounded by infection.

16.4 Risk Factors for Infection in Lower Limb Oedema

A systematic review on the risk factors, complications and predictors of complications of lower limb cellulitis in Africa over more than 30 years revealed that obesity was the only general risk factor [10]. Among the local risk factors, a break in the continuity of the skin barrier, chronic wounds, use of depigmentation drugs in addition to lower limb oedema or lymphedema were reported. Complications in infections were associated with nicotine addiction, chronic non-steroidal anti-inflammatory drugs (NSAIDs) use, delay in initiation of antibiotic therapy and increased erythrocyte sedimentation rate (ESR). Skin depigmentation products contain potent corticosteroids, prolonged use of which cause fragile skin with huge propensity to break. This in turn promotes penetration and colonization with pathogenic organisms. Over-the-counter use of inappropriate antibiotics especially in developing countries is also one of the most challenging issue for early diagnosis and treatment of infections [11]. Comorbid conditions like diabetes mellitus, peripheral arterial diseases, venous insufficiency and chronic tinea pedis increase the risk of developing cellulitis. Fungal infections in the toe webs, i.e. toe web dermatophytosis is also a common risk factor. In another study in 647 patients with lower limb infection, 77% had barrier defects the commonest being fungal infections [12]. It has been usually seen that a quarter of lymphoedema patients develop at least one episode of cellulitis or skin-related infections.

Development of cellulitis and lymphoedema is a vicious cycle each complementing one another for further damage. This vicious cycle is often multifactorial and unrelated to the primary aetiology of the infection. Early detection of the microbiological agent responsible for infection helps in deciding appropriate antibiotic therapy [4]. However, diagnosing cellulitis in lower limb oedema in early stages of infection is of low value by the commonly employed microbiological methods. While intact skin swabs are of no value, advanced ulcers and erosions often reveal colonization of wounds rather than the actual pathogen. In initial phases of cellulitis, blood cultures are of limited value as there is no overt bacteraemia unless the infection spreads as necrotizing fasciitis. It has been seen that blood cultures are positive in only 10% of the cases while swab culture is positive in only 30% of the cases [13]. Another study revealed that 31% of patients with cellulitis who were hospitalized were misdiagnosed [14].

16.5 Non-pharmacological Preventive Care for Protection Against Infection

Intensive self-care alone may significantly decrease the progression to infection. Majority of the studies on effectiveness of various antibiotic regimens have finally concluded that good foot care aids in decreasing infections in lower limb oedema [3]. Preventive approaches should encompass skincare, exudate management, care of wounds at initial stages and compression therapy. In this regard, the International

Table 16.2 Non-pharmacological measures for infection prevention in lower limb oedema

Skin changes	Non-pharmacological measures
Early stages of oedema that reduce on limb elevation Presence of varicose veins	Class 1 or 2 compression garments Skincare Emollients Simple exercises
Dermatitis with skin discoloration and occasional skin breaks	As above Limb elevation and short walks
Wounds with ulcerations and exudates	All above Full leg compression garments
Skin thickening with pigmentation and associated changes in limb shape	Full leg compression bandaging followed by class 2 or 3 compression garments Manual drainage by simple massage Skincare Emollients Limb elevation exercises
Dry, flaky hardened and fragile skin with skin folds due to prolonged oedema	All above

Lymphedema framework emphasizes the importance of lifelong treatment in cases of lower limb oedema with special importance of compression therapy and patient's own foot care education and enthusiasm [6]. The various non-pharmacological measures based on skin changes have been summarized in Table 16.2.

16.5.1 Skin Care

Care for one's skin is the pivot in the prevention of infection in all patients with chronic lower limb oedema irrespective of aetiology. Patients should pay attention to skin integrity and inspect daily for any areas of irritation or inflammation, drying, cracks, blistering or increased localized temperature [3]. Skincare consists of three main key components, i.e. cleansing, drying and moisturizing. Frequent washing of the limb, at least thrice weekly, is important for the removal of all the likely sources of infection like the dead cells of the skin, the assembly of emollients and the colonizing microorganisms. Normal soap can make the skin dry and disrupt the acidic mantle of the skin. To prevent this, a pH neutral cleanser or emollient can be used instead of soap [15]. If a wound is present, it needs proper caring and regular dressing. Make sure all of the limb is cleaned, not just the skin around the wound. Wound cleansing is important to maintain a healthy wound bed to optimize the chance of wound closure. Skin folds and web spaces should be specially cared for and ensured for complete dryness after cleaning as these are often the sites for fungal infections. Emollients should be applied along with the direction of the hair growth to prevent skin desquamation. Nail care is equally important to avoid scratches and infections from nails.

16.5.2 Manual Oedema Mobilization

Besides skincare, additional steps like belly breathing, light lymphatic massages, exercises involving elevation of limbs and compression garments should be considered. These help in improving lymphatic flow and clearance of fluid from tissues, improving venous return, reducing limb volumes and weight and increasing the range of movements. Infected areas should not be massaged as it helps in spread of infection [16].

Manual lymphatic drainage (MLD) is a type of specialized massage aimed at encouraging the flow of lymph around the body [17]. It can be useful to ease congestion and reduce limb volume in the intensive/decongestion phase of treatment. It helps to move extra lymph fluid from the tissues of the affected area so it can drain normally. It is usually used in conjunction with compression bandaging or hosiery to improve the efficacy of these treatments. Based on the initial skin changes, the following protective measures should be adopted at the earliest in order to prevent widespread infections [18, 19].

16.5.3 Compression Therapy

It is used to deliver external pressure to the limb so that on contraction of the calf-muscle pump, blood and lymph within the limb are squeezed from the tissue back into the circulation via the lymphatics [20]. It can be applied using bandaging, hosiery or wraps and should be applied in a graduated way, with pressure that is greatest at the ankle gradually decreasing towards the knee, with further reduction to the thigh if compression is applied to the full length of the leg. This graduation allows the venous blood to be pushed back up from the leg towards the heart [21]. Recently a single-centre, randomized, non-blinded trial, involving cases with chronic oedema of the leg and recurrent cellulitis in a 1:1 ratio compared leg the effects of compression therapy plus education (compression group) and education alone (control group) on cellulitis prevention. The study revealed that compression therapy resulted in a lower incidence of recurrence of cellulitis than conservative treatment [22].

16.5.4 Wound Care

Patient's skin condition and the effectiveness of the skincare regimen which is being followed should be monitored and assessed at regular intervals. Failure to do so might give rise to complications like leakage of lymph fluid through the skin in form of lymphorrhoea and recurrent cellulitis. Once cellulitis steps in and is diagnosed, prompt management is of utmost importance to prevent devastating complications. Such type of skin is more prone to infections and mechanical damage thus causing immense pain. In such painful situations, compression therapy should be temporarily discontinued. Once pain becomes less and bearable, therapy should be resumed to control oedema and prevent any further complications. The choices for treatment of cellulitis with oral antibiotics in mild cases and with intravenous antibiotics in severe cases have been discussed in later part of the chapter. Once cellulitis develops, risk of recurrent episodes of infections increases which can amount to repeated admissions in the hospital and its consequences associated with increasing economic burden for the patient [23, 24]. As repeated episodes of infections is a common entity accounting for nearly 2–3% of all hospital admissions [25]. It is a priority for the patient and the caregivers to break this vicious cycle of recurrent episodes of infection by adopting proper measures for skincare and being prompt for any breach in the continuity of the skin.

16.5.5 Lymphorrhoea

Lymphorrhoea is commonly perceived as 'wet leaky legs'. This entity is often mismanaged in the community due to lack of awareness on the causes responsible for the condition. In simple terms, cleaning up the leaking fluid is of immediate and utmost importance rather than trying to treat the underlying cause first. A better management approach is using compression therapy. If left untreated, the loss of fluid can be severe enough to debilitate the patient and he/she might be forced to use plastic bags and soaking incontinence pads to absorb the leaking fluid. Therefore, compression therapy is perhaps the only way to resolve this condition. Compression therapy in form of short-stretch compression bandaging can be used. Lymphorrhoea usually gets controlled once oedema reduces with compression therapy [26].

16.6 Management Protocol for Infection in Lower Limb Oedema

Management of infection in the vulnerable population is definitely laborious and time consuming. Therefore, it is very important to educate, counsel and encourage patients themselves for their own care as there has been evidence that this ultimately improves their outcomes [27]. The management protocol for infection prevention and treatment has been summarized in Fig. 16.2 a, b [28].

16.7 Antibiotic Therapy

Antibiotics should not be routinely used to treat the lower limb swelling until there is evidence of infection. Appropriate antibiotic therapy is essential for effective control of infections at early stages. Role of both empirical and target directed therapy should be kept in mind while prescribing antibiotics for infections. While there is no controversy on indications of antibiotics for acute episodes of cellulitis in lower limb oedema, opinions vary on the use of prophylactic low-dose antibiotics for prevention of recurrence [9]. However, recurrence in cellulitis is common and is most

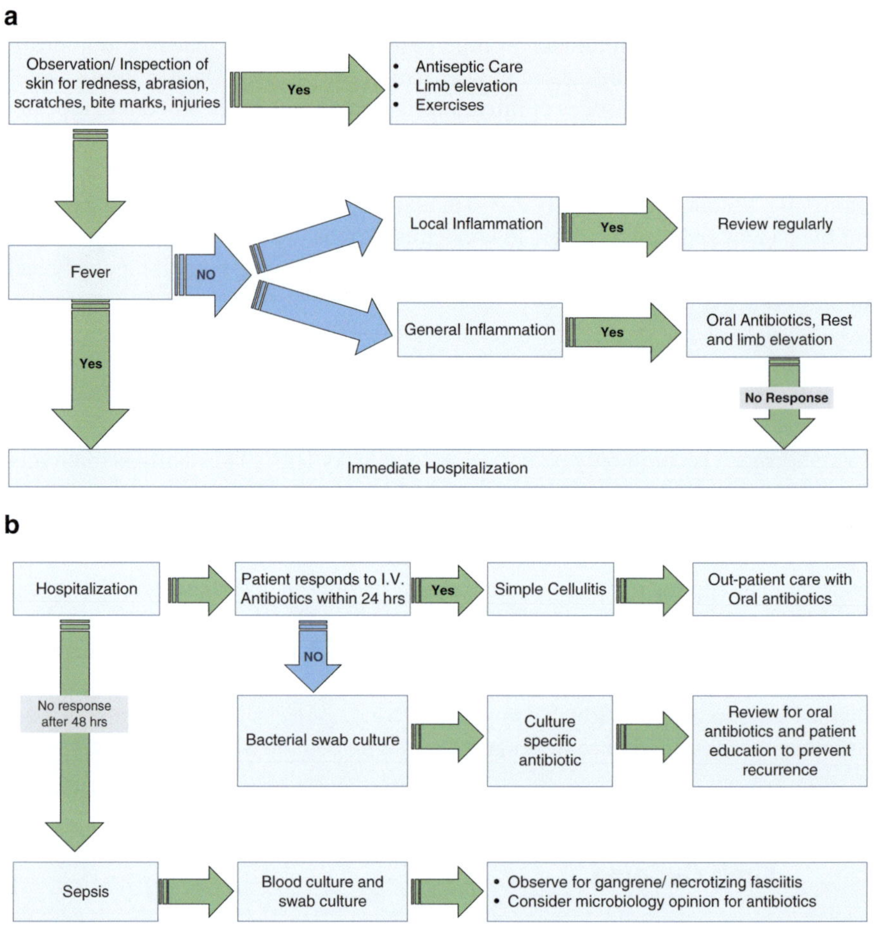

Fig. 16.2 Protocol for management of infection (**a**) prior to hospitalization and (**b**) after hospitalization

commonly caused by the *Streptococcus pyogenes*. Approximately 30% of admissions of cellulitis cases are for recurrent ones [29]. The recurrence rates progressively increase with time after the first episode of cellulitis [5]. Therefore, standard guidelines and randomized control trials provide guidance for appropriate antimicrobial therapy and prophylaxis. Of note, is the PATCH study conducted from June 2006 to January 2010, prior to which there were only a handful of studies inconclusive for prophylactic use of antibiotics in cases of lower limb oedema.

Majority of the studies have revealed the predominance of *Streptococcus pyogenes* and *Staphylococcus aureus* in these infections. Among other causes, *Streptococcus pneumoniae, Haemophilus influenzae*, Gram-negative bacilli and anaerobes are also responsible [30]. Therefore, the choice of antibiotic for prophylaxis should be based on the recent microbiological aetiology of the infection. Choice of the same antibiotic for both treatment and prophylaxis should be avoided.

The major recommendations from few of the listed trials and guidelines have been mentioned followed by the preferred choice of antibiotics in Tables 16.3 and 16.4, respectively [7, 30, 31].

While most of the international bodies from developed countries advocate the above choice of antibiotics, situations in developing countries are worrisome, which are often marked by the burden of multi-drug resistant pathogens. In this aspect, the Indian Council of Medical Research [11] has developed treatment guidelines on common syndrome approach in recognition with the problem of antimicrobial resistance. As per these guidelines following are the choice of antibiotics usually employed in regions of probability of infections with drug-resistant pathogens [11] as mentioned in Table 16.5.

Table 16.3 Recommendations for antibiotic prophylaxis in cellulitis

Name of the trial/body	Major inferences/guidelines
CREST	Recommended antibiotic prophylaxis for 1–2 years in patients with predisposing conditions who have had at least 2 episodes of cellulitis.
PATCH	Following first episode or recurrent cellulitis of lower limb, prophylactic low dose penicillin is effective and cost effective in preventing subsequent attacks.
NICE	Provided the choice of antibiotics for treatment and prophylaxis.

Table 16.4 Choice of antibiotics based on international guidelines

Indications	Antibiotics
Treatment of cellulitis	Flucloxacillin oral 500 mg 4 times daily for 7 days If not oral Flucloxacillin IV 2 gm 4 times daily, review after 48 h If allergic to penicillin Clarithromycin/Erythromycin oral 500 mg 4 times daily for 7 days
Prophylaxis	Phenoxymethyl penicillin 250 mg twice daily If allergic to penicillin Clarithromycin/Erythromycin oral 250 mg twice daily

Table 16.5 Choice of antibiotics in infections with drug-resistant pathogens

Indications	Antibiotics
Treatment of cellulitis	Cefazolin/cephalexin/amoxicillin-clavulanate +/– clindamycin for 7 days Doses: Cefazolin 1–2 g IV/8 hrly Cephalexin 750 mg BD, 500 mg TID Amoxicillin-clavulanate 1gm BD oral, 1.2 gm IV TDS Clindamycin 600–900 mg IV/8 hrly
Necrotizing fasciitis	Piperacillin-tazobactam +/– clindamycin for 14 days Ciprofloxacin + doxycycline for 14 days if *Aeromonas/Vibrio* spp. suspected Doses: Piperacillin-tazobactam (4.5 gm IV/ 6 hrly) + clindamycin (600 mg IV TDS) Ciprofloxacin 750 mg IV BD Doxycycline: 200 mg IV stat followed by 100 mg 1-0-1

16.8 State of the Art in Developing Countries

Developing countries like India are often challenged with the dual problem of unhygienic living conditions often promoting infections and the burden of multidrug-resistant organisms causing infection. Adding to this is the epidemiologic transition in the burden of non-communicable diseases from infectious diseases in most of the developing countries [19]. On one hand, among the major causes of limb oedema, the incidence of filariasis in India is on the decline. On the other hand, India has become the epicentre of many of the comorbid conditions like diabetes, hypertension and associated chronic kidney and liver diseases. Consequently, the challenges of addressing the management and effective control of lower limb oedema have also increased. Poor living conditions, lack of basic amenities, increased levels of malnourishment and undernourishment, inadequate health care facilities and above all lack of awareness and patient education have made infections in vulnerable patients a common entity.

Several cultural practices like walking barefoot, intake of raw salt with meals also compromise personal care. It should be emphasized that in this regard certain traditional practices definitely have a positive impact towards prevention of infection in these cases. While walking barefoot definitely predisposes to infection and provides an easy entry point for invasion by microorganisms, it should be acknowledged that on the contrary it facilitates better control of the foot position on striking the ground, improves balance, proprioception and muscle strength and develops better foot mechanics [32]. Similarly, integrative approaches involving dermatology therapy coupled with Indian medicine and a set of yoga exercises often addresses the issue of infection and lower limb oedema simultaneously in a much better way [33]. Whatever might be the situation, successful control of infection in any case of lower limb oedema can be done with an appropriate combination of self-care by the patient based on his/her training, education and a dedicated professional team.

16.9 Challenges and Future Directions

Despite considerable progress in our understanding and management of infection in lower limb oedema, several gaps in knowledge exist that require special attention and more scientific evidence. Our understanding of pathophysiology of infections in these cases with respect to skin microbiome alterations should be revealed for better care. While there have been studies revealing that skin commensals can affect the composition of the local microbiome and alter local immunity [34], further studies should clarify the relationships between the microbiome and infections. While microbiological diagnosis of infections is still challenging owing to lack of adequate resources and opinions on the methodologies in practice, exact causes of recurrent infections are not yet established. There has been no universal agreement on effective antibiotic regimens, the preferred antibiotics and the optimal duration of treatment in cases of cellulitis. Studies evaluating the effects of several of the newer regimens on treatment costs and hospitalizations should also be prioritized. The exact role of compression therapy is still debatable. However, there is enough evidence that successful control of infections in lower limb oedema requires a multidisciplinary team of expert physiotherapists, dieticians, specialized nurses, occupational therapists and psychologists to tackle these challenges.

Disclaimers and Disclosure of Conflicts of Interest None.

Prior Presentations None.

Sources of Support that Require Acknowledgement None.

References

1. Topham EJ, Mortimer PS. Chronic lower limb oedema. Clin Med. 2002;2(1):28.
2. Ely JW, Osheroff JA, Chambliss ML, Ebell MH. Approach to leg edema of unclear etiology. J Am Board Fam Med. 2006;19(2):148–60.
3. Fife CE, Farrow W, Hebert AA, Armer NC, Stewart BR, Cormier JN, Armer JM. Skin and wound care in lymphedema patients: a taxonomy, primer, and literature review. Adv Skin Wound Care. 2017;30(7):305–18.
4. Al-Niaimi F, Cox N. Cellulitis and lymphoedema: a vicious cycle. J Lymphoedema. 2009;4(2):38–42.
5. Cranendonk DR, Lavrijsen AP, Prins JM, Wiersinga WJ. Cellulitis: current insights into pathophysiology and clinical management. Neth J Med. 2017 Nov;75(9):366–78.
6. Atkin L. Lower-limb oedema: assessment, treatment and challenges. Br J Community Nurs. 2014;19(Suppl 10):S22–8.
7. NICE. Cellulitis and erysipelas: antimicrobial prescribing. [Internet]. National Institute for Health and care excellence. 2019. [Viewed 03 August 2020]. Available from: www.nice.org.uk/guidance/ng141
8. Banerjee T, Das A, Singh A, Bansal R, Basu S. The microflora of chronic diabetic foot ulcers based on culture and molecular examination: a descriptive study. Wound Manag Prev. 2019;65(5):16–23.
9. Sullivan T, de Barra E. Diagnosis and management of cellulitis. Clin Med. 2018;18(2):160.
10. Tianyi FL, Mbanga CM, Danwang C, Agbor VN. Risk factors and complications of lower limb cellulitis in Africa: a systematic review. BMJ Open. 2018;8(7):e021175.
11. ICMR. Treatment Guidelines for Antimicrobial Use in Common Syndromes. [Internet]. Indian Council of Medical Research. 2019. [Viewed 25 July 2020]. Available from: http://www.ijmm.org/documents/Treatment_Guidelines_2019_Final.pdf
12. Morris A. Cellulitis and erysipelas. Clin Evid. 2004;11:2133–9.
13. Eron LJ, Lipsky BA. Use of cultures in cellulitis: when, how, and why. Eur J Clin Microbiol Infect Dis. 2006;25:615–7.
14. Weng QY, Raff AB, Cohen JM, Gunasekera N, Okhovat JP, Vedak P, Joyce C, Kroshinsky D, Mostaghimi A. Costs and consequences associated with misdiagnosed lower extremity cellulitis. JAMA Dermatol. 2017;153(2):141–6.
15. Todd M. Self-management in chronic oedema. Br J Nurs. 2013;22(12):701–4.
16. Lehman LF, Geyer MJ, Bolton L. American leprosy missions — ten steps: a guide for health promotion and empowerment of people affected by neglected tropical diseases. [Internet]. Care for Swelling (Edema). [Viewed on 26 July 2020]. Available from: ALM-10Steps-Step8-021816.pdf (leprosy.org)

17. Bertelli DF, de Oliveira P, Gimenes AS, Moreno MA. Postural drainage and manual lymphatic drainage for lower limb edema in women with morbid obesity after bariatric surgery: a randomized controlled trial. Am J Phys Med Rehabil. 2013;92(8):697–703.
18. Bianchi J, Vowden K, Whitaker J. Chronic oedema made easy. Wounds UK. 2012;8(2):1–4.
19. Natarajan K. Practical approach to pedal Edema. J Assoc Physicians India. 2017;401–4.
20. Moffatt C, Martin R, Smithdale R. Leg ulcer management. Wiley-Blackwell; 2007.
21. Grey JE, Enoch S, Harding KG. ABC of wound healing: venous and arterial leg ulcers. BMJ. 2006;332(Suppl S4)
22. Webb E, Neeman T, Bowden FJ, Gaida J, Mumford V, Bissett B. Compression therapy to prevent recurrent cellulitis of the leg. N Engl J Med. 2020;383(7):630–9.
23. Anderson I. Aetiology, assessment and management of leg ulcers. Wound Essentials. 2006;1:20–36.
24. Cox NH. Management of lower leg cellulitis. Clin Med. 2002;2(1):23.
25. Posnett J, Franks P. The burden of chronic wounds in the UK. Nurs Times. 2008;104(3):44–5.
26. Anderson I. 'Leaky legs': strategies for the treatment and management of lower-limb lymphorrhoea. Nurs Times. 2017;113(1):50–3.
27. Department of Health. Equality and Excellence: Liberating the NHS. 2010. [Internet]. Viewed on25 July 2020. Available from: http://tinyurl.com/2dcyc82.
28. Eagle M. Understanding cellulitis of the lower limb. Wound Essentials. 2007;2:34–44.
29. Inghammar M, Rasmussen M, Linder A. Recurrent erysipelas-risk factors and clinical presentation. BMC Infect Dis. 2014;14(1):1–6.
30. UK Dermatology Clinical Trials Network's PATCH Trial Team. Prophylactic antibiotics for the prevention of cellulitis (erysipelas) of the leg: results of the UK dermatology clinical trials network's Patch II trial. Br J Dermatol. 2012;166(1):169–78.
31. Mason JM, Thomas KS, Crook AM, Foster KA, Chalmers JR, Nunn AJ, Williams HC. Prophylactic antibiotics to prevent cellulitis of the leg: economic analysis of the PATCH I & II trials. PLoS One. 2014;9(2):e82694.
32. Lindberg S. Does walking barefoot have health benefits?. [Viewed on 27 July 2020]. Available from: Does Walking Barefoot Have Health Benefits (medexpress.com).
33. Bose KS, Aggithaya GM. An integrative treatment for lower limb lymphoedema in India. Br J Community Nurs. 2011;16(Sup10):S22–7.
34. Christensen GJ, Brüggemann H. Bacterial skin commensals and their role as host guardians. Benef Microbes. 2014;5(2):201–15.

17 Dermatological Manifestations in Lower Limb Swelling

Tulika Rai

17.1 Manuscript Body

There can be many causes of lower limb swelling. The common causes of lower limb swelling from a dermatologist perspective can be broadly classified into-

1. Infectious causes
   (a) Bacterial skin infections—cellulitis, actinomycetoma
   (b) Deep fungal infections
      - Eumycetoma/Madura foot
2. Cellulitis mimics
   - Eosinophilic cellulitis
   - Pseudocellulitis
   - Venous disease
   - Lipodermatosclerosis
3. Dermatitis
   - Irritant contact dermatitis
   - Allergic contact dermatitis
   - Venous dermatitis
4. Thyroid dermopathy
5. Hansen's disease and lepra reactions
6. Drugs and adverse drug reactions
7. Malignancies

T. Rai (✉)
Department of Dermatology and Venereology, Institute of Medical Sciences, Banaras Hindu University, Varanasi, India

S. K. Tiwary (ed.), *Approach to Lower Limb Oedema*,
https://doi.org/10.1007/978-981-16-6206-5_17

17.2 Bacterial Skin Infections

17.2.1 Cellulitis

17.2.1.1 Introduction

Cellulitis is a common and painful skin infection caused by bacteria. Cellulitis may be defined as an acute infection of the skin involving the dermis and subcutaneous tissues. The predominant organisms causing cellulitis are Gram-positive bacteria such as *Streptococcus* species and *Staphylococcus aureus.* Positive blood cultures are found in less than 10% of cases. Wound or tissue cultures are negative in up to 70% cases [1], with *S aureus,* group A streptococci and group G streptococci being the most common isolates from wound cultures.

17.2.1.2 Clinical Features

The classic presentation of rubor (redness), dolor (pain), tumor (swelling), calor (heat) are the main features of cellulitis. Cellulitis of the legs may present with a painful, erythematous, localized swelling which is mostly unilateral. The spectrum of disease severity may range from localized erythema in a systemically well patient to the rapidly spreading erythema and fulminant sepsis seen with necrotizing fasciitis in few of the patients. If the pain is out of proportion to the clinical signs and is accompanied by a history of rapid progression, then one should consider a diagnosis of a necrotizing fasciitis [2]. Careful clinical examination may sometimes reveal a portal of entry such as insect bites, ulcers, trauma, eczema, or cutaneous mycosis in few patients [3]. The finding of bilateral lower limb erythema or edema in an afebrile patient with normal inflammatory markers should prompt the clinician to reconsider the diagnosis of cellulitis [4].

17.2.1.3 Differential Diagnosis

Few studies have concluded that approximately one-third of cellulitis patients are misdiagnosed [5]. The common differential diagnoses of cellulitis include venous dermatitis or stasis dermatitis, irritant contact dermatitis, allergic contact dermatitis, lymphoedema, and lipodermatosclerosis.

17.2.1.4 Management

It may be useful to carry out baseline assessment of liver and renal function for assessing end-organ dysfunction in patients who develop sepsis because of untreated cellulitis and also for appropriate dose of antimicrobials. Cultures of blood, aspirates, or biopsies are usually not recommended but should be considered in patients with systemic features of sepsis who are immunosuppressed or for cases associated with immersion injuries or animal bites [6].

Cellulitis is known to resolve slowly. Signs of inflammation and fever often persist during the first 72 h of treatment. Management should include limb elevation and continuing narrow-spectrum antimicrobial therapy alongside treatment of comorbid conditions exacerbating the cellulitis (lower limb oedema, diabetes mellitus, peripheral vascular disease) [7].

Non-purulent skin and soft tissue infections require treatment with systemic antimicrobials. Oral antimicrobial therapy is adequate for patients with no systemic signs of infection and no comorbidities, however few of such patients may require an initial period of intravenous (IV) antibiotic therapy if they do not respond adequately to oral antibiotics. Sometimes cellulitis may be accompanied by one or more pustules, folliculitis, furuncles, or abscesses with or without purulent drainage or exudate and is then referred to as purulent. Incision and drainage may be needed in purulent lesions. Intravenous agents should be used for those with evidence of systemic infection or those who do not respond to initial oral therapy.

The choice of antimicrobials may vary depending on the disease severity and from region to region according to local practice guidelines and resistance rates. Guidance from UK CREST recommends an agent with both anti-streptococcal and anti-staphylococcal activity, such as flucloxacillin [8]. For patients with mild disease, oral antibiotics like dicloxacillin 250 mg or cephalexin 500 mg 4 times a day for seven days works well. Cellulitis usually has a good prognosis with treatment. Patients with a known history of, or risk factors for, methicillin-resistant staphylococcal aureus (MRSA) colonization as well as in those with suspected necrotizing fasciitis spectrum should receive broad-spectrum antibiotics like linezolid for 7–14 days depending on the severity [9].

The optimal duration of antimicrobial therapy is not clear and 1–2 weeks of oral antibiotics is unnecessary. Recent evidence suggests that a 5-day course of oral antibiotics may be sufficient for uncomplicated cellulitis.

17.3 Mimics of Cellulitis

17.3.1 Well's Syndrome or Eosinophilic Cellulitis

17.3.1.1 Introduction

The term "eosinophilic cellulitis" was first introduced by Wells and Smith in the year 1971. Wells' syndrome, or eosinophilic cellulitis, is an uncommon dermatosis that is a recurrent, hypersensitivity reaction to an arthropod bite, drug, infections, Churg-Strauss syndrome, or an overlap with hypereosinophilic syndrome [10]. It has also been described in children after some vaccination. The etiopathogenesis is poorly understood, but aberrant and inadequate eosinophil skin homing may be one of the key mechanisms of the pathogenesis of Wells syndrome. There may a disturbed eosinophilic response.

17.3.1.2 Clinical Features

It is characterized by pruritic, erythematous, and edematous plaques that evolve rapidly over a period of 2–3 days. The lesions often regress spontaneously over a period of 2–8 weeks, leaving hyperpigmentation which may persist though scarring does not occur [11]. The disease may follow a waxing and waning, recurrent course, which may last for years [12]. The diagnosis should be considered in those with presumed cellulitis and eosinophilia who fail to respond to standard course of

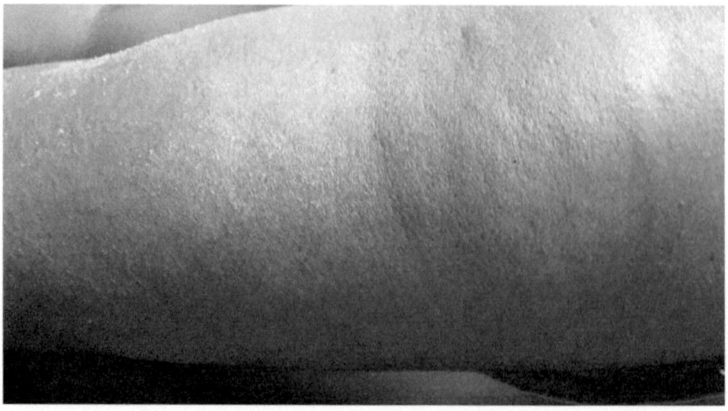

Fig. 17.1 An erythematous, edematous plaque seen on posterior aspect of the right thigh in a 30-year-old male—a case of eosinophilic cellulitis. (Picture contribution by Dr. Usha Chandra, KGMU)

antibiotics and also have pruritis as one of the symptoms [Fig. 17.1]. Sometimes such lesions may occur on the lower extremity and may present with localized lower limb erythema and edema [Fig. 17.1].

17.3.1.3 Histopathological Findings

The histopathological findings of skin lesions follow an evolutionary course through acute, subacute, and resolving stages. A 4 mm punch biopsy can be taken from the center of the lesion [11]. Dermal edema and an eosinophilic infiltrate in the upper and deep dermis characterize the acute stage. In the subacute stage, the hallmark is "flame figures," which are intense eosinophilic degranulation of major basic protein coating collagen bundles in the dermis. The histopathological findings will depend on the age of the lesion. There is a diffuse infiltrate composed predominantly of eosinophils with few lymphocytes and histiocytes. The hallmark "flame figures "may not be found in all skin biopsies.

17.3.1.4 Treatment

Oral antihistamines are effective in few cases. In refractory cases, oral corticosteroids may be given for a short course. Prednisolone may be given at a dose of 0.5–1 mg/kg/day for a period of 2–3 weeks in tapering doses. Other treatment options include topical corticosteroids, antimicrobials including minocycline and dapsone, colchicine, antimalarial drugs, and oral psoralen with ultraviolet A (PUVA), low dose cyclosporine, azathioprine, and interferon [12].

17.3.2 Pseudocellulitis

Pseudocellulitis is a noninfectious condition that can mimic cellulitis. Gemcitabine, a chemotherapeutic agent, has been known to cause a rash in thirty percent of patients [13]. Rashes seen with gemcitabine chemotherapy have been described as dermatitis, often from radiation recall, to myositis or erysipeloid reactions [14]. Radiation recall dermatitis reactions are known to occur on areas of the body that were radiated in the past. However, there are case reports in the literature of lower extremity pseudocellulitis in an area of the body that had never been radiated. Few authors believe that pseudocellulitis could occur in lower extremities due to drug accumulation in the subcutaneous tissues, especially where there may be impaired lymphatic drainage [15].

17.4 Deep Fungal Infections

17.4.1 Mycetoma

17.4.1.1 Introduction

Mycetoma is a localized, chronic, suppurative, infection affecting skin, subcutaneous tissue, and bones prevalent in tropical and subtropical regions. Gill first recognized mycetoma as a disease entity in 1842 in the southern province of Madura [16], from where the commonly used name "Madura foot" got prevalent. A formal classification was given by Chalmers and Archibald, who divided them into two groups [17].

- Group 1: Madura mycosis, caused by true fungi, and
- Group 2: Actinomycetoma, caused by actinomyces which are bacteria

17.4.1.2 Etiopathogenesis

Mycetomas are caused by various species of fungi and bacteria, which are commonly found as saprophytes in soil or on the plants. Actinomycotic mycetoma is caused by aerobic species of actinomycetes belonging to the genera *Nocardia, Streptomyces,* and *Actinomadura,* with *Nocardia brasiliensis, Actinomadura madurae, Actinomadura pelletieri*, and *Streptomyces somaliensis* being most common. Eumycotic mycetoma is caused by a variety of fungi, the most common being *Madurella mycetomatis* [18]. The causative organisms vary from region to region and also differ in various countries. In India, *Nocardia* species and *Madurella grisea* are the most common causative organisms of mycetoma [19].

17.4.1.3 Clinical Features

More than seventy-five percent of patients have a lesion of lower extremity, most commonly in the foot (70%), followed by hand involvement [Figs. 17.2 and 17.3]. The incubation period is variable, from 3 months to 9 years in natural infections. The patients often do not remember the preceding trauma [20]. The clinical features are fairly uniform, regardless of the organism involved. The pathognomonic feature is a triad of painless firm subcutaneous mass, multiple sinus formation, and a purulent or seropurulent discharge containing grains [18].

Mycetoma usually starts as a small, subcutaneous, painless nodular lesion that gradually increases in size, and the overlying skin usually ruptures to release seropurulent discharge and characteristic grains, which varies according to the causative organism. Mycetoma is usually localized but may extend slowly by direct contiguity along the fascial planes, invading the subcutaneous tissue, fat, ligaments, muscles, and bones [18]. In eumycotic mycetoma, there may be multiple punched-out

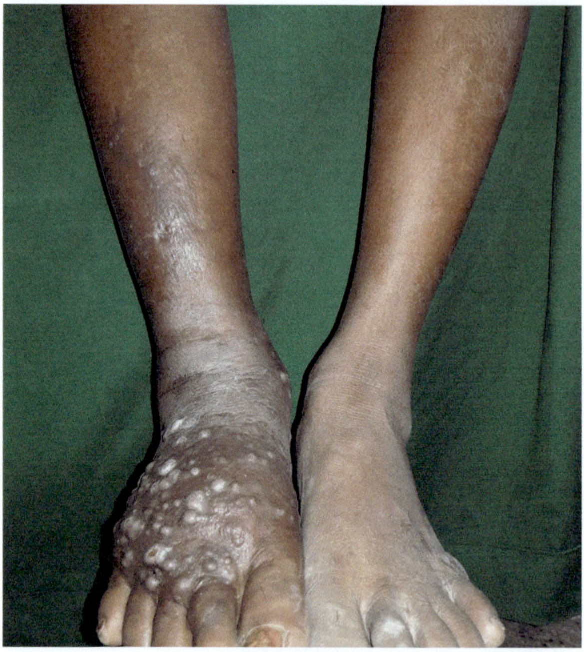

Fig. 17.2 An erythematous plaque present on dorsal aspect of right foot studded with pustular and nodular lesions with edema extending up to lower one-third of the right leg—a case of eumycetoma

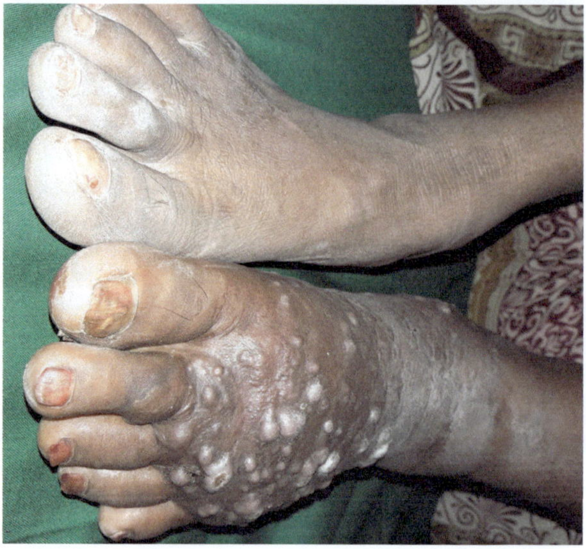

Fig. 17.3 An erythematous, edematous plaque with pustular and nodular lesions with draining sinuses on dorsal aspect of left foot with edema extending up to the ankle joint—a case of eumycetoma. (Picture contribution by Dr Usha Chandra, KGMU)

lytic lesions in bones, whereas actinomycotic mycetoma is characterized by both osteolytic and osteosclerotic lesions. Mycetoma leads to gross swelling of the affected part with deformity. Actinomycetoma tends to progress more rapidly than eumycotic mycetoma, with greater inflammation and tissue destruction and earlier invasion of bone.

17.4.1.4 Histopathology and Investigations

In all cases, histopathological and microbiological examination is important, but sometimes it is difficult to culture the causative organism. In the case of eumycetoma, suppurative granulomas composed of neutrophils are seen surrounding characteristic grains. In actinomycetoma, histopathology shows the homogeneous eosinophilic material around the grain in a star-shaped manner (Splendore-Hoeppli reaction). Serological tests exist but are not so reliable. The molecular techniques to identify relevant antigens have shown promise.

17.4.1.5 Treatment

The disease is notoriously difficult to treat. Eumycetoma may be unresponsive to standard antifungal therapy, which is usually given for 1–2 years. Oral itraconazole is quite effective and given as 400 mg/day in two divided doses with frequent monitoring of liver function tests. Actinomycetoma responds to antibiotic therapy, but prolonged treatment is necessary. The common consensus is that cotrimoxazole should be administered as a gold standard therapy in all actinomycetoma patients. The most commonly described regimens for actinomycetoma include streptomycin plus either TMP-sulfamethoxazole or dapsone. Combination antibiotic therapy is preferred to avoid the development of drug resistance and to eradicate any residual infection [18, 20].

17.4.2 Dermatitis

The word dermatitis and eczema are used as synonyms, but all dermatitis are not eczemas. Eczema is derived from a Greek word ekzem (meaning "to boil out"), is a reaction of the skin to various exogenous and endogenous causes and may present as acute, subacute, or chronic forms. Dermatitis is a group of noninfectious, inflammatory skin disorders in which there are pathological changes in the epidermis and dermis.

17.4.2.1 Introduction

Contact dermatitis (CD) is an inflammatory skin disease caused by chemicals or metal ions that exert irritant or toxic effects or by small reactive chemicals (contact allergens) that modify proteins and induce immune responses (predominantly by T-cell response) [21].

17.4.2.2 Classification

Contact dermatitis may manifest as irritant contact dermatitis and allergic contact dermatitis, which may occur in acute or chronic forms. Irritant contact dermatitis due to the application of any irritant is usually associated with erythema and pruritus and is usually localized to one limb. Dermatitis is therefore an important differential diagnosis to keep in mind whenever a patient presents with localized erythema, edema, scaling, and pruritus Fig. 17.4.

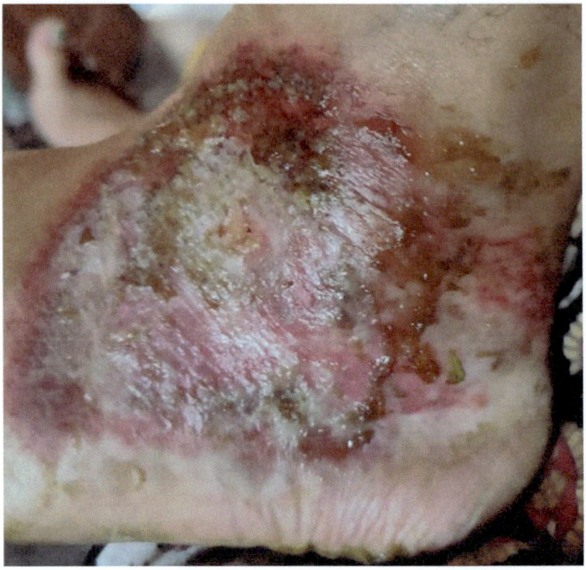

Fig. 17.4 A 45-year-old female presented with a localized, erythematous plaque with purulent discharge on lateral aspect of the left foot extending up to ankle joint with edema of the left foot—a case of irritant contact dermatitis due to camphor application

Irritant contact dermatitis (ICD) is a nonspecific skin response to direct chemical skin damage and there is release of inflammatory mediators, whereas allergic contact dermatitis is a delayed hypersensitivity reaction (type IV) to allergens, which includes immune responses (due to the interaction of T cells and cytokines) [21].

In irritant contact dermatitis, there are no immune reactions. There is no prior exposure to any substance (sensitization) as compared to allergic contact dermatitis, where sensitization is required. Most individuals exposed to such substance will manifest a similar reaction. Irritant contact dermatitis can occur as an acute or chronic disease. Lesions may occur anywhere but commonly appear on the hands.

17.4.2.3 Clinical Features of ICD

Acute irritant contact dermatitis is typically characterized by erythema, vesicles, pustules, hemorrhage, and erosions, and also with pruritus or even pain. Skin lesions in acute irritant contact dermatitis usually have a sharp border in the areas of contact (distant spread does not occur) and are usually asymmetric. Sometimes superficial bacterial infection may be superimposed on lesions of irritant contact dermatitis, leading to pain and edema. If ICD occurs on the lower limb, it may present with lower limb edema [Fig. 17.5].

One of the conditions frequently seen by dermatologists in India is **Paederus dermatitis**, an irritant contact dermatitis related to exposure to the rove beetle characterized by bullous lesions with surrounding erythema. Sometimes, very extensive lesions may be seen on the lower limbs with superadded bacterial skin infection. The causative toxin is pederin, which protects the beetle against predators and resides within the beetle's hemolymph, the equivalent of blood in most

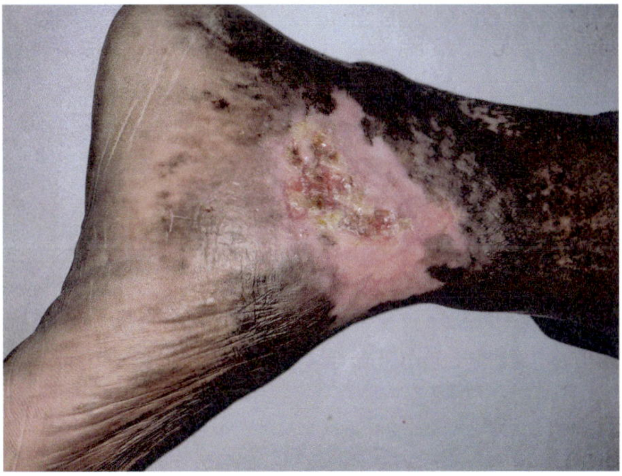

Fig. 17.5 A case of stasis dermatitis with surrounding 45-year-old skin changes

invertebrates. Exposure to pederin toxin occurs via direct contact with beetle secretions, usually via vigorous brushing or crushing of the beetle on the skin, and the patient will develop a rash at the site of inoculation an average of 12–72 h after initial exposure. The rash presents as linear vesicles with underlying erythema that forms over several days, which progresses into bullae. The distribution is often in areas of exposed skin, and the lesions may be associated with burning, pruritus, and pain, and the surrounding erythematous skin.

17.4.2.4 Clinical Features of Allergic Contact Dermatitis

In *allergic contact dermatitis*, a prior sensitization to the allergen occurs in all cases. In acute allergic contact dermatitis, the skin lesions develop after 24–48 h of exposure to the allergen. There may be erythema, vesiculation, and itching. The borders are not well demarcated, and skin lesions may develop at distant sites also. In chronic allergic contact dermatitis, skin lesions may persist and develop lichenification and fissuring.

17.4.3 Venous Eczema

This is also known as stasis dermatitis. It occurs secondary to venous hypertension and is a common condition that usually presents as eczematous lesions around the ankles and lower legs. Varicose veins are commonly associated with patches of dermatitis arising preferentially over them and around the ankle joint. Venous dermatitis is often the first manifestation of venous insufficiency and needs to be treated early. The condition is intensely pruritic, and other features of venous hypertension like leg edema (more towards evening), hemosiderin depositions, pigmented purpuric dermatoses, venous ulcerations, small patches of atrophic telangiectatic scarring and lipodermatosclerosis develop over a period of time [22].

The standard therapy includes the topical administration of highly potent corticosteroids and a long-term compression therapy. Few studies have shown benefit of oral doxycycline and ointment tacrolimus [23].

17.4.4 Thyroid Dermopathy

17.4.4.1 Introduction

There may be many causes of leg edema. Thyroid dermopathy may be a cause of leg edema, and there is always a delay in diagnosis, and this should be one differential diagnosis of nonpitting leg edema. Thyroid dermopathy can be readily diagnosed on clinical examination and by histopathologic examination of a skin biopsy specimen.

17.4.4.2 Clinical Features

Although thyroid dermopathy is rare, the treating physician should be alert when assessing patients with edema to establish the correct diagnosis and prevent unnecessary treatments, such as multiple courses of antibiotics. Most patients will have a preceding history of thyroid disease. It is characterized by localized nonpitting edema secondary to the deposition of dermal and subcutaneous hyaluronic acid.

The nonpitting edema form of thyroid dermopathy is the most prevalent presentation. The nodular form has been reported in 20% of cases, and the plaque-like form occurs in about 21% of cases. The elephantiasis form is a rare and extreme form of thyroid dermopathy, occurring in only 1 of 150 patients with skin involvement. Hyperpigmentation and progressive thickening usually accompany nonpitting edema, and the skin becomes thickened, woody, and firm, with a black-gray appearance. The combined incidence of the polypoid and elephantiasis types represents less than 1% of cases. More than one type can coexist. The shins are most commonly involved, but other sites may be affected [24].

17.4.4.3 Histopathology

Skin biopsy specimens from patients with thyroid dermopathy show normal collagen and wide separation of the superficial dermal collagen bundles with mucin deposition. Special stains such as Alcian blue indicate the presence of mucin between the separated collagen bundles. The etiopathogenesis is poorly understood. Patient should be investigated for thyroid disease.

17.4.4.4 Management

A thyroid profile test, anti-TPO (thyroid peroxidase), TSI (thyroid-stimulating immunoglobulin) should be done for all patients. Treatment options are limited with little efficacy. A high degree of clinical suspicion and careful evaluation may be important to diagnose such cases.

17.5 Hansen's Disease and Lepra Reactions

This is a chronic infectious and granulomatous disease caused by Mycobacterium leprae, which affects the skin and peripheral nerves. It causes social stigma and can cause disability in a small proportion of cases if not treated timely. The disease can have a spectrum of presentation depending on the immune status of the patient. Ridley and Jopling classification of leprosy is the most accepted classification system.

Ridley Jopling classification includes:

- Tuberculoid (TT)
- Borderline tuberculoid (BT)
- Mid-borderline (BB)
- Borderline lepromatous (BL)
- Lepromatous (LL)

The patients of Hansen's can develop lepra reactions due to change in the immune status of patients after giving MDT (Multidrug therapy) or if the patient downgrades during the course of the disease. Type 1 lepra reactions usually develop within 6 months of starting MDT in borderline leprosy patients. The existing skin lesions may develop erythema and swelling. Patients may present with oedema of hands and feet. Patients may have severe neuritis leading to nerve damage. In India, patients of Hansen's disease are commonly seen by dermatologists. Patients with Lepromatous leprosy may also present with bilateral pitting lower limb oedema. Patient with borderline leprosy may develop type 1 lepra reactions when they can present with lower limb swelling along with severe neuritis and inflammation of skin lesions.

Disclaimers and Disclosure of Conflicts of Interest None.

Prior Presentations None.

Sources of Support that Require Acknowledgment Image contribution by Dr. Usha Chandra.

References

1. Eron LJ, Lipsky BA. Use of cultures in cellulitis: when, how, and why? Eur J Clin Microbiol Infect Dis. 2006;25:615–7.
2. Keller EC, Tomecki KJ, Alraies MC. Distinguishing cellulitis from its mimics. Cleve Clin J Med. 2012;79:547–52.
3. Eriksson B, Jorup-Rönström C, Karkkonen K, Sjöblom AC, Holm SE. Erysipelas: clinical and bacteriolo gic spectrum and serological aspects. Clin Infect Dis. 1996;23:1091–8.

4. Weng QY, Raff AB, Cohen JM, et al. Costs and consequences associated with misdiagnosed lower extremity cellulitis. JAMA Dermatol. 2017;153:141–6.
5. Levell NJ, Wingfield CG, Garioch JJ. Severe lower limb cellulitis is best diagnosed by dermatologists and managed with shared care between primary and secondary care. Br J Dermatol. 2011;164:1326–8.
6. Stevens DL, Bisno AL, Chambers HF, et al. Practice guidelines for the diagnosis and management of skin and soft tissue infections: 2014 update by the Infectious Diseases Society of America. Clin Infect Dis. 2014;59:e10–52.
7. Sullivan T, de Barra E. Diagnosis and management of cellulitis. Clin Med (Lon).2018;18(2):160–3.
8. Fulton R, Doherty L, Gill D, et al. Guidelines on the management of cellulitis in adults. CREST: Northern Ireland; 2005.
9. Eron LJ, Lipsky BA, Low DE, et al. Managing skin and soft tissue infections: expert panel recommendations on key decision points. J Antimicrob Chemother. 2003;52(Suppl 1):i3–17.
10. Fujimoto N, Wakabayashi M, Kato T, Nishio C, Tanaka T. Wells syndrome associated with Churg–Strauss syndrome. Clin Exp Dermatol. 2011;36:46–8.
11. Moossavi M, Mehregan DR. Wells' syndrome: A clinical and histopathologic review of seven cases. Int J Dermatol. 2003;42:62–7.
12. Gilliam AE, Bruckner AL, Howard RM, Lee BP, Wu S, Frieden IJ. Bullous "cellulitis" with eosinophilia: Case report and review of Wells' syndrome in childhood. Pediatrics. 2005;116:e149–55.
13. Ohtsuka T. Oral tacrolimus treatment for refractory eosinophilic cellulitis. Clin Exp Dermatol. 2009;34:e597–8.
14. Tan DHS, Bunce PE, Liles WC, Gold WL. Gemcitabine-related "pseudocellulitis": Report of 2 cases and review of the literature. Clin Infect Dis. 2007;45:e72–6.
15. Korniyenko A, Lozada J, Ranade A, Sandhu G. Recurrent lower extremity pseudocellulitis. Am J Therapeut. 2012;19(4):e141–2.
16. Carter HV. On a new and striking form of fungus disease principally affecting the foot and prevailing endemically in many parts of India. Trans Med Phys Soc Bombay. 1860;6:104–42.
17. Chalmers AJ, Archibald RG. A Sudanese maduromycoses. Ann Trop Med. 1916;10:169.
18. Relhan V, Mahajan K, Agarwal P, Garg VK. Mycetoma: an update. Indian J Dermatol. 2017;62:332–40.
19. Maiti PK, Ray A, Bandyopadhyay S. Epidemiological aspects of mycetoma from a retrospective study of 264 cases in West Bengal. Trop Med Int Health. 2002;7:788–92.
20. Fahal AH. Mycetoma: a thorn in the flesh. Trans R Soc Trop Med Hyg. 2004;98:3–11.
21. Przybilla B, Rueff F. Contact dermatitis. In: Burgdorf WHC, Plewig G, Wolf HH, Landthaler M, editors. Braun-Falco's dermatology. Berlin: Springer-Verlag; 2009. p. 377–401.
22. Jindal R, Sharma NL, Mahajan VK, Tegta GR. Contact sensitization in venous eczema: preliminary results of patch testing with Indian standard series and topical medicaments. Indian J Dermatol Venereol Leprol. 2009;75:136–41.
23. Maroo N, Choudhury S, Sen S, Chatterjee S. Oral doxycycline with topical tacrolimus for treatment of stasis dermatitis due to chronic venous insufficiency: a pilot study. Indian J Pharmacol. 2012;44(1):111–3.
24. Fatourechi V, Pajouhi M, Fransway AF. Dermopathy of Graves disease (pretibial myxedema); review of 150 cases. Medicine (Baltimore). 1994;73:1–7.

18 Overview of Management in Lower Limb Edema

Satyendra K. Tiwary and Vivek Kumar Katiyar

18.1 Introduction

Lower limb swelling is one of the most common manifestation in clinical practice in many local and systemic diseases. Usually, the condition may be due to trivial cause most of the time but sometimes delayed clinical consultation and irreversibility of the changes due to disease may lead to difficulty in management. A good clinical history with proper clinical examination is essential to confirm the diagnosis and plan further management of the disease.

18.2 Clinical Examination

Clinical examination should be carried out in both the limbs irrespective of their involvement. Examination starts with the inspection mainly to check for any color changes, asymmetry, scars, ulcers, etc. (Fig. 18.1).

Chronic diseases usually present with thickened and discolored skin. Skin changes are also evident in varicose veins. In erysipelas, local edema is often present in addition to skin redness and tenderness. Elevated temperature is present in acute conditions like cellulitis. Pitting edema may be caused by deep vein thrombosis, venous insufficiency, and early stages of lymphedema as well as systemic causes like CHF, edema due to renal etiologies, etc. Non-pitting edema can be seen in cases of filariasis and hypothyroidism. Tenderness of affected area points toward more local causes.

S. K. Tiwary (✉) · V. K. Katiyar
Department of General Surgery, Institute of Medical Sciences, Banaras Hindu University, Varanasi, India

S. K. Tiwary (ed.), *Approach to Lower Limb Oedema*,
https://doi.org/10.1007/978-981-16-6206-5_18

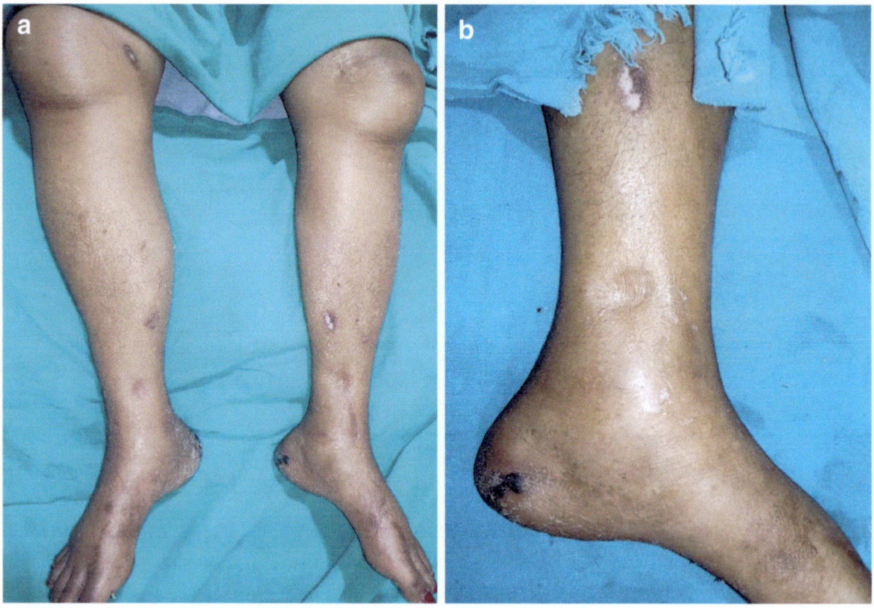

Fig. 18.1 (**a**), (**b**) Post-traumatic lower limb Edema

Clinical examination of both limbs is essential. The Leg-O-Meter (François Zuccarelli, MD, Hospital St-Michel, Service de Chirurgie Vasculaire, Départment de Phlébologie et d'Angeiologie, Paris, France) designed to measure the circumference of the ankle or calf [1]. it is simple to apply for assessing the limb swelling related to venous disease but not related to lymphedema.

Water displacement volumetry is more accurate to assess the limb volume than the circumferential measurements with a tape [2]. The tissue tonicity can also be used to assess the disease but it is more useful in assessing the response of treatment [3]. Bioelectrical impedance is one of the efficient methods to evaluate the swelling but has not yet been evaluated for leg edema [4]. Cesarone [5] developed the edema measuring device.

A plastic plate with protrusions or holes is applied over the swollen limb which applies the pressure and measures the edema. It can differentiate between primary and secondary edema and can be used as a screening tool.

18.3 Radiologic Investigation

18.3.1 Lymphangiogram

This technique was mainly used for visualizing the anatomy of lymphatics. It is an invasive technique. In this technique, direct cannulation of lymphatic through a small incision in skin is carried out. It is painful and time consuming and leads to infection, local inflammation, and fibrosis. This also increases the risk of hypersensitivity reaction and emboli [6].

So, this technique is not used largely. It is only useful in operative interventions like bypass procedure [7].

18.3.2 Lymphoscintigram

Lymphoscintigram is the gold standard technique, and was introduced in 1953. In this technique, radiolabeled protein is used to assess the lymphatic function, lymph movement, lymph drainage, and response to treatment [8].

The radioisotope, usually technetium Tc 99 m-labeled colloid including antimony sulfur and albumin [9] are used. The heptaminol adenosine phosphate is used to increase the lymph flow and measurement [10].

The sensitivity and specificity of the lymphoscintigram are 73% to 97% and 100% [11], respectively. Contrast lymphangiogram can also be used to elucidate the lymphatic anatomy.

After the isotope injection, the lymphatics may or may not be visualized within the first hour. Some patients may show normal lymphatics or missed diagnosis. Only delayed film (2–24-hour post-isotope injection) shows the real eccentricities [12].

Condensed image processing using a modified Kleinhans score and time-activity curves [13] are used to enhance the detection of abnormalities of the lymphatic system.

Lymphoscintigram can differentiate between lymphedema and edema of venous origin [14].

In case of varicose veins and deep vein incompetence [7], lymphoscintigraphy reveals significantly reduced lymph drainage. This is suggestive of association between chronic venous insufficiencies with lymphatic insufficiency.

Both epifascial and subfascial lymphatics are abnormal in lymphedema, while in post-thrombotic disease, there is a decrease in the subfascial lymphatic flow whereas the epifascial flow remains normal [15], it can differentiate between post-thrombotic disease and lymphedema [15].

In lipedema patients, lymphoscintigraphy will confirm that peripheral lymphatics remain normal. Asymmetry may be appearing in bilateral lipedema disease suggestive of the dynamic nature of the lymphoscintigram. Lymphoscintigraphy also depicts the impairment of lymphatic drainage or lymphatic disruption after arterial reconstruction.

18.3.3 Indocyanine Green Lymphography

In this technique, fluorescence lymphography using contrast ICG leads to the diagnosis of lymphedema [16]. Indocyanine Green Lymphography (ICG-LG) clearly visualizes superficial lymph flow without radiation exposure, and recently has found its way to the evaluation of lymphedema.

18.3.4 Ultrasound

Volume changes in dermis, subcutaneous layer, and an increase/decrease in the muscle mass along with structural changes like hyperechogenic dermis and hypoechogenic subcutaneous layer may appear in limb swelling on ultrasound. It does not give information about the anatomy of lymphatics [17].

18.3.5 Duplex Ultrasound

Duplex USG uses two modalities—Doppler and B-mode to assess the speed of blood flow and visualize the structure of leg vessels. Duplex ultrasonography is a noninvasive, cheap, and reliable investigation to establish a diagnosis of DVT. A combination of a duplex scan and lymphoscintigram might be able to diagnose the cause of limb edema in majority of the patients (Fig. 18.2a and b). However, some authors refute the correlation between chronic limb edema and increased venous reflux [18]. Intraluminal blood clot appears hypoechoic or anechoic in acute cases whereas in chronic DVT, it appears hyperechoic with peripheral revascularization on color Doppler imaging.

18.3.6 Computed Tomography

Computed tomography scan can be used to confirm the diagnosis and to assess the effect of treatment. The CT scan imaging show skin and subcutaneous compartment thickening increased fat density, thickened perimuscular aponeurosis [19] and honeycomb appearance. Honeycomb appearance is not seen in venous disease but subcutaneous compartment and skin thickening may appear. In lipedema, there is

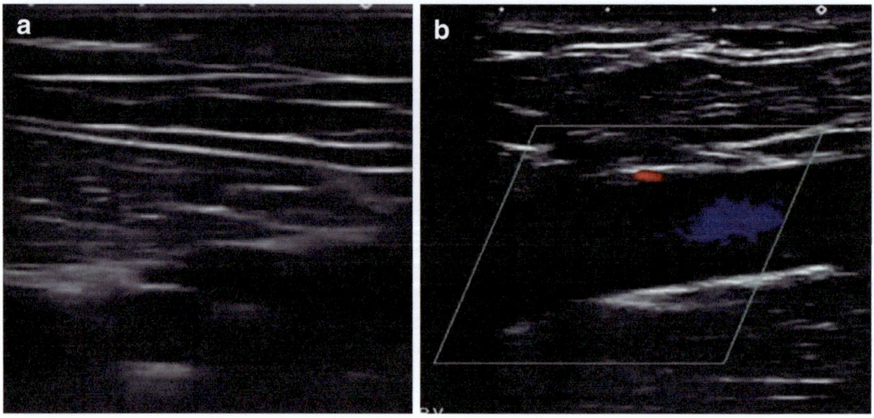

Fig. 18.2 (**a**) Color Doppler showing increased subcutaneous tissue thickness in edema. (**b**) Color Doppler showing blood flow in lower limb

thickened subcutaneous compartment, normal skin thickness with normal subfascial compartment.

In DVT thickened subcutaneous layer, with signs of lymphedema, enlarged muscle area and enlarged superficial veins may be seen. CT scan is unreliable in DVT.

18.3.7 Magnetic Resonance Imaging

To differentiate among lymphedema, lipedema, and phlebedema [20] Magnetic Resonance Imaging (MRI) can be used [21].

Lymphedema appears as increased subcutaneous tissue volume, circumferential edema, honeycomb appearance between the muscle and subcutis with marked thickening of the dermis [20]. MRI cannot differentiate the primary and secondary lymphedema. MRI can also prove useful to assess the result of reconstructive surgery.

In case of DVT, MRI shows the edema of leg muscles mainly in posterior compartments and soft tissue swelling consists only of fat with normal lymphatics in lipedema.

18.4 Management of Pedal Edema

Management of limb edema depends upon its etiology.

A. Venous Insufficiency Mild cases of venous insufficiency can be improved by limb elevation only. In chronic cases, compression stocking is useful. Compression stocking should not be used in peripheral vascular disease as it may aggravate the symptoms. Pneumatic compression stocking may be used in patients where stockings are contraindicated. Topical steroids and emollients can be used for skincare and prevention of ulceration, dryness, etc. Diuretics can cause metabolic derangement so should be avoided.

B. Congestive Heart Failure and Chronic Liver Disease In case of CHF in mild cases, limb elevation fluid restriction and salt restriction can improve the mild stage of limb edema. Diuretics can be used in non-responding cases. If liver failure is present, chronic hypoalbuminemia can be corrected by albumin infusion. It can provide temporary relief from the symptoms.

C. Chronic Renal Failure In case of renal failure fluid, salt restriction is the primary line of management.

Diuretics can be used in refractory cases. Hyperkalemia can be caused by aldosterone antagonist and so, should be avoided.

D. Obstructive Sleep Apnea Due to pulmonary hypertension limb edema may occur it can be controlled by weight reduction and positive pressure ventilation.

E. Deep Vein Thrombosis Chronic bedridden patients are prone to DVT. For prevention of DVT pneumatic compression, bandages, and stockings can be used. Anticoagulant therapy should be started prophylactically as well as therapeutically.

F. Lymphedema Mild lymphedema can be managed by limb exercise, limb massage, limb elevation, compression bandages, stockings, etc., in chronic and symptomatic cases, surgical procedures can be performed.

G. Lipedema Weight loss can improve the symptoms. It has no definitive treatment.

H. Idiopathic Edema It can be improved by treatment with aldosterone antagonists like spironolactone.

18.5 Treatment

18.5.1 Lifestyle Modification

Lifestyle modifications are essential for prevention as well as treatment of lower limb edema.

Exercise/movement: The contraction and relaxation of muscle may lead to decrease the edema by pumping the excess fluid back toward the heart.

Massage: On stroking the affected area pressure may change and help the drainage of excessive fluid toward the heart. Precaution should be taken as massage should not be vigorous as it can be painful.

Elevation: Elevation of limb above the level of the heart may lead to resolution of swelling/edema of the limb due to gravity.

Protection and skincare: The swollen area is susceptible to infection and injury. Always protect the affected area from injury and keep it dry and clean.

Reduce salt intake: Excessive salt intake may lead to retention of fluid and worsen edema.

Heat therapy produces some benefits to limb swelling but the mechanism is not fully known. It can be done using hot water, microwave, or electromagnetic radiation. It produces dilatation of blood capillaries, increases venous return and decreases dermal inflammation.

Balneotherapy is the use of thermal or mineral water (1 gm/L conc.) for treatment of disease. It acts through mechanical, chemical, and physical mechanisms to treat and reduce pain and edema. It improves circulation and muscle relaxation. It also improves the immune system.

Chronic lymphedema can persist lifelong. So, results can improve by fully understanding and committing to all therapeutic measured and psychological support. Weight reduction also has a positive impact on limb swelling.

Aggressive antibiotic therapy helps when needed like in the case of cellulitis. The infection can cause lymphatic deterioration. For filariasis, prevention and treatment are important because it affects a large population in a country like India.

In areas where compression therapy is not feasible, Kinesio taping can be used which improves lymphatic drainage by skin traction during movements.

18.5.2 Physical Modalities and Compression

The first-line treatment for lymphedema is complex physical therapy.

Compression Stockings The compression stockings are used in the management of long-term chronic edema. It can be used as a prophylaxis in a high-risk patient who is prone to develop limb edema. The stocking is based on the patient's general condition, mobility, and limb size. The stocking is applied from foot with padding of all bony prominences excluding the toes. The stocking should be worn from the morning before leaving the bed till the time to go to bed.

Graduated Compression Bandages It is used in chronic forms of severe edema. The bandage is made of various materials applied in overlapping layers. The effect depends upon pressure exerted, number of layers, components used in bandage, and elastic properties.

According to pressure exerted near the ankle joint, stocking is classified as class I–class IV. The type of stockings depends upon the length and circumference of the leg and the pressure required (Table 18.1).

Table 18.1 Selection criteria for compression bandages [22]

Stage	Pressure	Lower limb disease/condition
Class I	15–23 mmHg	• Mild venous insufficiency or in cases where higher pressure cannot be used due to other existing conditions • Prevention of venous thrombosis • Prevention of varicose veins, e.g., during pregnancy
Class II	24–34 mmHg	• Venous insufficiency • Varicose eczema and venous leg ulcers • Mild lymphatic edema and edema post-cancer surgery • Follow-up care after varicose vein surgery and erysipelas • Treatment and prevention of deep vein thrombosis and superficial venous thrombophlebitis
Class III	35–49 mmHg	• Severe edema not managed with lower pressure
Class IV	50+ mmHg	• Very severe lymphatic edema or severe venous insufficiency

Pneumatic Compression Pump Pneumatic compression devices are made up of air pump and inflatable garment to create compression for legs or other body parts [23]. The functional aim of the device is to squeeze fluid from the underlying tissue and veins, and displace it proximally. When the inflatable sleeves deflate, the veins fill up with blood. The intermittent compressions device will ensure the movement of fluid and venous blood.

Complex Physical Therapy or Complete Decongestive Therapy CPD is the one of the effective approaches for lymphedema treatment. It improves the lymphatic function and reduction of fluid accumulation. Lifelong compression therapy can be used. It has two components, manual lymph drainage (MLD) and compression therapy [24].

The therapy depends upon phases of edema. In phase I of decongestion 1–3 MLD per decompression and exercises for 2–5 weeks.

18.5.3 Manual Lymphatic Drainage

There are two methods to achieve interstitial fluid movement to manage subcutaneous edema of the leg and foot [25]. One way is by encouraging fluid movement in the extra vascular space and second by stimulating fluid movement from the extra vascular space into the venous system. The edematous fluid is redirected through collaterals toward normally functioning pathway or by increasing the activity of the normal lymphatics [26]. The procedure is performed proximally to distally in a lying down position for up to 30–60 minutes daily, weekly or monthly, depending on the stage and severity [20, 27].

The treatment can be accentuated by the lymph fluoroscopy mapping [28].

The techniques are Leduc et al. Földi [29] and Casley-Smith methods, both being equally efficient. Even still, there have been no exclusive evidences for MLD and its efficacy for edema.

Compression Therapy Compression stockings improve symptoms by providing graduated compression therapy to control leg swelling and discomfort [30].

It is a simple and effective measure to increase the blood flow activity in the lower limbs and strengthening the vein support. It applies gentle pressure to the ankles and legs which promotes venous return and impedes stasis. It stretches out vein walls and improves the limb circulation, which helps in eliminate the swelling.

18.6 Medical Management

18.6.1 Benzopyrones

Benzopyrones are effective for treatment of lymphedema. The drug acts by reducing the edema fluid, increasing the softness of tissue and decreasing the elevated temperature [31]. It also increases the number of macrophages and enhances the proteolysis which helps in removal of protein and edema with reduction of the inflammation and infection [32]. It also improves the symptoms like hardness, heaviness and swelling. The adverse effects of this drug are nausea, vomiting, and diarrhea which are relatively uncommon and resolve spontaneously. The drug can be used with physical measures [33].

This drug is banned for use in the United Kingdom, Australia and France due to reports of hepatotoxicity [33].

Micronized Purified Flavonoid Fraction(MPFF) It is said to decrease the limb swelling by aiding the chronic venous insufficiency by decreasing the venous stasis and also improves the post-surgery edema [34]. The mechanism of action of Micronized Purified Flavonoid Fraction is to reduce the capillary permeability and inflammation of the tissue. This drug is under trial for lower limb lymphedema.

Immunotherapy Role of immunotherapy is not well understood. Activated antilogous lymph infused into arteries by injection activates macrophages in the interstitial tissue, which decomposes the excess protein. The activated macrophages and CD4T cells play a role in proliferation of lymphatic endothelial cells and aberrant lymphangiogenesis. The role of activated lymph still remains unclear.

Gene Therapy Gene abnormality is reported in primary lymphedema. Hepatocyte growth factor (HGF) neovascularization related to lymph vessels neogenesis is suggested. It is reported that peripheral vascular growth in limbs with severe ischemia is related to HGF in rat breast cancer model [35, 36].

9-Cis Retinoic Acid Retinoic acids (RAs) regulating genes have an essential role in cell proliferation, differentiation, apoptosis, and metabolism. They induce lymphangiogenesis through fibroblast growth factor (FGF) receptor-dependent pathway. Some studies have found that 9-*cis* retinoic acid aids lymphangiogenesis and improves lymphedema [37]. Further experiments are required to establish a strong consequence.

18.7 Surgical Treatment

The recommendations of the American Venous Forum on the principles of the surgical treatment of chronic lymphedema are summarized in Table 18.2 [38].

The surgical treatment is only considered after failure of all the nonsurgical measures in chronic and symptomatic cases for more than 6 months of therapy. Surgical interventions in lymphatic are very difficult and require a trained surgical team. The goal is reconstruction and restoration of the functional continuity with reduction of edema volume by excision surgery causing the handicapping.

Table 18.2 Guidelines of the American Venous Forum on the principles of the surgical treatment of chronic lymphedema [38]

Guideline	Grade of recommendation 1. Strong 2. Weak	Grade of evidence A - High quality B - Moderate quality C - Low or very low quality
All interventions for chronic lymphedema should be preceded by at least 6 months of non-operative treatment	1	C
Excisional operations or liposuction only to patients with late-stage non-pitting lymphedema who fail conservative measurement	2	C
Microsurgical lymphatic reconstruction in Centre of excellence for selected patients with secondary lymphedema if performed early in the course of disease	2	C

Preoperative evaluation and postoperative outcome cannot be overemphasized. Optimizing the limb before surgery is necessary. To prevent the chances of recurrence, it is important for the patient to wear a compression stocking.

Surgical management can be divided into the following types [39]:

1. Bypass procedures and lymphovascular anastomoses
2. Debulking or excisional surgery
3. Prophylactic surgery

18.8 Surgical Bypass Procedures

It is useful in selective cases of chronic limb edema after failure of medical therapy where the venous system is competent and intact lymphatic structures, such as regional lymphatics and lymph nodes, are present.

Lymphovenous anastomosis for the treatment of chronic lymphedema was first attempted by Nielubowicz and Olszewski. It is the anastomoses of lymph vessel or lymph node to the vein distal to the obstructing segment [40, 41].

.End-to-end or end-to-side lymphatic-venous anastomosis can be performed [42]. It can have complications such as venous thrombosis at the anastomotic site blockage of lymphatics [42].

End-to-end technique avoids venous reflux into the lymphatics and thus decreases the risk of venous thrombosis. The risk of anastomotic stricture formation can be avoided by using a secondary tributary of the main vein as the site of anastomoses. The lymphatic capsule-venous anastomosis can be performed in pediatric patients.

Ipsen concluded that lymphovenous bypass decreased limb circumference by 0.8 to 4.1 cm in secondary lymphedema but no change was noted in primary lymphedema cases.

Lymphatic autotransplantation: Lymphatic grafting introduced by Baumeister is used for secondary lymphedema [43]. In this procedure, the normal, functionally unaffected vessels are used to bypass the obstruction area. It can be performed successfully even with coexisting venous disease.

Autologous Interposition Vein Grafting can also be used in coexisting venous disease. The procedure involves lymphatic-venous-lymphatic anastomoses directly. The contraindications of the surgery are severe hypoplasia, aplasia of lymphatics or lymph nodes, and extensive damage to the superficial as well as deep lymphatics. The patient who is contraindicative for bypass procedure can be considered for debulking procedure.

Adipo lymphaticovenous transfer was performed by Tanaka with the use of long saphenous vein along with its lymphatics. Free autografts of the greater omentum have also been used. It has satisfactory results in short series. Necrosis is the main complication in this procedure.

Vascularized lymph node transplantation was described by Backer [44, 45].

Lymph nodes from the inguinal region were transplanted microsurgically to the axillary region in mastectomy lymphedema patients. It can be done in selected patients and necessitates monitoring. The procedure can also be used in congenital prophylactic lymphedema [46]. The results are not well established. The skill of the surgeon and timing of intervention is a crucial factor along with lifelong medical therapy [47].

18.9 Debulking Procedures

This procedure is not truly debulking. In this procedure, the **subcutaneous drainage of lymphedema** fluid is achieved by using multi-perforated silicon tubes, which are linked to a chamber by a one-way valve. The chamber is connected to the venous drainage system via the long saphenous vein in the same manner as a peritoneovenous shunt. In this procedure, up to 70% reduction in size has been reported. However, it has a limited role in long-term patency due to high protein content of edema fluid blocking the system.

Charles procedure is a well known procedure in which en bloc removal of the skin, subcutaneous tissue, and deep fascia is done. The radical excision of subcutaneous tissue is followed by primary or staged skin grafting. In primary skin grafting, either skin from the excised tissue or from a non-affected area is used. Staged skin grafting also reports good results. There was no difference in results in primary or secondary edema. Skin and subcutaneous excision combination with liposuction improve symptoms but can develop into foot edema. In Charles' procedure, only the affected part of the limb is treated and the cosmetic outcome is poor.

Servelle described a technique of two-stage reduction where the first stage involves the medial aspect and the second stage involves the lateral aspect of the limb. This procedure is *total superficial lymphangiectomy* and is a modification of the Homan procedure.

The complications of debulking procedure include infection, necrosis, scarring, difficult wound healing of the skin graft, and poor cosmetic and functional results [48].

18.9.1 Liposuction

It is useful in lymphedema secondary to adipose tissue deposits and in selective cases with non-fibrotic primary or secondary lymphedema which causes up to a 23% reduction in volume. Cellulitis is the main complication.

18.10 Prophylactic Surgery

Patients who require extensive lymph node dissection in pelvic region are prone to developing edema. In these patients, **prophylactic lymphatic tissue transplant** via omentoplasty may prove useful. The concept of omentoplasty was evaluated by Logmans and coworkers [49] and the concept of prophylactic lymphovenous anastomoses after ilioinguinal dissection was given by Orefice and coworkers [49]. Prophylactic bypass has reduced the frequency of edema and hospital stay.

18.11 Conclusion

In approaching lower limb edema, a variety of etiologies must be considered (Figure 18.3). History and physical examination are required for differentiation of causes and subsequent selection of cost-effective and appropriate diagnostic testing and management. Treatment mainly emphasizes on treating the etiology and systemic disease along with symptomatic treatment for the edema. Lifestyle modification physical exercise and compression bandaging can improve the condition. Medical treatment is not effective in every case and cannot cure completely. Surgical management is required in selective cases and has a limited outcome. Surgery cannot resolve the disease completely.

Some newer modalities have also evolved for the treatment of lower limb swelling but require further research to provide better outcomes. However, till now lifestyle modifications and physical modalities are the mainstay of treatment for lower limb swelling.

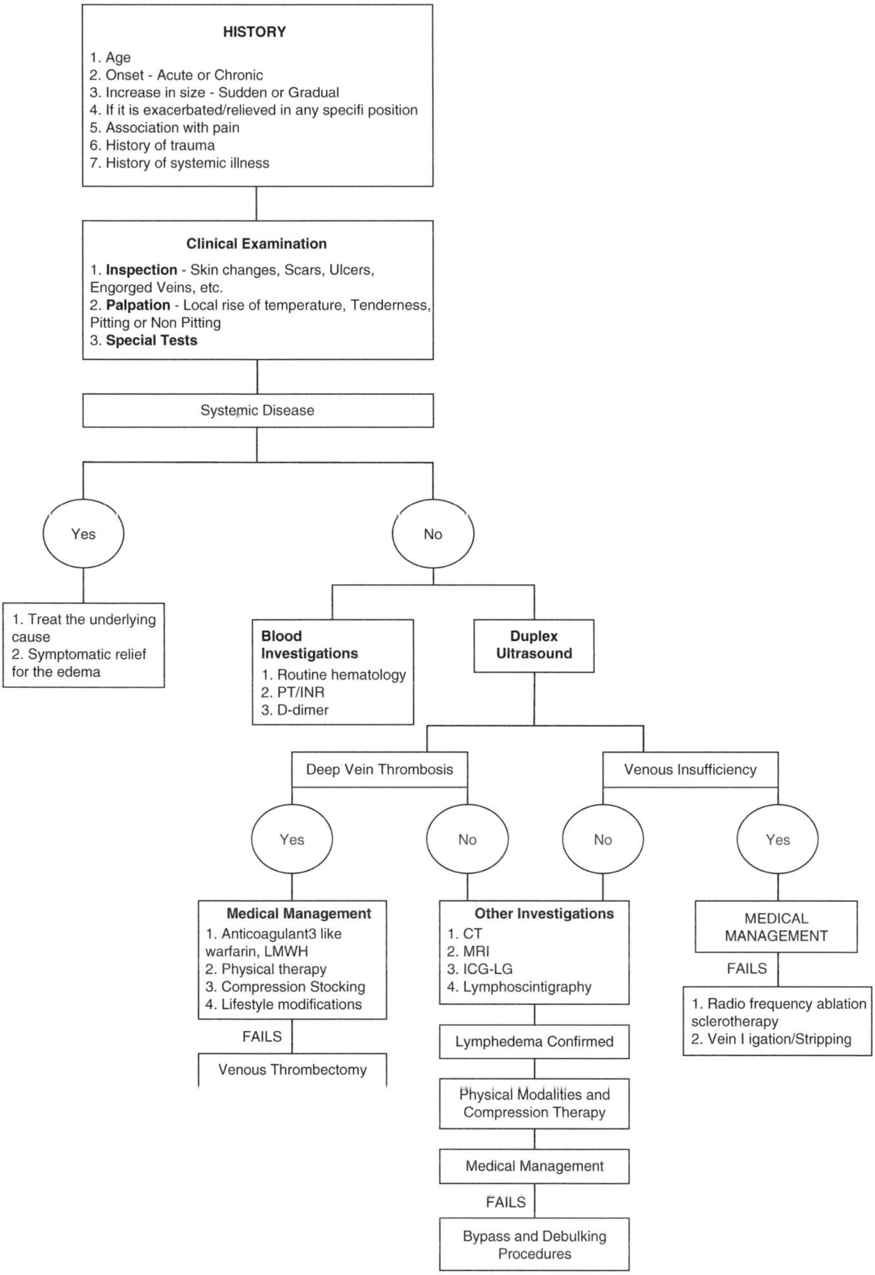

Fig. 18.3 Algorithm for evaluation and management of limb edema

References

1. Berard A, Zuccarelli F. Test-retest reliability study of a new improved leg-O-meter, the leg-O meter II, in patients suffering from venous insufficiency of the lower limbs. Angiology. 2000;51:711–7.
2. Casley-Smith JR. Measuring and representing peripheral oedema and its alterations. Lymphology. 1994;27:56–70.
3. Liu NF, Olszewski W. Use of tonometry to assess lower extremity lymphedema. Lymphology. 1992;25:155–8.
4. Ward LC. Regarding Edema and leg volume: methods of assessment. Angiology. 2000;51:615–6.
5. Cesarone MR, Belcaro G, Nicolaides AN, et al. The edema tester in the evaluation of swollen limbs in venous and lymphatic disease. Panminerva Med. 1999;41:10–4.
6. Weissleder H, Weissleder R. Interstitial lymphangiography: initial clinical experience with a dimeric nonionic contrast agent. Radiology. 1989;170:371–4.
7. Burnand KG, McGuinness CL, Lagattolla NR, Browse NL, El Aradi A, Nunan T. Value of isotope lymphography in the diagnosis of lymphoedema of the leg. Br J Surg. 2002:8974–8.
8. Williams WH, Witte CL, Witte MH, McNeill GC. Radionuclide lymphangioscintigraphy in the evaluation of peripheral lymphedema. Clin Nucl Med. 2000;25:451–64.
9. Wheatley DC, Wastie ML, Whitaker SC, Perkins AC, Hopkinson BR. Lymphoscintigraphy and colour Doppler sonography in the assessment of leg oedema of unknown cause. Br J Radial. 1996;69:1117–24.
10. Thibaut G, Durand A, Follignoni P, Bertrand A. Measurement of lymphatic flow variation by non-invasive method cases of lymphedema. Angiology. 1992;43:567–71.
11. Ter SE, Alavi A, Kim CK, Merli G. Lymphoscintigraphy: reliable test for the diagnosis of lymphedema. Clin Nucl Med. 1993;18:646–54.
12. Larcos G, Foster DR. Interpretation of lymphoscintigrams in suspected lymphoedema: contribution of delayed images. Nucl Med Commun. 1995;16:683–6.
13. Rijke AM, Croft BY, Johnson RA, de Jongste AB, Camps JA. Lymphoscintigraphy and lymphedema of the lower extremities. J Nucl Med. 1990;31:990–8.
14. Proby CM, Gane JN, Joseph AE, Mortimer PS. Investigation of the swollen limb with isotope lymphography. Br J Dermatol. 1990;123:29–37.
15. Brautigam P, Vanscheidt W, Foldi E, Krause T, Moser E. The importance of the subfascial lymphatics in the diagnosis of lower limb edema: investigations with semiquantitative lymphoscintigraphy. Angiology. 1993;44:464–70.
16. Mihara M, Hara H, Araki J, Kikuchi K, Narushima M, Yamamoto T, Iida T, Yoshimatsu H, Murai N, Mitsui K, et al. Indocyanine green (ICG) lymphography is superior to lymphoscintigraphy for diagnostic imaging of early lymphedema of the upper limbs. PLoS One. 2012;7:e38182. https://doi.org/10.1371/journal.pone.0038182.
17. Doldi SB, Lattuada E, Zappa MA, Pieri G, Favara A, Micheletto G. Ultrasonography of extremity lymphedema. Lymphology. 1992;25:129–33.
18. Valentin LI, Valentin WH. Comparative study of different venous reflux duplex quantitation parameters. Angiology. 1999;50:721–8.
19. Marotel M, Cluzan R, Ghabboun S, Pascot M, Alliot F, Lasry JL. Transaxial computer tomography of lower extremity lymphedema. Lymphology. 1998;31:180–5.
20. Gordon K, Mortimer PS. Decongestive lymphatic therapy. In: Lee BB, Rockson SG, Bergan J, editors. Lymphedema. A concise compendium of theory and practice. 2nd ed. Cham, Switzerland: Springer International Publishing AG; 2018. p. 413–29.
21. Werner GT, Scheck R, Kaiserling E. Magnetic resonance imaging of peripheral lymphedema. Lymphology. 1998;31:34–6.
22. Stockport JC, Groarke L, Ellison DA, McCollum C. Single-layer and multilayer bandaging in the treatment of venous leg ulcers. J Wound Care. 1997;66(10):485–8.

23. International Society of Lymphology The diagnosis and treatment of peripheral lymphedema. Consensus document of the international society of lymphology. Lymphology. 2013;46:1–11.
24. Dean SM. Lymphedema: physical and medical therapy. In: Gloviczki P, editor. Handbook of venous and lymphatic disorders. Guidelines of the American venous forum. 4th ed. Boca Raton: CRC Press; 2017. p. 725–35.
25. Watanabe Y, Koshiyama M, Yanagisawa N. Treatment of leg and foot edema in women. Women's Health Open J. 2017:68–73. https://doi.org/10.17140/WHOJ-3-124.
26. Best Practice for the Management of Lymphoedema International Consensus. [(accessed on 17 July 2019)].
27. Foldi E, Foldi M, Rockson S. Complete decongestive physiotherapy. In: Lee BB, Rockson SG, Bergan J, editors. Lymphedema. A concise compendium of theory and practice. 2nd ed. Cham, Switzerland: Springer International Publishing AG; 2018. p. 403–11.
28. Johansson K, Karlsson K, Nikolaidis P. Evidence-based or traditional treatment of cancer-related lymphedema. Lymphology. 2015;48:24–7.
29. Földi E. The treatment of lymphedema. Cancer. 1998;83(12 Suppl):2833–4.
30. Badger CM, Peacock JL, Mortimer PS. A randomized, controlled, parallel-group clinical trial comparing multilayer bandaging followed by hosiery versus hosiery alone in the treatment of patients with lymphedema of the limb. Cancer. 2000;88:2832–7.
31. Casley-Smith JR, Morgan RG, Piller NB. Treatment of lymphedema of the arms and legs with 5,6-benzo-[alpha] pyrone. N Engl J Med. 1993;329:1158–63.
32. Casley-Smith JR, Casley-Smith JR. Modern treatment of lymphoedema, II: the benzopyrones. Australas J Dermatol. 1992;33:69–74.
33. Badger CMA, Preston N, Seers K, Mortimer P. Benzopyrones for reducing and controlling lymphoedema of the limbs. Cochrane Database Syst Rev. 2004;2:CD003140.
34. Olszewski W. Clinical efficacy of micronized purified flavonoid fraction (MPFF) in edema. Angiology. 2000:5125–9.
35. Shigematsu H, Yasuda K, Iwai T, et al. Randomized, double-blind, placebo-controlled clinical trial of hepatocyte growth factor plasmid for critical limb ischemia. Gene Ther. 2010;17:1152–61.
36. Shigematsu H, Yasuda K, Sasajima T, et al. Transfection of human HGF plasmid DNA improves limb salvage in Buerger's disease patients with critical limb ischemia. Int Angiol. 2011;30:140–9.
37. Choi I, Lee S, Kyoung Chung H, et al. 9-cis retinoic acid promotes lymphangiogenesis and enhances lymphatic vessel regeneration: therapeutic implications of 9-cis retinoic acid for secondary lymphedema. Circulation. 2012;125:872–82.
38. Al-Ajam Y, Mohan AT, Saint-Cyr M. Principles of the surgical treatment of chronic lymphedema. In: Gloviczki P, editor. Handbook of Venous and Lymphatic Disorders. 4th ed. Guidelines of the American Venous Forum. Boca Raton: CRC Press; 2017. p. 737–746.
39. Tiwari A, Hamilton G, Myint F. Management of lower limb lymphoedema. Beard J Murray Seds. Pathways in vascular surgery Shrewsbury. England TFM Publishing. 2002:71–6.
40. Boccardo F, Fulcheri E, Villa G, Molinari L, Campisi C, Dessalvi S, et al. Lymphatic microsurgery to treat lymphedema: Techniques and indications for better results. Ann Plast Surg 2013;71:191–5.
41. Damstra RJ, Voesten HG, van Schelven WD, van der Lei B. Lymphatic venous anastomosis (LVA) for treatment of secondary arm lymphedema. A prospective study of 11 LVA procedures in 10 patients with breast cancer related lymphedema and a critical review of the literature. Breast Cancer Res Treat. 2009;113:199–206.
42. Campisi C, Boccardo F, Tacchella M. Reconstructive microsurgery of lymph vessels: the personal method of lymphatic venous lymphatic (LVL) interpositioned grafted shunt. Microsurgery. 1995;16:161–6.
43. Baumeister RG. Lymphedema: surgical treatment. In: Cronenwett JL, Johnston KW, editors. Rutherford's vascular surgery. 8th ed. Philadelphia: Sauder's; 2014. p. 1028–42.
44. Becker C. Autologous lymph node transfers. J Reconstr Microsurg. 2016;32:28–33.

45. Batista BN, Germain M, Faria JC, Becker C. Lymph node flap transfer for patients with secondary lower limb lymphedema. Microsurgery. 2017;37:29–33.
46. Becker C, Arrive L, Saaristo A, Germain M, Fanzio P, Batista BN, et al. Surgical treatment of congenital lymphedema. Clin Plast Surg. 2012;39:377–84.
47. Lee BB, Andrade M, Antignani PL, Boccardo F, Bunke N, Campisi C, et al. Diagnosis and treatment of primary lymphedema. Consensus document of the international union of phlebology (IUP)-2013. Int Angiol. 2013;32:541–74.
48. International Society of Lymphology The diagnosis and treatment of peripheral lymphedema: 2016 consensus document of the International Society of Lymphology. Lymphology 2016; 49:170–184.
49. Logmans A, Kruyt RH, de Bruin HG, Cox PH, Pillay M, Trimbos JB. Lymphedema and lymphocysts following lymphadenectomy may be prevented by omentoplasty: a pilot study. Gynecol Oncol. 1999;75:323–7.

Pregnancy and Lower Limb Swelling 19

Marcelo Bellini Dalio, Leandro Augusto Gardenghi, and Nei Rodrigues Alves Dezotti

19.1 Introduction

Lower limb swelling is present in about 80% of all pregnancies [1, 2]. Healthy women without any evidence of venous disease often present oedema during late pregnancy [3]. The so-called physiologic gestational oedema is not in itself dangerous, but it can cause significant anxiety. Pregnant women frequently seek consultations with obstetricians, clinicians, and also vascular specialists [4].

In some common situations, lower limb swelling can be a manifestation of a pathological condition. Leg oedema is one of the core features of preeclampsia, together with raised blood pressure and proteinuria [5]. Painful leg oedema is a manifestation of deep venous thrombosis [6]. Chronic venous disease is also a cause of severe leg swelling in pregnant women, associated with varicose veins and skin changes [7].

This chapter aims to discuss the physiology, causes, and management of lower limb swelling in pregnancy.

19.2 Physiologic Gestational Oedema

Most pregnant women present pitting oedema of the ankles and legs, especially at the end of the day (Figs. 19.1 and 19.2). Commonly, they require increased shoe sizes. Symptoms such as pain, feeling of heaviness, night cramps, and paraesthesiae are also reported. Usually, the symptoms are mild, and there is neither redness nor severe pain on physical examination. These latter findings may raise the suspicion

M. B. Dalio (✉) · L. A. Gardenghi · N. R. A. Dezotti
University of São Paulo, Ribeirão Preto Medical School, Department of Surgery and Anatomy, Division of Vascular and Endovascular Surgery, São Paulo, Brazil
e-mail: mbdalio@usp.br

S. K. Tiwary (ed.), *Approach to Lower Limb Oedema*,
https://doi.org/10.1007/978-981-16-6206-5_19

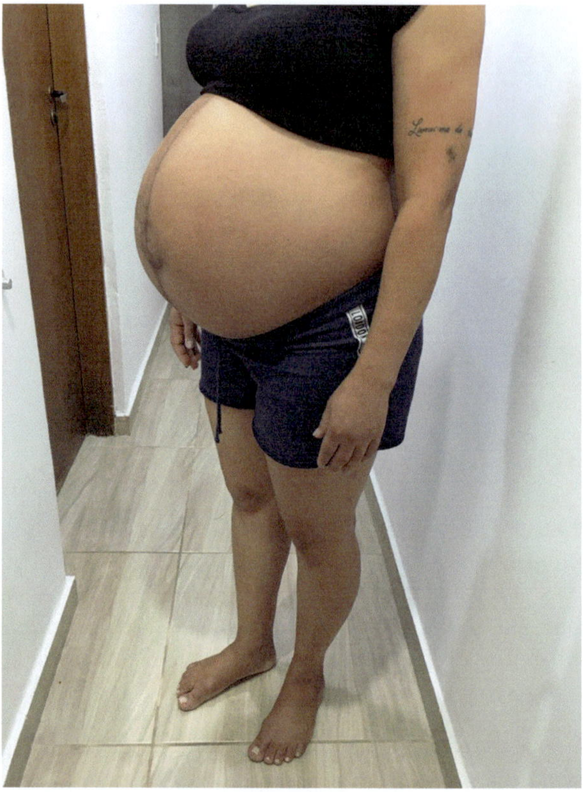

Fig. 19.1 Digital image of a young primigravida in her third trimester with physiologic gestational oedema. There are mild foot and ankle oedema in both limbs. The oedema is pitting, cold, symmetrical, and there is neither redness nor severe pain

of a pathological cause. Typically, the oedema is more pronounced in the last trimester [8]. Gestational oedema can be monitored in the prenatal care through maternal weight gain. The average weight gain during pregnancy approximates 12.5 kg or 27.5 Ib [9]. Physiologic gestational oedema generally resolves in the postpartum [10].

Two key factors cause gestational oedema: the hormonal and the mechanical:

- The **hormonal factor** consists of the effects of pregnancy hormones. Oestrogen and progesterone trigger many systemic changes, leading to alterations in the venous system [11, 12]. The volume and the pressure are increased, causing venous distension and stasis. The venous wall also has an increased distensibility [7]. Furthermore, a surge of corticotrophin and oestrogen produces vasodilatation [13]. To prevent maternal immunoreactivity to the foetus, hypertrophic adrenal glands create a transient, physiologic hypercortisolism [14]. A nitric oxide-mediated vessel engorgement also increases the oedematous effect [13].
- The **mechanical factor** involves the compression generated by the enlarged uterus, which is more present during late pregnancy [15]. The compression is exerted over the inferior vena cava and the pelvic veins, causing an elevation in hydrostatic pressure, venous dilatation, stasis, and oedema [12, 15]. When the

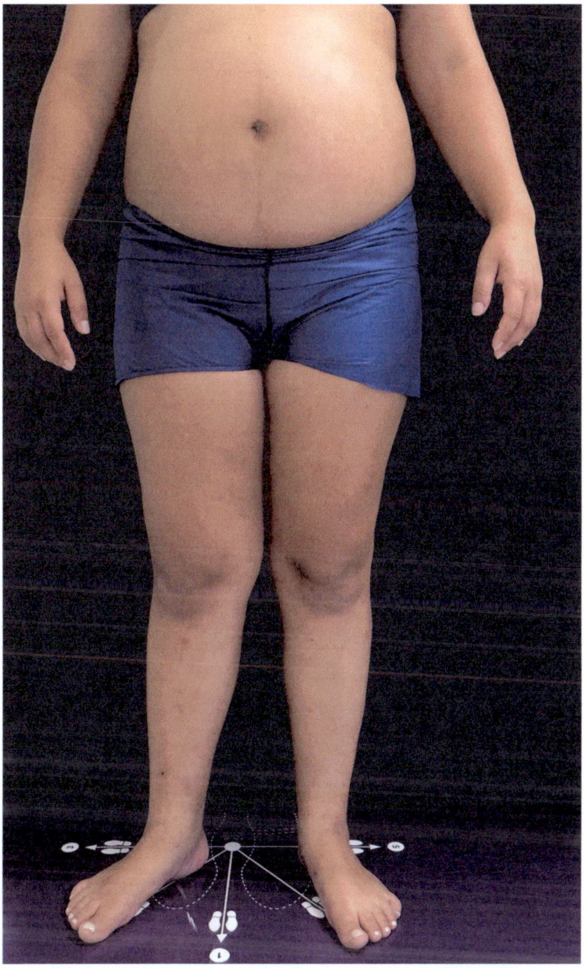

Fig. 19.2 Digital image of a 22-week primigravida exhibiting typical physiologic gestational oedema: pitting foot and ankle oedema in both limbs

pregnant woman lies on her left side, the uterus moves left, and the compressive effect is suppressed [16]. The mechanical factor also predisposes to deep venous thrombosis [6].

All these factors contribute to cause dilatation of lower limb veins and oedema. Venous dilatation, rather than reflux, is the most common vascular alteration during pregnancy [17, 18]. However, pregnancy-induced venous dilatation also causes valvular incompetence and reflux in healthy gravidae [7]. As occurs with gestational oedema, this novel venous reflux often resolves in the postpartum [17, 19, 20]. It is not well established if venous reflux that appears during pregnancy causes worsening of lower limb oedema [8].

A clinical investigation conducted by our group employed duplex scan to analyse the association of lower limb oedema with venous reflux in healthy primigravidae

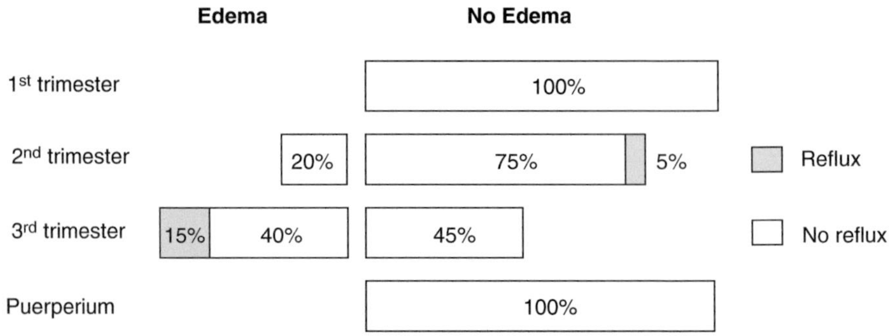

Fig. 19.3 Occurrence of lower limb oedema and reflux during the three trimesters of pregnancy and the postpartum. (Data from Gardenghi LA, Dezotti NR, Dalio MB, Joviliano EE, Piccinato CE (2017) Gestational lower limb edema and venous reflux in healthy primigravidae. Int Angiol 36:569–573)

during pregnancy and in the postpartum [21]. We found that no woman presented with oedema or reflux in the first trimester. In the second trimester, reflux was found in 5% of patients and oedema was found in 20%. In the third trimester, 15% developed reflux and 55% developed oedema. Both in the second and in the third trimester, reflux and oedema were not associated. In the postpartum, neither reflux nor oedema was found (Fig. 19.3). Almost all reflux was in the superficial venous system. Only one patient developed reflux in the deep venous system. The superficial system is more subjected to develop reflux than the deep system [22]. Curiously, all new reflux developed only on the left side. This could be explained by the anatomic relationships between the left common iliac vein and the right common iliac artery. The iliac bifurcation is usually a site of physiologic compression, and the presence of a gravid uterus may exacerbate it [15]. We concluded that lower limb oedema was not associated with venous reflux. Both were present in the second and in the third trimesters and resolved spontaneously in the postpartum. Both are products of the same physiological changes that occur in pregnancy, which are discussed above.

19.3 Management of Physiologic Gestational Oedema

The basis of management of lower limb swelling in pregnancy is adequate prenatal care. During prenatal visits, clinical history, physical examination, and maternal weight gain should be assessed to exclude any pathological condition. Routine and specific laboratory exams help to monitor normal conditions. Imaging investigations are usually not necessary in physiologic oedema. The pathological causes of oedema during pregnancy and their management are discussed below. Gravidae with physiologic gestational oedema should be informed that the swelling is expected and may worsen as the pregnancy progresses. They should be reassured that oedema will improve within a few months after giving birth [23].

Some simple measures help to control oedema. These interventions are low-cost and are unlikely to be harmful [24]:

- Avoid standing or sitting for a prolonged time;
- Periodic calf flexion-extension movements;
- Daytime and night rest, with legs, elevated 15–20 cm;
- In the third trimester, rest lying on the left side;
- Physical activity;
- If it is a planned pregnancy, organize to have the last trimesters during the cold season.

Treatments used for lower limb oedema during pregnancy include compression therapy, venoactive drugs, water immersion, and reflexology [25].

Compression therapy continues to be the standard therapy in the treatment of gestational oedema [10]. It works by exerting a contact pressure on the tissue, leading to superficial venous system compression. Consequently, the deep venous system flow accelerates, the venous return improves, the insufficient venous valves regenerate, and venous hypertension decreases. When used during pregnancy, compression therapy leads to a lesser increase in lower leg volume. It is well tolerated by pregnant women and there is an improvement in their subjectively perceived symptoms [26]. There is no consensus regarding the type of compression. Both class I (15–20 mmHg) and class II (20–30 mmHg) compression materials can be used. Women may use maternity pantyhose, above-knee or below-knee compression stockings. The choice must be made on an individual basis. Compression therapy should be initiated at the start of oedema and continued until four weeks after the childbirth [24].

O-Beta-hydroxyethyl rutoside is a semi-synthetic compound that relieves leg symptoms of varicose veins. The mode of action is probably based on a direct effect on the capillary wall and capillary functions [27]. In a recent study, rutosides reduced oedema and also feeling of heaviness, night cramps, and paraesthesiae in late pregnancy, without causing neonatal mortality or congenital malformation. However, there is not enough data to assess its safety in pregnancy. The study had less than 100 patients [25].

Water immersion has been proposed to control gestational oedema. During immersion, water pressure is exerted uniformly from all sides and drives the extravascular fluid into the intravascular space, decreasing oedema. A single, safe, and well-tolerated 45 min water exercise session significantly decreased severe bilateral lower leg oedema in uncomplicated pregnancies [28].

Reflexology and other types of leg massage have also been used to control leg swelling in pregnant women. In a recent review, reflexology showed a trend in improving leg oedema and could be recommended in women with troublesome leg symptoms. However, the sample size was too small to be able to draw conclusions [4]. It is important to consider that professional massage requires specialist training, and it is likely to be a costly treatment [23].

19.4 Pathological Causes of Lower Limb Swelling During Pregnancy

Although present in 80% of normal pregnancies, lower limb oedema can indicate a pathological condition in some situations. Adequate prenatal care is crucial to detect these pathological conditions. When evaluating pregnant women with severe bilateral oedema, physicians should consider systemic diseases such as preeclampsia, malnutrition, diabetes, renal and hepatic disease, or congestive heart failure [29]. Severe unilateral or asymmetric oedema should raise the suspicion of deep venous thrombosis or infection. Chronic venous disease is a common cause of leg swelling during pregnancy and can cause unilateral and bilateral oedema.

Preeclampsia is one of the most dangerous obstetric condition, and cannot be ignored in pregnant women who complain of leg swelling [25]. A placental dysfunction triggers a cascade of events that lead to systemic inflammation and hypoxia. Preeclampsia can progress rapidly to severe complications, including the death of both mother and foetus [5]. It is diagnosed during the third trimester by the presence of lower limb oedema, new-onset hypertension, and either proteinuria or signs and symptoms of end-organ dysfunction [30]. Early diagnosis is essential. The current management of preeclampsia includes perinatal blood pressure control and monitoring, prenatal aspirin therapy in high-risk women, betamethasone for patients <34 weeks, parenteral magnesium sulphate, and careful follow-up of postpartum blood pressures. Timely delivery of the foetus and the placenta remains the only definitive treatment [5].

Deep venous thrombosis and its most severe complication, pulmonary embolism, cause significant maternal mortality [31]. The hormonal factor creates a natural prothrombotic state. The mechanical factor causes decreased venous flow velocity, venous dilatation, and stasis. Both factors promote the formation of blood clots in the deep venous system. Vascular trauma during delivery, especially with assistive devices and caesarean section, further increases postpartum thrombotic risk. The most important risk factors for deep venous thrombosis in pregnancy are previous thrombosis, thrombophilia, and age >35 years [6].

Pregnancy-associated deep venous thrombosis manifests as painful unilateral leg oedema. Sometimes it is difficult to establish a diagnosis since oedema is widespread during pregnancy. D-dimers levels are largely unreliable because they continuously increase during normal pregnancy. Duplex scan is the standard of care for diagnosing pregnancy-associated deep venous thrombosis [32].

All pregnant women diagnosed with deep venous thrombosis should be treated with systemic anticoagulation. For those with contraindication to anticoagulation, an inferior vena cava filter may be an option. Low-molecular-weight heparin is the preferred choice in patients with a normal kidney function. It can be administered subcutaneously once or twice a day. In patients with a glomerular filtration rate <30 ml/min, unfractionated heparin can be used. It is typically started with a continuous intravenous infusion and transitioned to dose-adjusted twice-a-day subcutaneous doses. The therapeutic ranges can be monitored by partial thromboplastin time or anti-Xa levels [6]. Following delivery, therapeutic anticoagulation can be restarted 24 h after epidural catheter removal, 6 to 12 h after a vaginal delivery, or 12 to 24 h after caesarean section, if there is no bleeding. Therapeutic anticoagulation should be continued in the postpartum for six weeks. In the postpartum, breast-feeding mothers can either continue the antepartum anticoagulant or switch to warfarin [33]. Direct oral anticoagulants (DOACs) are not recommended in pregnancy because they have not been extensively studied, and safety data are not established [34].

Chronic venous disease is present in about 60% of the population. In nonpregnant women, primary vein wall abnormalities cause venous reflux, which determines chronic venous hypertension. Clinical manifestations are varicose veins, oedema, eczema, hyperpigmentation, lipodermatosclerosis, and ulcers (Fig. 19.4). During pregnancy, the hormonal and the mechanical factors further increase venous hypertension. Gravidae usually report worsening of pre-existent oedema and enlargement of their varicose veins, mainly in the third trimester [35]. As with gestational oedema, varicose veins typically regress in the postpartum [10]. The management of chronic venous disease during pregnancy is generally conservative. The objective is to control symptoms (oedema, pain, heaviness, cramps, and paraesthesiae) and avoid complications (thrombophlebitis, bleeding). The measures discussed above for gestational oedema (rest, leg elevation, lie on the left side, exercises,

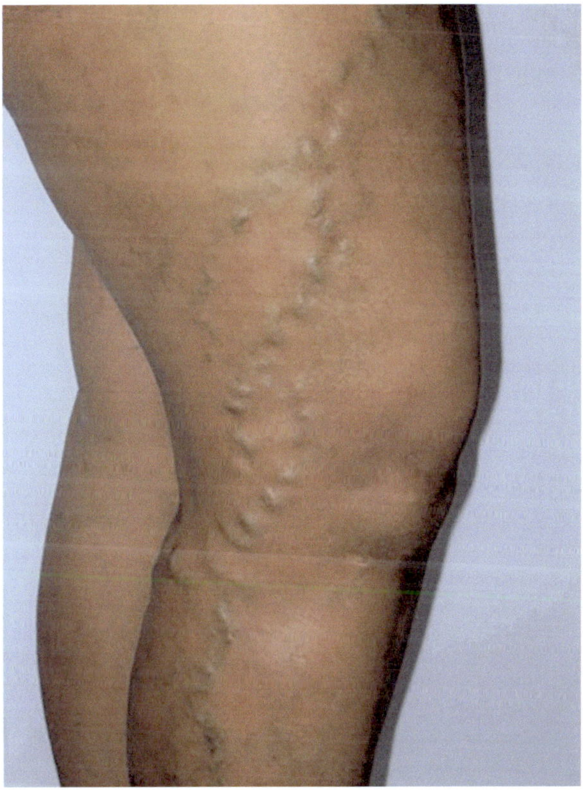

Fig. 19.4 Digital image of a multigravida during the last trimester. She complained of worsening of pre-existent oedema and enlargement of their varicose veins

compression therapy) should be offered on an individual basis. In many cases, varicose veins decrease, but not disappear entirely in the postpartum. The current recommendation is to wait at least three months before performing any surgical procedure to remove the varicose veins. If a new pregnancy is planned for soon, the surgical treatment should be delayed after the last pregnancy [36]. The surgical treatment offers excellent results in chronic venous disease [37].

Other pathological causes of lower limb swelling during pregnancy, such as malnutrition, diabetes, renal and hepatic disease, congestive heart failure, and infection can be diagnosed with adequate prenatal care. Their management is beyond the objective of this chapter.

19.5 Conclusion

Lower limb swelling is expected in pregnancy. Pitting oedema of the ankles and legs, at the end of the day, and more intense in the third trimester is the typical clinical picture. Physiologic gestational oedema usually resolves in the postpartum. Pregnancy hormones and enlarged uterus are the main causative factors. Management of gestational oedema includes rest, leg elevation, lie on the left side, exercises, compression therapy, and other measures. Several pathological conditions in pregnancy can manifest as lower limb swelling: preeclampsia, malnutrition, diabetes, renal and hepatic disease, congestive heart failure, chronic venous disease, deep venous thrombosis and infection. Adequate prenatal care can diagnose these conditions. Their management is specific.

References

1. Robertson EG. The natural history of oedema during pregnancy. J Obstet Gynaecol Br Commonw. 1971;78:520–9.
2. Thomson AM, Hytten FE, Billewicz WZ. The epidemiology of oedema during pregnancy. J Obstet Gynaecol Br Commonw. 1967;74:1–10.
3. Skudder PA, Farrington DT. Venous conditions associated with pregnancy. Semin Dermatol. 1993;12:72–7.
4. Bamigboye AA, Hofmeyr GJ. Interventions for leg edema and varicosities in pregnancy. Eur J Obstet Gynecol Reprod Biol. 2006;129:3–8. https://doi.org/10.1016/j.ejogrb.2006.03.008.
5. Rana S, Lemoine E, Granger J, et al. Preeclampsia: pathophysiology, challenges, and perspectives. Circ Res. 2019;124:1094–112. https://doi.org/10.1161/CIRCRESAHA.118.313276.
6. Nichols KM, Henkin S, Creager MA. Venous thromboembolism associated with pregnancy: JACC focus seminar. J Am Coll Cardiol. 2020;76:2128–41. https://doi.org/10.1016/j.jacc.2020.06.090.
7. Lohr JM, Bush RL. Venous disease in women: epidemiology, manifestations, and treatment. J Vasc Surg. 2013;57:37S–45S. https://doi.org/10.1016/j.jvs.2012.10.121.
8. Ponnapula P, Boberg JS. Lower extremity changes experienced during pregnancy. J Foot Ankle Surg. 2010;49:452–8. https://doi.org/10.1053/j.jfas.2010.06.018.
9. Jebeile H, Mijatovic J, Louie JCY, et al. A systematic review and metaanalysis of energy intake and weight gain in pregnancy. Am J Obstet Gynecol. 2016;214:465–83. https://doi.org/10.1016/j.ajog.2015.12.049.

10. Stansby G. Women, pregnancy, and varicose veins. Lancet. 2000;355:1117–8.
11. Goulart VB, Cabral ACV, Reis ZS, et al. Anatomical and physiological changes in the venous system of lower limbs in pregnant women and findings associated with the symptomatology. Arch Gynecol Obstet. 2013;288:73–8. https://doi.org/10.1007/s00404-013-2728-9.
12. Ouzounian JG, Elkayam U. Physiologic changes during normal pregnancy and delivery. Cardiol Clin. 2012;30:317–29. https://doi.org/10.1016/j.ccl.2012.05.004.
13. Dørup I, Skajaa K, Sørensen KE. Normal pregnancy is associated with enhanced endothelium-dependent flow-mediated vasodilation. Am J Physiol. 1999;276:H821–5.
14. Genazzani AR, Fraioli F, Hurlimann J, et al. Immunoreactive ACTH and cortisol plasma levels during pregnancy. Detection and partial purification of corticotrophin-like placental hormone: the human chorionic corticotrophin (HCC). Clin Endocrinol (Oxf). 1975;4:1–14.
15. Benninger B, Delamarter T. Anatomical factors causing oedema of the lower limb during pregnancy. Folia Morphol (Warsz). 2013;72:67–71. https://doi.org/10.5603/FM.2013.0011.
16. McLennan CE. Antecubital and femoral venous pressure in normal and toxemic pregnancy. Am J Obstet Gynecol. 1943;45:568–91. https://doi.org/10.1016/S0002-9378(43)90832-4.
17. Sparey C, Sissons G, Haddad N, et al. Serial colour flow duplex scanning of the veins of the lower limb throughout pregnancy. Br J Obstet Gynaecol. 1999;106:557–62.
18. Gardenghi LA, Dezotti NRA, Dalio MB, et al. Lower limb venous diameters and haemodynamics during pregnancy and postpartum period in healthy primigravidae. Phlebology. 2016:26835551667158. https://doi.org/10.1177/0268355516671586.
19. Boivin P, Cornu-Thenard A, Charpak Y. Pregnancy-induced changes in lower extremity superficial veins: an ultrasound scan study. J Vasc Surg. 2000;32:570–4. https://doi.org/10.1067/mva.2000.107991.
20. Sparey C, Haddad N, Sissons G, et al. The effect of pregnancy on the lower-limb venous system of women with varicose veins. Eur J Vasc Endovasc Surg. 1999;18:294–9. https://doi.org/10.1053/ejvs.1999.0870.
21. Gardenghi LA, Dezotti NR, Dalio MB, et al. Gestational lower limb edema and venous reflux in healthy primigravidae. Int Angiol. 2017;36:569–73. https://doi.org/10.23736/S0392-9590.17.03865-2.
22. Labropoulos N, Tiongson J, Pryor L, et al. Definition of venous reflux in lower-extremity veins. J Vasc Surg. 2003;38:793–8. https://doi.org/10.1016/S0741-5214(03)00424-5.
23. World Health Organization. WHO recommendation on interventions for the relief of varicose veins and oedema during pregnancy. WHO Reprod Heal Libr. 2018; https://extranet.who.int/rhl/topics/preconception-pregnancy-childbirth-and-postpartum-care/antenatal-care/general-antenatal-care/who-recommendation-interventions-relief-low-back-and-pelvic-pain-during-pregnancy
24. Ramelet AA, Perrin M, Kern P. Prévention - Grossesse. Les varices télangiectasies. 2e édition, Issy-Les-Moulineaux: Elsevier Masson; 2010, p. 186.
25. Smyth RMD, Aflaifel N, Bamigboye AA. Interventions for varicose veins and leg oedema in pregnancy. Cochrane Database Syst Rev. 2015;10:CD001066. https://doi.org/10.1002/14651858.CD001066.pub3.
26. Adamczyk A, Krug M, Schnabl S, et al. Compression therapy during pregnancy: bane or boon? Phlebologie. 2013;42:301–7. https://doi.org/10.12687/phleb2165-6-2013
27. Nicolaides AN, Allegra C, Bergan J, et al. Management of chronic venous disorders of the lower limbs guidelines according to scientific evidence. Int Angiol. 2008;27:1–59.
28. Hartmann S, Huch R. Response of pregnancy leg edema to a single immersion exercise session. Acta Obstet Gynecol Scand. 2005;84:1150–3. https://doi.org/10.1111/j.0001-6349.2005.00829.x.
29. Reynolds D. Severe gestational edema. J Midwifery Women's Heal. 2003;48:146–8. https://doi.org/10.1016/S1526-9523(02)00419-1.
30. Dharlwal NK, Lynde GC. Update in the Management of Patients with Preeclampsia. Anesthesiol Clin. 2017;35:95–106. https://doi.org/10.1016/j.anclin.2016.09.009.
31. Ozsvath KJ, Moore CJ. Venous occlusive diseases in women. J Vasc Surg. 2013;57:46S–8S. https://doi.org/10.1016/j.jvs.2012.10.120.

32. Kearon C, Aki EA, Ornelas J, et al. Antithrombotic Therapy for VTE Disease: CHEST Guideline. Chest. 2016:7–20. https://doi.org/10.1016/j.physa.2010.10.017.
33. McLintock C, Brighton T, Chunilal S, et al. Recommendations for the diagnosis and treatment of deep venous thrombosis and pulmonary embolism in pregnancy and the postpartum period. Aust New Zeal J Obstet Gynaecol. 2012;52:14–22. https://doi.org/10.1111/j.1479-828X.2011.01361.x.
34. Burnett AE, Mahan CE, Vazquez SR, et al. Guidance for the practical management of the direct oral anticoagulants (DOACs) in VTE treatment. J Thromb Thrombolysis. 2016;41:206–32. https://doi.org/10.1007/s11239-015-1310-7.
35. Wittens C, Davies AH, Bækgaard N, et al. Management of chronic venous disease. Eur J Vasc Endovasc Surg. 2015;49:678–737. https://doi.org/10.1016/j.ejvs.2015.02.007.
36. Ramelet AA, Perrin M, Kern P. Choix du traitement en fonction du sexe du patient. Les varices télangiectasies. 2e édition, Issy-Les-Moulineaux: Elsevier Masson; 2010, p. 305.
37. Uema RT, Dezotti NRA, Joviliano EE, et al. A prospective study of venous hemodynamics and quality of live at least five years after varicose vein stripping. Acta Cir Bras. 2013;28:794–9. https://doi.org/10.1590/S0102-86502013001100009.

20 Lymphedema

Takumi Yamamoto and Nana Yamamoto

20.1 Etiology and Clinical Manifestations of Lymphedema

Lymphedema is an edematous disease caused by abnormal lymph circulation [1–5]. There are various types of lymphedemas, and most of them are intractable and progressive. Lymphedema is largely classified into primary lymphedema and secondary lymphedema [1, 3, 4, 6–8]. Secondary lymphedema has an evident cause of the disease such as infection, trauma, and surgical intervention to lymphatic system, and lymphedema other than secondary lymphedema is called primary lymphedema [1, 2, 8]. Majority of lymphedema cases are secondary lymphedema [2–4, 9–11]. In tropical areas, filaria infection is a major cause of secondary lymphedema; filarial lymphedema. In developed countries, cancer treatments are major causes of secondary lymphedema; cancer-related lymphedema or cancer treatment-related lymphedema [3, 7–9].

As the lymphatic system plays important role in fluid balance, immune system, and lipid metabolism, various clinical manifestations can be seen in lymphedema [1, 8, 12]. Lymph retention causes edematous changes in various tissues especially subcutaneous fat tissue [1–4, 9, 13]. Abnormal lymph circulation deteriorates immune system and lipoprotein profile [1, 3, 9, 10, 14]. Long-lasting inflammation may lead to development of angiosarcoma; Stewart–Treves syndrome [5, 10, 15, 16]. As lymph flow deterioration progresses subclinically, appropriate evaluations including lymph flow visualization are important for lymphedema management [1, 2, 9, 11, 17–21].

T. Yamamoto (✉) · N. Yamamoto
Department of Plastic and Reconstructive Surgery, Center Hospital of National Center for Global Health and Medicine, Tokyo, Japan
e-mail: tyamamoto-tky@umin.ac.jp

S. K. Tiwary (ed.), *Approach to Lower Limb Oedema*,
https://doi.org/10.1007/978-981-16-6206-5_20

20.1.1 Etiology of Primary Lymphedema

Various conditions cause primary lymphedema. Although specific gene mutations are reported in familial lymphedema cases, most primary lymphedema cases are sporadic and their causes are unknown [1, 2, 8, 9]. Various abnormalities during development of the lymphatic system can cause primary lymphedema.

One of the most genetic mutations causing primary lymphedema is VEGFR3 causing Milroy disease. Others include GJC2 (Meige disease), FOXC2 (lymphedema distichiasis syndrome), KIF11/VEGFC (Milroy-like disease), RASA1 (Parkes-Weber syndrome), AKT/PIK3/mTOR (CLOVE/fibroadipose hyperplasia), AKT1 (Proteus syndrome), CCBE1 (Hennekam syndrome), GATA2, and several genes causing syndromic lymphedema such as Turner syndrome, Fabry disease, and yellow nail syndrome [1, 2, 8, 12].

Most primary lymphedema cases are sporadic and their causes are unknown [1, 2, 8]. Some are clarified to be associated with malformation and/or dysfunction of lymph nodes and lymph vessels including the collecting lymph vessels, the pre-collecting lymph vessels, and the lymphatic capillaries.

20.1.2 Etiology of Secondary Lymphedema

Majority of lymphedema cases are secondary lymphedema [3–7, 9, 10, 22, 23]. Secondary lymphedema has obvious causes of development of the disease such as trauma, surgery, radiation, infection, tumor, malformation, and venous diseases. Any injury to the lymphatic system can cause secondary lymphedema [3, 4, 6, 7, 10, 22]. The most common causes are parasite infection in tropical regions, and cancer treatments in developed countries.

Filarial infection is the commonest cause of secondary lymphedema in the world [3, 5, 12]. Infection by the filaria, *Wuchereria bancrofti*, causes multi-site inflammation in the lymph vessels and nodes, resulting in lymph flow obstructions. In spite of effective antimicrobial agents to the parasite, there are still many new filarial lymphedema cases because of limited availability of the drug and neglect of the disease's significance in developing tropical countries.

Cancer treatments are the leading cause of secondary lymphedema in most developed countries [3, 6, 10, 12, 22]. Surgical resection and/or irradiation of regional lymph nodes causes lymph flow obstruction. Extensive lymph node dissection with radiation has a higher risk of developing secondary lymphedema. Extensive intra-lymphatic metastasis of tumor cells can also cause lymph flow obstruction and subsequent lymphedema.

Venous stasis ultimately causes abnormal lymph circulation, as lymph flows into venous circulation [2, 12, 24]. Advanced venous congestion can be associated with lymphedema; phlebolymphedema. Phlebolymphedema manifests as more progressive edematous disease with frequent inflammatory episodes of cellulitis and ulceration complicated with lymphorrhea.

20.1.3 Clinical Manifestations and Prognosis of Lymphedema

Abnormal lymph circulation causes dysfunction in fluid balance, lipid metabolism, and immune system [1, 3, 9, 10, 12]. Clinical manifestations are caused by edematous changes, poor lipid metabolism, and local immune-insufficiency in affected regions.

Lymph retention leads to volume changes mostly in the adipose tissue via edematous changes [4, 10, 11, 23]. Lymph, protein-rich fluid, retains in the interstitial tissue, manifesting pitting edema. Protein-rich fluid in the interstitial tissue causes subclinical inflammation and adipose tissue deposition, manifesting non-pitting edema with significant duration after lymphedema development. Long-lasting inflammation finally leads to fibrotic changes of the dermis and the adipose tissue, manifesting elephantiasis. In advanced lymphedema, dermal lymphatic capillaries are dilated in the very superficial layer in the dermis, manifesting lymphocyst. Lymphocyst is likely to be ruptured spontaneously, causing leakage of lymph called lymphorrhea [4, 9, 12, 20, 25, 26].

Inflammation is caused either by interstitial lymph retention itself or by infectious conditions [1, 10, 16, 25]. Clinically evident inflammation can be seen in lymphedematous regions, called lymphangitis or cellulitis. Bacterial infection is more frequently seen in progressed lymphedema complicated with lymphorrhea or phlebolymphedema, and is sometimes life-threatening because of sepsis. Decades-long inflammation eventually causes malignant mutation of the lymph vessels' cell gene, causing life-threatening lymphangiosarcoma or angiosarcoma called Stewart–Treves syndrome [6, 10, 15].

Lymphedema starts from subclinical conditions with abnormal lymph circulation, and progresses to clinically evident edematous changes; first with pitting edema, then non-pitting edema [3, 9, 11, 17, 25, 27]. Although the progression is gradual and not rapid in most cases, lymphedema is progressive and non-curable in nature, and its treatment requires life-long time. Lower hemi-body lymphedema, lower extremity lymphedema, and genital lymphedema have poorer prognosis compared with upper extremity lymphedema.

20.2 Diagnosis and Evaluation of Lymphedema

The most important point in lymphedema evaluation is to understand that clinical manifestations can be confirmed only after abnormal lymph circulation significantly progresses [10, 11, 27]. Lymph flow obstruction leads to distal lymphatic hypertension and dilatation of lymph vessels, causing retrograde lymph flows as lymphatic valvular insufficiency takes place due to lymphatic dilatation. Only after significant retrograde lymph flow takes places, lymph retains in the interstitial spaces, which is manifested as clinically evident pitting edema. Long history of lymph retention in the interstitial spaces and inflammation in the soft tissue causes fat deposition, manifested as non-pitting edema and skin fibrosis. Classical physical examinations, such as Stemmer sign, can be useful only for already significantly progressed cases [1, 3, 12, 21, 27].

20.2.1 Conventional Examinations and Gene Testing

History taking helps a medical staff to suspect lymphedema. When an edematous patient has a past history of treatment for malignancy with lymph node dissection and/or radiation, travel to or residence in tropical regions where filarial infection is common, trauma or surgical intervention to major lymphatic pathways, or family history of lymphedema, probability of lymphedema becomes higher as a cause of the edema [1, 2, 5–7, 12, 22, 23]. Other medical and social history, which may influence edematous conditions such as several organs failure and hormonal conditions, should be assessed to rule out other edematous diseases. Systemic involvement can be seen in some primary lymphedema cases, and non-edematous body parts and related symptoms should also be assessed, such as the eyelid (lymphedema distichiasis), nail (yellow nail), skin color change (Stewart–Treves syndrome), and diarrhea (protein-losing enteropathy due to intestine lymphangiectasia) [1, 2, 8, 12]. Blood tests, X-ray, and electrocardiogram may be used to rule out other edematous diseases. Specific gene testing is needed for definitive diagnosis of above-mentioned primary lymphedema due to gene mutation.

20.2.2 Volumetry

As fluid retention is the most evident clinical manifestation of lymphedema, volume evaluation is the most common routine assessment for lymphedema [3, 9, 10, 12, 28]. There are various volume evaluations, including circumference measurements, water displacement method, image-based volumetry, and other volumetric methods. Although objective measurement, volumetry cannot evaluate lymph circulation itself which is the most important for lymphedema evaluation.

Circumference measurement is the most commonly applied lymphedema evaluation. Various extremity parts are measured with tape, and followed to assess therapeutic courses of lymphedema. A major drawback of circumference measurement is that it is 1-dimensional evaluation in spite that lymphedematous volume change is 3-dimensional (3D). Therefore, circumference measurement data should be used to calculate 3D volume using truncated cone model or lymphedema index formula (Fig. 20.1) [28–31].

Water displacement method is used to directly measure limb volume. A limb is inserted into water-container fulfilled with fixed volume of water, and water volume overflowed from the container is measured to represent the limb volume. Although used as a gold standard for volumetry, water displacement method is time consuming and non-convenient, which is not practical in most daily lymphedema clinics [3, 28, 30].

Computed tomography (CT) and magnetic resonance imaging (MRI) can be used to calculate volume. Although reconstruction of images and calculation of limb volume take some time, CT- and MRI-based volumetry allows accurate and reproducible volume measurement. A major drawback is high cost for CT and MRI, and they are not practical for routine follow-up methods [3, 21, 31].

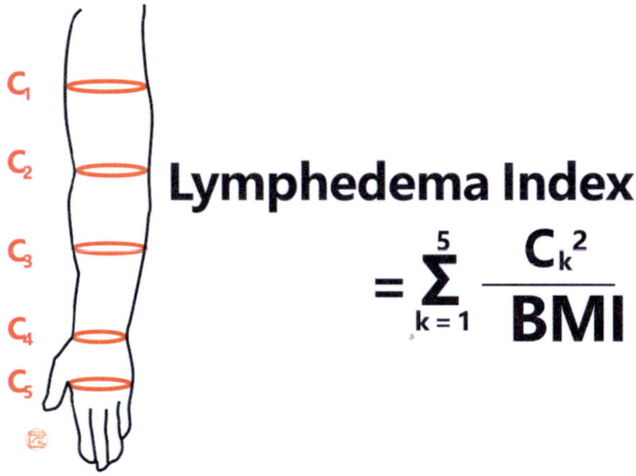

Fig. 20.1 Formula for lymphedema index

Other volumetry methods include specialized volumetry measures such as laser-scan volumetry and 3-dimensional photography [3, 21, 32]. Laser-scan volumetry and 3D photography-based volumetry allow limb volume measurement via laser scanning and 3D reconstructed image, respectively. Unlike CT-based volumetry, laser scanning and 3D photograph are free from radiation exposure.

20.2.3 Bio-Impedance Spectroscopy

Bio-impedance spectroscopy (BIS) quantifies fluid balance in the human body by measuring various parts' impedance to calculate fluid components in the muscle and the fat tissues of various body parts. BIS is not invasive and its data is easily available, allowing clinically practical routine evaluation method. BIS can detect small changes of fluid retention, and allows early diagnosis of lymphedema [3, 11, 28, 33]. A major drawback is that BIS only quantifies fluid balance and cannot assess lymph circulation which is crucial for lymphedema evaluation. Small change of fluid balance can occur in daily activity or physiological and non-pathological leg edema. Therefore, it is necessary for definitive diagnosis of lymphedema to rule out other edematous conditions with other modalities.

20.2.4 Imaging Studies Other than Lymph Flow Imaging

Edematous changes can be detected by CT, MR, and ultrasound (US). Fluid retention is represented as higher density area in CT, higher intensity area in T2 weighted MRI, and hypoechoic area in US [3, 12, 21, 22]. Typically, fluid retention is seen mostly in the deep fat layer above the deep fascia in lymphedema, whereas venous edema shows fluid retention also in the deeper tissues such as the muscles. CT and MRI have an advantage that edema distribution is visualized three-dimensionally. CT allows quick scanning to obtain images, but has a risk of radiation exposure.

MRI visualizes 3D distribution of fluid and fat without radiation exposure, but requires longer scanning time than CT. US allows real-time visualization and sometimes visualizes the collecting lymphatic vessels, but its image quality largely depends on an examiner [10, 22, 34].

20.2.5 Lymph Flow Imaging Studies

Lymph flow visualization is the most important for lymphedema evaluation, and basically necessary for definitive diagnosis. There are several lymphography methods, including direct oil-contrast lymphangiography (LAG), lymphoscintigraphy (LSG) and single photon-emission computed tomography-computerized tomography (SPECT-CT), magnetic resonance lymphography (MRL), and indocyanine green fluorescent lymphography (ICG-L) [3, 8, 9, 17, 19, 21, 35–39].

Direct LAG using oil-contrast such as lipiodol used to be a gold standard for direct lymphatic visualization [3, 36, 39]. Oil-contrast is injected directly into the collecting lymphatic vessel via a small skin incision and cannulation, and radiographic images are taken. Although anatomy of the collecting lymphatic vessels proximal to the injection site is clearly visualized, LAG has a risk of lymphedema worsening because oil-contrast evokes inflammation and subsequent obstruction of the enhanced lymph vessels. Therefore, LAG is not currently used for lymphedema evaluation, and mainly used for diagnosis and treatment for lymph leakage diseases such as lymphorrhea, chyloabdomen, and chylothorax (Fig. 20.2) [3, 39].

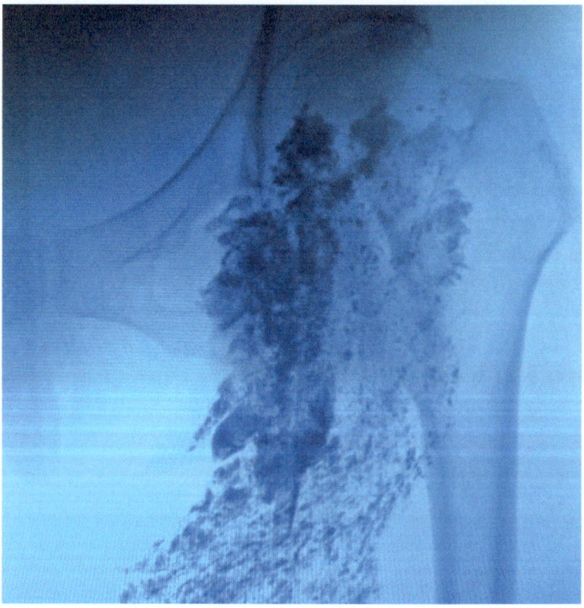

Fig. 20.2 LAG showing the inguinal lymph nodes and lymphatic leakages

LSG is currently considered a gold standard for lymph flow evaluation [2, 3, 8, 12, 17, 22, 36]. Contrast agent combined with radioisotope is subcutaneously injected at the distal limb, and scintigram scan images are obtained after injection. LSG visualizes superficial and deep lymph flows in a whole body, and is necessary for primary lymphedema evaluation with systemic involvement. Major drawbacks include obscure image and a risk of radiation exposure (Fig. 20.3) [3, 20, 36]. LSG can be combined with CT image; SPECT-CT. SPECT-CT allows 3D evaluation of lymph circulation (Fig. 20.4). With advancement of lymphatic reconstructive surgeries, LSG or SPECT-CT images are not enough for precise localization of lymph vessels suitable for lymphatic surgery, and the following new modalities are becoming popular [36, 39–41].

Contrast-agent for MRI, gadolinium, can be injected subcutaneously, which visualizes lymph vessels on MRI; MRL. MRL allows both fluid/fat balance evaluation on non-enhanced images and lymph flow visualization on MRL images. Unlike LSG or SPECT-CT, MRL images are clear enough to consider indication and design of lymphatic surgeries [3, 21, 36, 39]. Major drawbacks include obscure image and a risk of radiation exposure (Fig. 20.5). Although MRL gives abundant information of lymphedema, subcutaneous injection of gadolinium has a risk of injected site skin necrosis which may result in severe sequela of cellulitis worsening lymphedema, and is contraindicated for patients with renal failure.

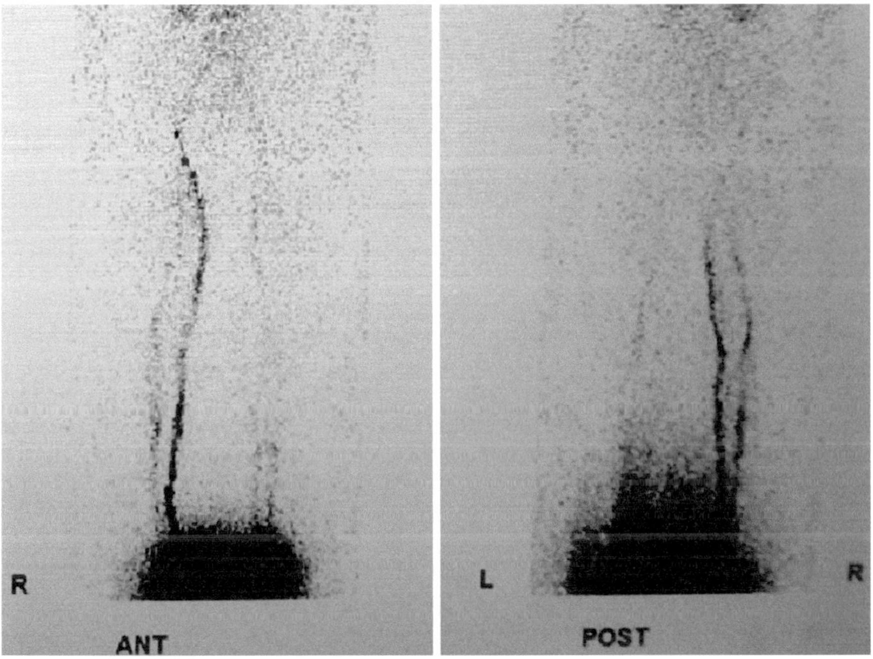

Fig. 20.3 LSG images showing lower extremity lymph flows

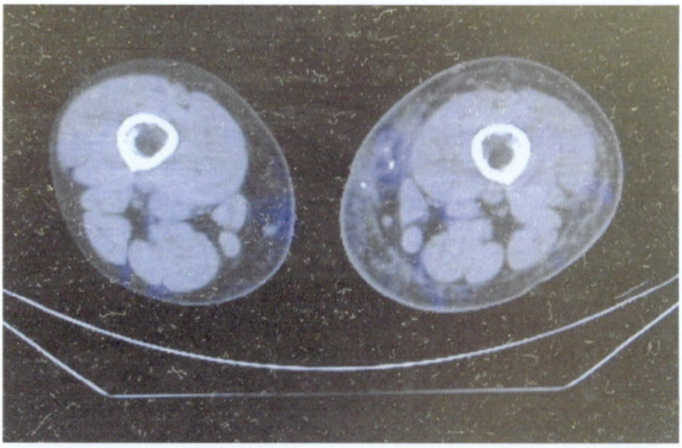

Fig. 20.4 SPECT/CT image showing 3D location of the lymph vessels

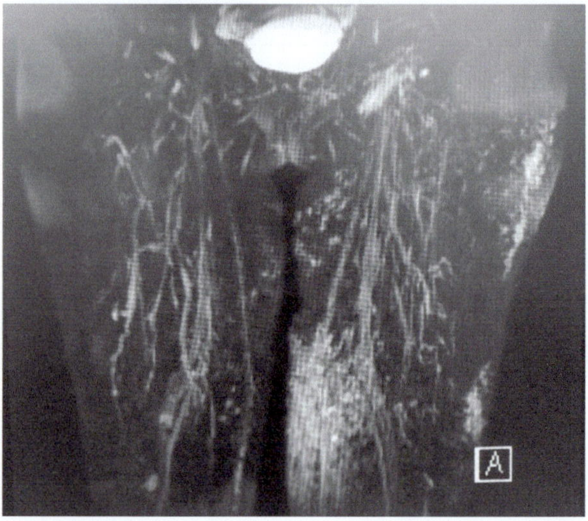

Fig. 20.5 MRL showing the lymph vessels and DB; veins are also shown

ICG-L images are obtained using a near-infrared camera after subcutaneous injection of ICG. Superficial lymph circulation is clearly visualized without a risk of ionized radiation exposure [3, 17, 20, 35, 38] (Fig. 20.6). Unlike any other lymph flow imaging methods, ICG-L allows real-time imaging, which is clinically useful for intra-interventional evaluation of lymph circulation; a surgeon can evaluate lymph flow conditions intraoperatively and use it for intraoperative navigation, and a physiotherapist can evaluate efficacy of manual lymph drainage (MLD) [17, 23, 40–48]. Compared with other modalities, ICG-L allows the earliest detection of abnormal lymph circulation, dermal backflow (DB), leading to diagnosis of subclinical lymphedema and possible radical prophylactic intervention. With its usefulness and convenience, ICG-L is becoming popular and one of the most important evaluation for lymphedema management in most advanced lymphedema centers. A major drawback is that ICG-L visualizes only superficial lymph flows 2-cm in depth from the skin surface and cannot directly visualize deep lymph flows.

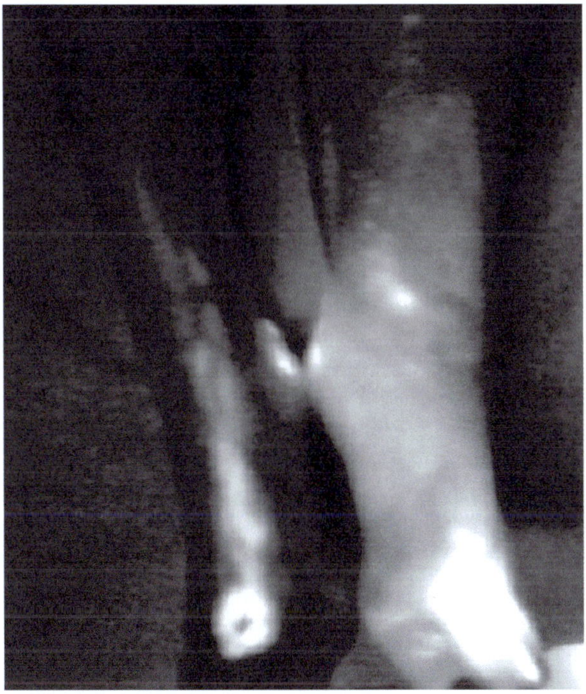

Fig. 20.6 ICG-L showing superficial lymph flows. Linear pattern is seen in the right leg and DB pattern in the left leg

20.3 Classification and Severity Evaluation

As various conditions take place with progression of lymphedema, various classification and severity staging systems are reported. Most classifications are based on physical findings such as edematous conditions and volume changes, and on lymph circulation. Although most commonly applied in daily clinics, physical finding-based classifications does not always represent pathophysiological conditions of lymphedema, and lymph flow-based classifications should be utilized as possible.

20.3.1 Staging Based on Physical Examination

Physical finding-based stages utilize edematous conditions such as temporary edema, pitting and non-pitting edema, and fibrotic changes such as elephantiasis. The most popular and widely used classification is International Society of Lymphology (ISL) stage [3, 5, 45]. ISL stage consists of stage 0, stage I, stage II, and stage III. ISL stage 0 represents no edema but with impaired lymphatic transport, ISL stage I mild temporary edema which can be resolved with limb elevation, ISL stage II pitting or non-pitting edema which cannot be subsided with limb elevation, and ISL stage III elephantiasis. There are several clinical stages similar to ISL stage, and some include limb volume change as criteria.

20.3.2 Primary Lymphedema Classification

Onset age is most commonly used classification for primary lymphedema, and primary lymphedema is classified into congenital lymphedema, lymphedema praecox, and lymphedema tarda [1, 2, 8]. Cutoff values of age are 0 and 35 years; congenital lymphedema represents primary lymphedema seen at birth, lymphedema praecox from 0 to 35 years old, and lymphedema tarda after 35 years old. Although the most popular classification, onset age-based classification does not represent its pathophysiology and is not useful to predict prognosis. For some primary lymphedema with specific gene mutation, gene-based classification or diagnosis can be used for clinical evaluation and management [8, 12].

Image-based classification has been reported useful for pathophysiology-based classification and prognosis prediction. ICG lymphography classification consists of proximal DB (PDB), distal DB (DDB), less enhancement (LE), no enhancement (NE) types (Table 20.1) (2). DB pattern is seen predominantly in the proximal region in PDB type, and in the distal region in the DDB type. In LE type, Linear pattern is seen in the distal region, but no enhancement is observed in the proximal region. In NE type, no enhancement is observed other than ICG injected sites. PDB type has similar prognosis to secondary lymphedema, and DDB type is more frequently associated with cellulitis. LE type has better prognosis, and compression therapy alone is enough to control lymphedema. NE type is clinically most severe form and has the worst prognosis against physiotherapy or lymphatic bypass surgery.

20.3.3 Secondary Lymphedema Staging

Various lymphatic images are used to classify secondary lymphedema severity. US, MRI, and CT-based classification utilizes fluid retention and its contribution/extension as criteria. These images-based volumetry is also used to classify secondary lymphedema severity [3, 9, 10, 21, 36, 38]. As mentioned before, they just represent fluid retention and do not represent pathophysiological conditions.

Table 20.1 ICG classification for primary lymphedema

ICG classification	Lymphography findings
PDB type	DB pattern mainly in the proximal region
DDB type	DB pattern mainly in the distal region
LE type	Linear pattern only in the distal region (no DB pattern)
NE type	No enhancement (no linear or DB pattern)

ICG indocyanine green, *DB* dermal backflow, *PDB* proximal, *DB*. DDB, distal DB. *LE* less enhancement, *NE* no enhancement

LSG is a widely used lymphatic imaging study to evaluate pathophysiological conditions of secondary lymphedema [3, 36, 37]. Based on visibility of lymphatic image and extension of DB, LSG stage and transport index are determined. LSG is clarified useful for secondary lymphedema diagnosis, and there are several reports of usefulness of LSG for prognosis prediction and considering surgical indication.

ICG-L stages are reported for secondary lymphedema of the various body parts; upper extremity, lower extremity, genitalia, face/head/neck, and breast [17, 20–25]. ICG-L findings are divided into normal Linear pattern and abnormal Splash (mild DB) pattern, Stardust (moderate DB) pattern, and Diffuse (severe DB) pattern (Fig. 20.7) [17, 27]. ICG stage consists of stage 0 (Linear pattern only), stage I (Linear and Splash pattern), stage II (Linear and Stardust/Diffuse pattern in 1 region), stage III (Linear and Stardust/Diffuse pattern in 2 regions), stage IV (Linear and Stardust/Diffuse pattern in 3 regions), and stage V (Stardust/Diffuse pattern only) (Table 20.2) [18, 27, 46, 49]. Using ICG-L, ISL stage 0 can be divided into 3 stages; ICG stage 0 (no lymphedema) with no risk of progression, ICG stage I

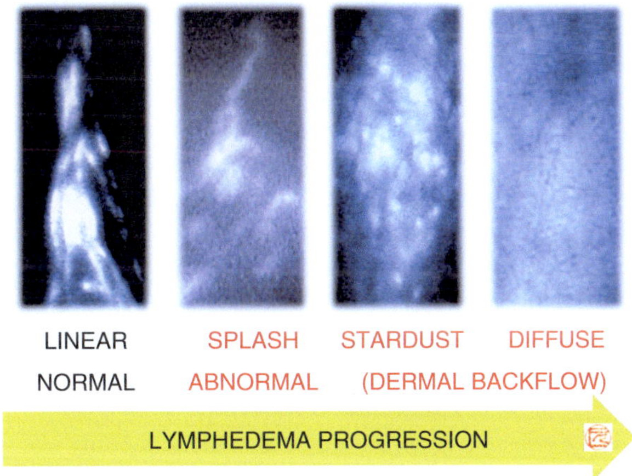

Fig. 20.7 Characteristic ICG lymphography findings. Normal Linear pattern and abnormal DB patterns (Splash, Stardust, and Diffuse pattern)

Table 20.2 ICG stage for secondary lymphedema

ICG stage	Lymphography findings
Stage 0	Linear pattern only (no dermal backflow pattern)
Stage I	Linear pattern + splash pattern[a]
Stage II	Linear pattern + stardust/diffuse pattern (1 region)[b]
Stage III	Linear pattern + stardust/diffuse pattern (2 regions)[b]
Stage IV	Linear pattern + stardust/diffuse pattern (3 regions)[b]
Stage V	Stardust/diffuse pattern only (no linear pattern)

ICG indocyanine green

[a] Splash pattern is usually seen around the axilla/groin

[b] Upper/lower extremity are divided into 3 regions; the upper-arm/thigh, the forearm/lower-leg, and the hand/foot. Face/head/neck is divided into 3 regions; the neck, and the lower/upper hemiface below/above the eye level. Genitalia is divided into 3 regions; the lower abdomen above the mons pubis, the scrotum/labia majora, and the penis/labia minora

(subclinical lymphedema) with 10–30% risk of progression, and ICG stage II (early lymphedema) with 30–100% risk of progression; lower extremity and genital lymphedema have higher risks, whereas upper extremity, breast and face/head/neck lymphedema have lower risks. ICG stage III-V represent progressed lymphedema with 100% risk of progression.

20.4 Management of Lymphedema

Mainstays of lymphedema management are conservative treatments, and surgical treatments are considered for compression-refractory cases [3–5, 9, 10, 15, 22, 23]. Prophylactic lymphatic reconstructive surgery may be considered for primary prevention of lymphedema after cancer treatments. Multidisciplinary approach is essential for management of this challenging disease.

20.4.1 Conservative Treatments

Complete decongestive therapy (CDT), consisting of skin care, compression therapy, appropriate exercise, and MLD, is performed by specialized lymphedema therapists. Compression therapy using lymphedema-specialized garment is the most important one among CDT [3, 5, 9, 10, 12, 22, 26, 50]. Although mainstay for lymphedema management, CDT is basically anti-symptomatic therapy and does not address pathophysiology of lymphedema; abnormal lymph circulation is not improved by CDT. Therefore, conservative treatments are required basically for a life-long period.

Several medications have been used to treat lymphedema, but most of them are abandoned due to adverse effects without therapeutic efficacy; for example, diuretics are now contraindicated for lymphedema. Some advanced medical treatments can be considered for limited cases. Gene therapy and growth factor therapy may be applied in some primary lymphedema cases, but would be contraindicated for cancer-related lymphedema because of risks of facilitating cancer metastasis [1, 3, 8, 12]. Some herbal medicines are undergoing clinical trials.

20.4.2 Surgical Treatments

Surgical treatments are divided in to debulking surgery and reconstructive surgery [3, 7, 9, 10, 12, 13, 16, 26, 40–44, 50]. Debulking surgery, including surgical resection and liposuction, aims to remove edematous tissue, resulting in immediate volume reduction but deterioration of lymph circulation. Surgical resection is associated with high postoperative wound complication rates and morbidities, and liposuction requires even more strict compression therapy for a life-long period.

Reconstructive surgery aims to improve lymph circulation by diverting congested lymph flow via bypass or by implanting an intact lymphatic tissue [7, 9, 26, 40, 42, 43]. Lymphatic bypass surgeries include lymphaticolymphatic bypass and

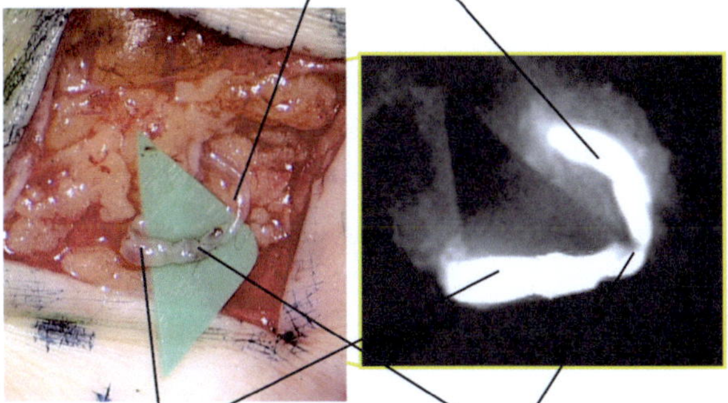

Fig. 20.8 Supermicrosurgical LVA. A collecting lymphatic vessel is anastomosed to a nearby venule or a small vein in an intima-to-intima coaptation manner. Intraoperative ICG-L shows patency of the anastomosis

lymphaticovenous bypass. Lymphaticolymphatic bypass requires a long lymph vessel graft which may cause donor site lymphedema [3, 9, 16]. Lymphaticovenous bypasses include lymph node-to-venous coaptation, lymphaticovenous implantation (telescopic anastomosis), and supermicrosurgical lymphaticovenular anastomosis (LVA); former 2 procedures are done with microsurgical technique, and tissues other than the endothelium are exposed inside the lumen, which would result in anastomosis site thrombosis when venous reflux occurs [9, 10, 22, 26, 40, 44, 50]. On contrary to microsurgical implantations, intima-to-intima coaptation is utilized in LVA, which has a far less risk of anastomosis site thrombosis even with venous reflux. LVA is becoming popular with its efficacy and minimally invasiveness (Fig. 20.8).

Lymphatic tissue transfers include lymph node transfer (LNT), lymph vessel transfer (LVT), and lymph-interpositional-flap transfer (LIFT) [7, 9, 10, 22, 43]. Lymph node/vessel and its surrounding tissue are transferred with microvascular anastomosis in LNT/LVT. In LVT, additional LVA is basically required to optimize its efficacy. In LIFT, vascularized soft tissue including lymph vessels is transferred with microvascular anastomosis, and its lymph vessels' stumps are approximated to recipient lymph vessels' stump to bridging lymphatic gaps. LNT and LVT are indicated for severe lymphedema cases where LVA hardly works due to lymphosclerosis, and LIFT is indicated for soft tissue defect cases associated with defects of major lymph pathways (Fig. 20.3) [7, 9, 10, 43, 46].

20.5 Summary of Recent Advancements

Significant achievements have been established recently regarding diagnosis and treatment of lymphedema. Many genes related to primary and secondary lymphedema are identified, and some of them are applied in gene therapy mainly for primary lymphedema. ICG-based lymphography has been widely applied in evaluation and navigation of lymphedema interventions, including near-infrared imaging and photoacoustic imaging. Combined surgical approach using debulking and reconstructive surgery is becoming popular to achieve lymphedema cure with complete lymphedematous volume reduction and compression-free conditions.

Disclaimers and Disclosure of Conflicts of Interest None.

Prior Presentations None.

Sources of Support that Require Acknowledgement None.

References

1. Lee BB, Villavicencio JL. Primary lymphoedema and lymphatic malformation: are they the two sides of the same coin? Eur J Vasc Endovasc Surg. 2010;39(5):646–53.
2. Yamamoto T, Yoshimatsu H, Narushima M, Yamamoto N, Hayashi A, Koshima I. Indocyanine green lymphography findings in primary leg lymphedema. Eur J Vasc Endovasc Surg. 2015;49:95–102.
3. Murdaca G, Cagnati P, Gulli R, et al. Current views on diagnostic approach and treatment of lymphedema. Am J Med. 2012;125(2):134–40.
4. Warren AG, Brorson H, Borud LJ, Slavin SA. Lymphedema: a comprehensive review. Ann Plast Surg. 2007;59(4):464–72.
5. Simmonds JC, Mansour MK, Dagher WI. Cervical lymphatic Filariasis in a pediatric patient: case report and database analysis of lymphatic Filariasis in the United States. Am J Trop Med Hyg. 2018;99(1):104–11.
6. Siotos C, Sebai ME, Wan EL, et al. Breast reconstruction and risk of arm lymphedema development: a meta-analysis. J Plast Reconstr Aesthet Surg. 2018;71(6):807–18.
7. Yamamoto T, Iida T, Yoshimatsu H, Fuse Y, Hayashi A, Yamamoto N. Lymph flow restoration after tissue replantation and transfer: importance of lymph axiality and possibility of lymph flow reconstruction using free flap transfer without lymph node or supermicrosurgical lymphatic anastomosis. Plast Reconstr Surg. 2018 Sep;142(3):796–804.
8. Connell FC, Gordon K, Brice G, et al. The classification and diagnostic algorithm for primary lymphatic dysplasia: an update from 2010 to include molecular findings. Clin Genet. 2013;84(4):303–14.
9. Yamamoto T, Yamamoto N, Kageyama T, Sakai H, Fuse Y, Tsuihiji K, Tsukuura R. Technical pearls in lymphatic supermicrosurgery. Glob Health Med. 2020;2(1):29–32. https://doi.org/10.35772/ghm.2019.01010.
10. Brahma B, Yamamoto T. Breast cancer treatment-related lymphedema (BCRL): an overview of the literature and updates in microsurgery reconstruction. Eur J Surg Oncol. 2019; Jan 4 [epub ahead of print]
11. Yamamoto T, Koshima I. Subclinical lymphedema: understanding is the clue to decision making. Plast Reconstr Surg. 2013;132(3):472e–3e.
12. Oliver G, Kipnis J, Randolph GJ, Harvey NL. The lymphatic vasculature in the 21st century: novel functional roles in homeostasis and disease. Cell. 2020;182(2):270–96.
13. Yamamoto T, Yamashita M, Furuya M, Hayashi A. Lymph preserving lipectomy under indocyanine green lymphography navigation. J Plast Reconstr Aesthet Surg. 2015;68(1):136–7.
14. Yamamoto T, Yamamoto N, Yamashita M, Furuya M, Hayashi A, Koshima I. Relationship between lymphedema and arteriosclerosis: higher cardio-ankle vascular index in lymphedematous limbs. Ann Plast Surg. 2015 Feb 18; [Epub ahead of print]
15. Sharma A, Schwartz RA. Stewart-Treves syndrome: pathogenesis and management. J Am Acad Dermatol. 2012;67(6):1342–8.
16. Yamamoto T, Koshima I. Supermicrosugical anastomosis of superficial lymphatic vessel to deep lymphatic vessel for a patient with cellulitis-induced chronic localized leg lymphedema. Microsurgery. 2015;35(1):68–71.

17. Yamamoto T, Narushima M, Doi K, Oshima A, Ogata F, Mihara M, Koshima I, Mundinger GS. Characteristic indocyanine green lymphography findings in lower extremity lymphedema: the generation of a novel lymphedema severity staging system using dermal backflow patterns. Plast Reconstr Surg. 2011;127(5):1979–86.
18. Yamamoto T, Yamamoto N, Doi K, Oshima A, Yoshimatsu H, Todokoro T, Ogata F, Mihara M, Narushima M, Iida T, Koshima I. Indocyanine green (ICG)-enhanced lymphography for upper extremity lymphedema: a novel severity staging system using dermal backflow (DB) patterns. Plast Reconstr Surg. 2011;128(4):941–7.
19. Yamamoto T, Iida T, Matsuda N, Kikuchi K, Yoshimatsu H, Mihara M, Narushima M, Koshima I. Indocyanine green (ICG)-enhanced lymphography for evaluation of facial lymphoedema. J Plast Reconstr Aesthet Surg. 2011;64(11):1541–4.
20. Yamamoto T, Yamamoto N, Yoshimatsu H, Hayami S, Narushima M, Koshima I. Indocyanine green lymphography for evaluation of genital lymphedema in secondary lower extremity lymphedema patients. J Vasc Surg Venous Lym Dis. 2013;1(4):400–5.
21. Liu NF, Yan ZX, Wu XF. Classification of lymphatic-system malformations in primary lymphoedema based on MR lymphangiography. Eur J Vasc Endovasc Surg. 2012;44(3):345–9.
22. Yamamoto T. Onco-reconstructive supermicrosurgery. Eur J Surg Oncol. 2019 Jul;45(7):1146–51.
23. Yamamoto T, Yamamoto N, Kageyama T, Sakai H, Fuse Y, Tsuihiji K, Tsukuura R. Supermicrosurgery for oncologic reconstructions. Glob Health Med. 2020;2(1):18–23. https://doi.org/10.35772/ghm.2019.01019.
24. Lerman M, Gaebler JA, Hoy S, et al. Health and economic benefits of advanced pneumatic compression devices in patients with phlebolymphedema. J Vasc Surg. 2019;69(2):571–80.
25. Yamamoto T, Yamamoto N, Furuya M, Hayashi A, Koshima I. Genital lymphedema score: genital lymphedema severity scoring system based on subjective symptoms. Ann Plast Surg. 2016;77(1):119–21.
26. Yamamoto T, Koshima I, Yoshimatsu H, Narushima M, Mihara M, Iida T. Simultaneous multisite lymphaticovenular anastomoses for primary lower extremity and genital lymphoedema complicated with severe lymphorrhea. J Plast Reconstr Aesthet Surg. 2011;64(6):812–5. Epub2010 Nov 17
27. Yamamoto T, Matsuda N, Doi K, Oshima A, Yoshimatsu H, Todokoro T, Ogata F, Mihara M, Narushima M, Iida T, Koshima I. The earliest finding of indocyanine green (ICG) lymphography in asymptomatic limbs of lower extremity lymphedema patients secondary to cancer treatment: the modified dermal backflow (DB) stage and concept of subclinical lymphedema. Plast Reconstr Surg 2011;128(4):314e–321e.
28. Yamamoto T, Matsuda N, Todokoro T, Yoshimatsu H, Narushima M, Mihara M, Uchida G, Koshima I. Lower extremity lymphedema index: a simple method for severity evaluation of lower extremity lymphedema. Ann Plast Surg. 2011;67(6):637–40.
29. Yamamoto T, Yamamoto N, Hayashi N, Hayashi A, Koshima I. Practicality of lower extremity lymphedema index: lymphedema index versus volumetry-based evaluations for body-type corrected lower extremity volume evaluation. Ann Plast Surg. 2016 Jan;30. [epub ahead of print]
30. Yamamoto T, Yamamoto N, Hara H, Mihara M, Narushima M, Koshima I. Upper extremity lymphedema (UEL) index: a simple method for severity evaluation of upper extremity lymphedema. Ann Plast Surg. 2013;70(1):47–9.
31. Yamamoto N, Yamamoto T, Hayashi N, Hayashi A, Iida T, Koshima I. Arm volumetry versus upper extremity lymphedema index: validity of upper extremity lymphedema index for body-type corrected arm volume evaluation. Ann Plast Surg. 2016 Jun;76(6):697–9.
32. Naoum GE, Roberts S, Brunelle CL, et al. Quantifying the Impact of Axillary Surgery and Nodal Irradiation on Breast Cancer Related Lymphedema and Local Tumor Control: Long Term Results From a Prospective Screening Trial [published online ahead of print, 2020 Jul 30]. J Clin Oncol. 2020;JCO2000459
33. Koelmeyer LA, Borotkanics RJ, Alcorso J, et al. Early surveillance is associated with less incidence and severity of breast cancer-related lymphedema compared with a traditional referral model of care. Cancer. 2019;125(6):854–62.

34. Hayashi A, Yamamoto T, Yoshimatsu H, Hayashi N, Furuya M, Harima M, Narushima M, Narushima M, Koshima I. Ultrasound visualization of the lymphatic vessels in the lower leg. Microsurgery 2015Apr 8 [epub ahead of print].
35. Yamamoto T, Narushima M, Yoshimatsu H, Yamamoto N, Oka A, Seki Y, Todokoro T, Iida T, Koshima I. Indocyanine green velocity: lymph transportation capacity deterioration with progression of lymphedema. Ann Plast Surg. 2013;71(5):59–594.
36. Szuba A, Shin WS, Strauss HW, Rockson S. The third circulation: radionuclide lymphoscintigraphy in the evaluation of lymphedema. J Nucl Med. 2003;44(1):43–57.
37. Baulieu F, Bourgeois P, Maruani A, et al. Contributions of SPECT/CT imaging to the lymphoscintigraphic investigations of the lower limb lymphedema. Lymphology. 2013;46(3):106–19.
38. Yamamoto T, Narushima M, Yoshimatsu H, Yamamoto N, Kikuchi K, Todokoro T, Iida T, Koshima I. Dynamic indocyanine green lymphography for breast cancer-related arm lymphedema. Ann Plast Surg. 2014;73(6):706–9.
39. Sommer CM, Pieper CC, Itkin M, et al. Conventional Lymphangiography (CL) in the Management of Postoperative Lymphatic Leakage (PLL): A Systematic Review [published online ahead of print, 2020 Mar 26]. Konventionelle Lymphangiografie (KL) beim Management postoperativer Lymphleckagen (PLL): Eine Systematische Übersicht [published online ahead of print, 2020 Mar 26]. Rofo. 2020;https://doi.org/10.1055/a-1131-7889.
40. Yamamoto T, Yamamoto N, Azuma S, Yoshimatsu H, Seki Y, Narushima M, Koshima I. Near-infrared illumination system-integrated microscope for supermicrosurgical lymphaticovenular anastomosis. Microsurgery. 2014;34(1):23–7.
41. Yamamoto T, Yamamoto N, Numahata T, Yokoyama A, Tashiro K, Yoshimatsu H, Narushima M, Kohima I. Navigation lymphatic supermicrosurgery for the treatment of cancer-related peripheral lymphedema. Vasc Endovasc Surg. 2014;48(2):139–43.
42. Yamamoto T, Yoshimatsu H, Koshima I. Navigation lymphatic supermicrosurgery for iatrogenic lymphorrhea: supermicrosurgical lymphaticolymphatic anastomosis and lymphaticovenular anastomosis under indocyanine green lymphography navigation. J Plast Reconstr Aesthet Surg. 2014;67(11):1573–9.
43. Yamamoto T, Yoshimatsu H, Yamamoto N. Complete lymph flow reconstruction: a free vascularized lymph node true perforator flap transfer with efferent lymphaticolymphatic anastomosis. J Plast Reconstr Aesthet Surg. 2016;69(9):1227–33.
44. Yamamoto T, Narushima M, Yoshimatsu H, Seki Y, Yamamoto N, Oka A, Hara H, Koshima I. Minimally invasive lymphatic supermicrosurgery (MILS): indocyanine green lymphography-guided simultaneous multi-site lymphaticovenular anastomoses via millimeter skin incisions. Ann Plast Surg. 2014;72(1):67–70.
45. Executive Committee of the International Society of Lymphology. The diagnosis and treatment of peripheral lymphedema: 2020 consensus document of the international society of lymphology. Lymphology. 2020;53(1):3–19.
46. Yamamoto T, Yamamoto N, Yoshimatsu H, Narushima M, Koshima I. Factors associated with lymphosclerosis: an analysis on 962 lymphatic vessels. Plast Reconstr Surg. 2017;140(4):734–41.
47. Yamamoto T, Narushima M, Koshima I. Lymphatic vessel diameter in female pelvic cancer-related lower extremity lymphedematous limbs. J Surg Oncol. 2018;117(6):1157–63.
48. Yamamoto T, Yamamoto N, Yoshimatsu H, Narushima M, Koshima I. Factors associated with lower extremity dysmorphia caused by lower extremity lymphedema. Eur J Vasc Endovasc Surg. 2017 Jul;54(1):126.
49. Yamamoto T, Yamamoto N, Fuse Y, Narushima M, Koshima I. Optimal sites for supermicrosurgical lymphaticovenular anastomosis: an analysis of lymphatic vessel detection rates on 840 surgical fields in lower extremity lymphedema. Plast Reconstr Surg. 2018;142(6):924e–30e.
50. Yamamoto T, Narushima M, Kikuchi K, Yoshimatsu H, Todokoro T, Mihara M, Koshima I. Lambda-shaped anastomosis with intravascular stenting method for safe and effective lymphaticovenular anastomosis. Plast Reconstr Surg. 2011;127(5):1987–92.

Lipedema

21

Dave Harnanan, Lemuel Pran, Patrick Harnarayan,
and Vijay Naraynsingh

21.1 Introduction

Lipedema is a condition where there is abnormal, increased deposition of adipose tissue in the subcutaneous tissues. This distinct clinical entity which affects the lower limbs, was initially described by Allen and Hines [1]. The longstanding and progressive nature of this disease condition often results in discomfort, pain, and disfiguration, which can each affect an individual's quality of life.

There is a preponderance of women compared to men and it most frequently affects the age groups from puberty to mid-30s. Lipedema can affect both lower and upper limbs (30% of cases) [2], with symmetrical bilateral distribution. One particular distinguishing feature is sparing of the hands and feet which is seen only in lipedema as compared to lymphedema. Due to the misdiagnosis of lipedema as obesity or lymphedema, the true prevalence is significantly under-reported. Although the precise prevalence is evasive, it is estimated that 1 in 10 women can develop lipedema [1, 3, 4].

As such by the time the diagnosis has been obtained, chronic irreversible changes such as pain, tightness and a bruising tendency are already present, which result in significant challenges to effective treatment.

There are several proposed contributary factors resulting in hyperplasia and hypertrophy of adipose tissue seen in lipedema. These include genetic, hormonal, and cellular factors which are summarized in Table 21.1.

D. Harnanan · P. Harnarayan · V. Naraynsingh (✉)
Department of Clinical Surgical Sciences, University of the West Indies,
Trinidad and Tobago

L. Pran
Vascular/General Surgeon, Eric Williams Medical Sciences Complex,
Trinidad and Tobago

S. K. Tiwary (ed.), *Approach to Lower Limb Oedema*,
https://doi.org/10.1007/978-981-16-6206-5_21

Table 21.1 Pathophysiology

Factor	Pathological effect
Hormonal	Estrogen modulation of lipid metabolism by signaling the Alpha and Beta estrogen receptors. There is decreased ER-Alpha expression and increased ER-Beta expression
Genetic	Familial predilection in 60% (first-degree relative also affected) [5–7]
Cellular	Adipogenesis is a main feature due to augmented adipose stem cell proliferation resulting in adipose cellular hypertrophy and hyperplasia. Excessive adipogenesis results in primary endothelial dysfunction as a consequence of hypoxia lead to microangiopathy, angiogenesis, and increased capillary permeability. Changes in the lymphatic system also occur with chronic disease and may have similar findings to lymphedema on lymphoscintigraphy [3].

Table 21.2 Clinical features of lipedema

Clinical features of lipedema
• Bilateral, symmetrical, disproportionate fatty tissue hypertrophy on the limbs
• Sparing of the hands and feet (cuff phenomenon)
• Approximately 30% involvement of the arms
• Negative Stemmer sign[a]
• A feeling of heaviness and tension in the affected limbs
• Pain on pressure and touch
• Marked tendency to form hematomas
• Stable limb circumference with weight reduction or caloric restriction
• Worsening of symptoms over the course of the day
• Telangiectases and visible vascular markings around fat deposits
• Hypothermia of skin

[a]Positive Stemmer sign (in case of secondary lymphedema: the skin fold between the second and the third toe is thickened and cannot be lifted)

21.2 Diagnostic Evaluation

The diagnosis of lipedema is one of exclusion, having eliminated all other possible medical causes. The diagnosis is easily missed since the presenting symptoms can be quite heterogenous and can coexist with other conditions with similar modes of presentation.

Persons suffering from lipedema often have a positive family history and the onset of the disease is typically triggered by hormonal changes (puberty, pregnancy, menopause). Differentiating between obesity, lymphedema, and lipedema can be difficult since they may all coexist to varying degrees and may have similar presentations [8]. Even in an obese person, the characteristic symptoms of pain, a feeling of tightness, and a tendency toward bruising (hematoma formation) indicate that lipedema is present as well. Table 21.2. In some situations, lipedema may be unmasked following bariatric surgery for obesity. After marked weight loss, the persistence of abnormal patterns of fat distribution heralds the diagnosis of lipedema [9, 10].

The clinical constellation (Table 21.2) of the major manifestations of the disorder appearing together (tissue tenderness, a feeling of tightness, and an excessive tendency toward hematoma formation), in a patient with a bilaterally symmetrical, disproportionate proliferation of fatty tissue on the limbs but not on the hands/ feet— is pathognomonic for the diagnosis of lipedema.

21.3 Clinical Examination

The distribution of the abnormal fatty tissue in lipedema of gynoid type, with typical involvement of the hips, buttocks, thighs, and lower legs, resulting in a disproportion between the upper and lower body (waist-hip ratio <1). One clinical feature of lipedema is a sharp separation between normal and abnormal tissue at the ankle ("cuff sign") and disproportion in circumference between the hips and waist ("riding breeches"). Based on this distribution, five types of lipedema have been described [11]:

- TYPE I—Lipedema fat tissue accumulates around the hips and buttocks
- TYPE II—Lipedema fat accumulation involves the area from hips to knees
- TYPE III—hip to ankle phenotypic distribution
- TYPE IV—involvement of arms
- TYPE V—involvement of the calf only (rare)

Four stages of the disease have been described (Fig. 21.1) and are characterized by progressive changes in the structure of the skin surface and findings on (Fig. 21.2) palpation [11]:

- STAGE 1—skin may be smooth and soft, but the underlying hypodermis is enlarged.
- STAGE 2—skin may be indented over palpable pearl-sized nodules ("peaud'orange").
- STAGE 3—characterized by folds and divots over deforming, larger fat masses (Fig. 21.3)
- STAGE 4—development of concomitant lymphedema (Fig. 21.4) (Lipo-lymphedema)

Lipedema progression is heterogeneous and highly variable from one individual to the other. Some patients develop minor lipedema, stabilizing over time, while

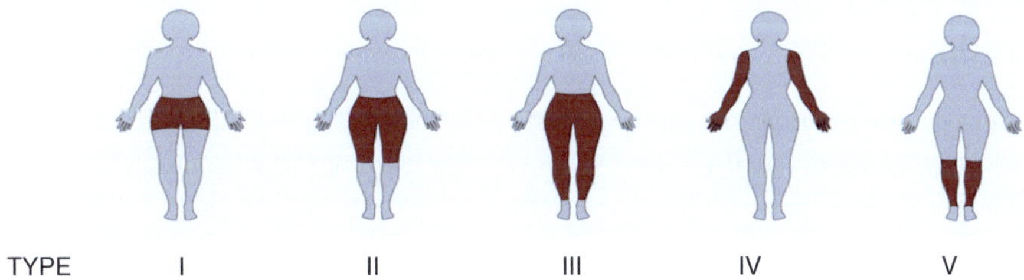

Fig. 21.1 Lipedema types

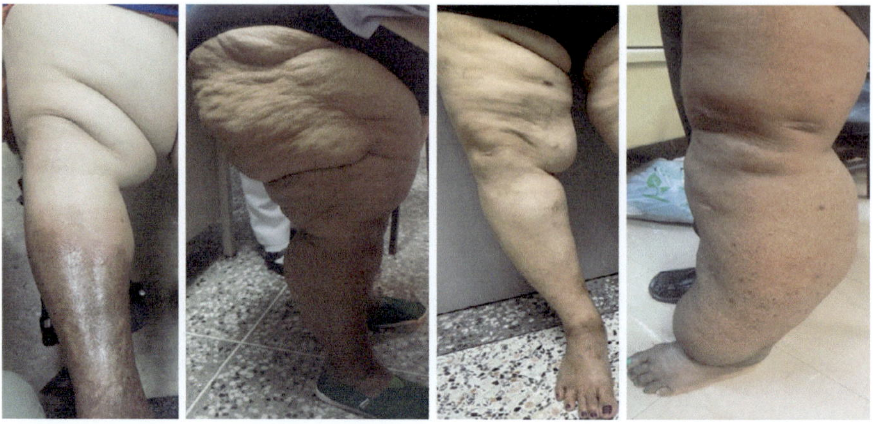

STAGE

I II III IV

Fig. 21.2 Lipedema stages

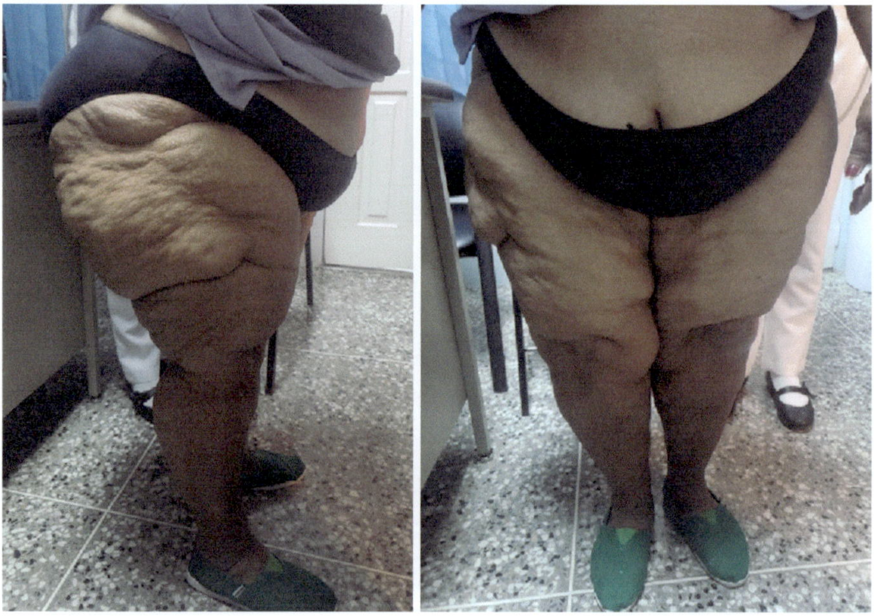

Fig. 21.3 Type II/Stage 3 Lipedema

others exhibit gradual disease progression with sudden stress-induced exacerbation (pregnancy or surgery) [6]. Easy bruisability and moderate to severe pain on digital pressure of the affected limbs and orthostatic edema are cardinal signs of lipedema. Excessive fat on the buttocks, hips, thighs, and lower legs also impacts the gait of patients with consequent mal-alignment of the mechanical leg axis, thus resulting in

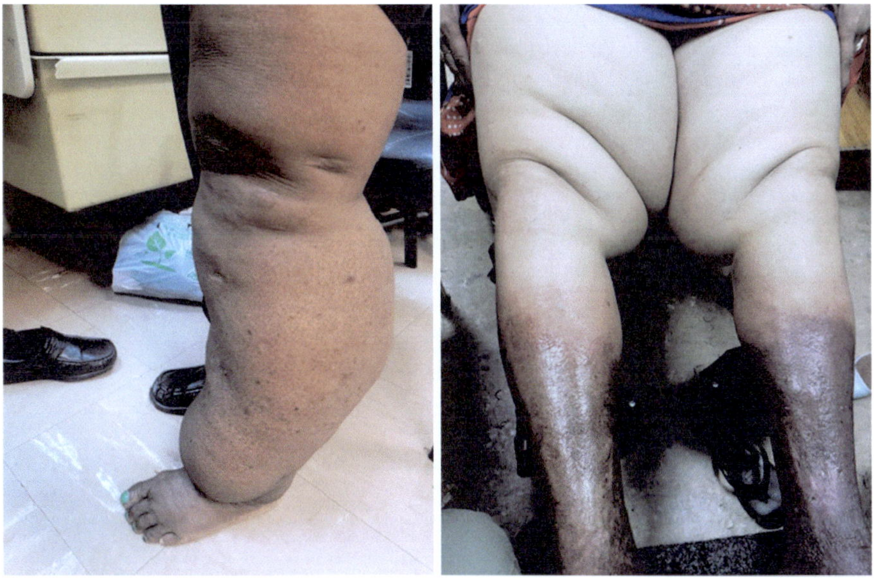

Fig. 21.4 Lipo-lymphedema with "cuffing sign" and Veno-lipedema with lipodermatosclerosis

joint stress [12]. This often provokes knee valgus, osteoarthritis, antalgic gait, and feet overpronation.

Routine evaluation of these patients should be tailored toward eliminating other causes; however, once the diagnosis of lipedema is entertained, evaluation should include standard anthropometric measurements (body weight, body mass index, waist-to-hip ratio, waist-to-height ratio, limb volume and circumference). In addition to this, a pain perception score (Visual Analog Score, Schmeller questionnaire and indices of daily activities), and tissue tenderness or capillary fragility scores which are rarely done in clinical practice, can be utilized. The skin and subcutaneous tissue can be studied qualitatively and quantitatively with ultrasonography, computed tomography, or magnetic resonance imaging.

Structural and functional evaluation of the lymphatic system can be performed and may include a combination of indirect lymphography, fluorescence microlymphography, functional lymphatic scintigraphy, and magnetic resonance lymphangiography. However, these do not reveal any specific or pathognomonic findings of lipedema [5].

21.4 Treatment

21.4.1 Conservative

Because of its rarity and the confusion with morbid obesity, compounded by its cohabitance with venous and lymphatic conditions, lipedema treatment is devoid of conclusive, effective management modalities. Based on its link to lymphatic dysfunction and adipocyte hypertrophy and the propagation to lipo-lymphedema in later stages, most of the conservative options in management are aligned to that of management of lymphedema. The consensus medical recommendation has been that patients should be advised to accept the condition and modify their mode of living accordingly [1].

A strategic treatment plan should be initiated with the extent and duration of therapy agreed upon by all parties involved, with specific reference to the goals of this treatment plan. The patient must understand that the aim of treatment is geared at improving symptomatology and not at changing the appearance of the limb. This modality of treatment will also have the additional benefit of preventing skin lesions and progression of disease. The classic components of conservative management are the following:

- Manual lymph drainage
- Appropriate compression therapy with custom-made compressive garments (compression classes II–III)
- Physiotherapy and exercise therapy
- Psychosocial therapy
- Dietary counseling and weight management
- Patient education on self-management

While the benefits of conservative therapy result in a minimal reduction in tissue volume, various reports have demonstrated improvements in edema, lymph drainage, and capillary fragility leading to a reduction in tenderness and tightness of limb [4, 6].

21.4.2 Patient Education

Lipedema is a chronic, progressive disorder and it is crucial that the patient is educated about the condition and its anticipated sequelae. It is quite common that the patient may develop depression and anxiety issues which can further catapult them into sedentary lifestyles and eating disorders. As a result, seeking professional assistance in dealing with emotional conditions plays a vital role in the management strategy for this debilitating condition. While there are many emotional and physical detriments to this condition, De la Torre et al. in 2018 detailed the pros and cons of lipedema which can be utilized in counseling patients about this condition [8].

21.4.3 Weight Control

Lipedema patients are at increased risk of developing morbid obesity which can worsen the manifestations of lipedema [8, 13]. The pathological subcutaneous fat in lipedema is considered to be diet-resistant but weight modification can improve symptoms [14, 15].

21.4.4 Dietary Modification

There is no specific, evidence-based diet for lipedema patients. However, dietary approaches should be designed to lower body weight through hypocaloric nutrition [14], inhibition of systemic inflammation with anti-oxidative/inflammatory components [16], and fluid removal [17].

21.4.5 Decongestive Therapy

Szolnoky et al. investigated the role of complex decongestive therapy as a treatment option for patients suffering from lipedema [18]. The authors measured capillary fragility (CF) before and after complex decongestive physiotherapy (CDP) to determine whether CDP may reduce CF. A total of 38 women were included in the study; 21 were patients treated with CDP and 17 with moisturizers as a control. CDP consisted of daily manual lymph drainage, intermittent pneumatic compression, and multilayered short stretch bandaging throughout a 5-day course. Results demonstrated that CDP significantly reduced the number of petechiae in the treatment group, in addition to significantly reducing CF in such patients. Thus, CDP was demonstrated as a management option for reducing hematoma formation in patients with lipedema [18]. In a subsequent study, Szolnoky et al. studied whether CDP alone or combined with intermittent pneumatic compression (IPC) could improve treatment outcomes in women with lipedema [19]. In both groups, there was a significant reduction in mean lower extremity volume, demonstrating that although IPC is safe in such patients [19].

Exercise therapy should be tailored to the patient's individual needs and disease stage and should be aimed at controlled, cyclical walking or running movements that activate the calf-muscle pump but do not cause any excessive tissue trauma [19, 20]. Aqua-therapy is particularly useful in aiding with reducing edema and minimizing joint stresses in overweight patients.

21.4.6 Surgery

If there is a progression of disease, despite appropriate conservative management, resulting in significant symptomatology and impairment of quality of life, the potential indication for liposuction should be evaluated [21].

(a) Lymph Sparing Liposuction

In five observational studies of liposuction for the lasting reduction of fatty tissue, with follow-up for up to 8 years, significant relief of symptoms was found. Surgery brought about improvement both in subjective criteria (pain perception, a feeling of tightness, tendency to form hematomas, quality of life) and in objectively measured variables, such as leg circumference and the frequency and extent of conservative treatment. Complication rates were low and corresponded to the reported rates after liposuction in larger cohorts of patients who did not have lipedema (1% hemorrhage, 4% erysipelas, 4.5% wound infection) [22–29]. Patients in any stage of the disease whose weight exceeds 120 kg or whose BMI exceeds 32 kg/m^2 should be treated for obesity in conformity with current guidelines before the potential indication for liposuction is considered [12, 21, 24, 30].

(b) Surgical Debulking

In highly advanced stages of the disease, with accompanying lymphedema, the involved tissue is so fibrotic that liposuction cannot adequately reduce its volume. In such cases, open surgical debulking (dermato-fibro-lipectomy) may be indicated. Nevertheless, it has to be noted that this technique may be associated with the development of secondary lymphedema [31].

21.5 Conclusion

Lipedema is an under-diagnosed medical condition that is frequently misdiagnosed as morbid obesity or lymphedema. While these conditions may coexist, their management strategies remain uniquely different. The clinical features of lipedema can significantly affect patients' quality of life and effective management of this condition can result in improved symptomatology. Stratification of the disease allows for tailoring of management strategies to the stage of the disease. While there are no evidence-based management guidelines available at this time, effectively diagnosing this condition will allow for improved patient acceptance, realistic management strategies, and clearly defined treatment goals.

References

1. Allen EV, Hines EA. Lipedema of the legs: a syndrome characterized by fat legs and or- thostatic edema. Proc Staff Mayo Clinic. 1940:184–7.
2. Herpertz U. Lipedema. Z Lymphol. 1995;19:1–11.
3. Meier-Vollrath I, Schneider W, Schmeller W. Lipödem: VerbesserteLebensqualitätdurch-Therapiekombination. DtschArztebl. 2005;102:A-1061–7.
4. Forner-Cordero I, Szolnoky G, Forner-Cordero A, Kemeny L. Lipedema: an overview of its clinical manifestations, diagnosis and treatment of the disproportional fatty deposition syndrome—systematic review. Clin Obes. 2012;2:86–95.
5. Lohrmann C, Foeldi E, Langer M. MR imaging of the lymphatic system in patients with lipedema and lipo-lymphedema. Microvasc Res. 2006;30:688.
6. Langendoen SI, Habbema L, Nijsten TE, Neumann HA. Lipoedema: from clinical presentation to therapy. A review of the literature. Br J Dermatol. 2009;161:980–6.
7. Szolnoky G, Borsos B, Barsony K, Balogh M, Kemeny L. Complete decongestive physiotherapy with and without pneu- matic compression for treatment of lipedema: a pilot study. Lymphology. 2008;41:40–4.

8. Torre YS, Wadeea R, Rosas V, Herbst KL. Lipedema: friend and foe. Horm Mol Biol Clin Investig. 2018;33:1–10.
9. Pouwels S, Huisman S, Smelt HJM, Said M, Smulders JF. Lipoedema in patients after bariatric surgery: report of two cases and review of literature. Clin Obes 2018; 8: 147–50. Presentation to therapy. A review of the literature. Br J Dermatol. 2009;161:980–6.
10. Bast JH, Ahmed L, Engdahl R. Lipedema in patients after bariatric surgery. Surg Obes Relat Dis. 2016;12:1131–2.
11. Marshall MS-SC. Prevalence of lipoedema in professional women in Germany. Phlebologie. 2011;40:127–34.
12. Stutz J. Liposuction in lipedema to prevent later joint complications. Vasomed. 2011;23:6.
13. Child AH, Gordon KD, Sharpe P, et al. Lipedema: an inherited condition. Am J Med Genet A. 2010;152a:970–6.
14. Faerber G. ErnährungstherapiebeiLipödem und Adipositas – Er- gebnisseeinesleitlinien-gerechtenTherapiekonzepts. Vasomed. 2017;29:176–7.
15. Warren AG, Janz BA, Borud LJ, Slavin SA. Evaluation and management of the fat leg syndrome. Plast Reconstr Surg. 2007;119:9e–15e.
16. Ehrlich C, Iker E, Herbst K, et al. Lymphedema and lipedema nutrition guide: foods, vitamins, minerals, and supplements. San Francisco, USA: Lymph Notes; 2016.
17. Coetzee O, Filatov D. Lipidema and lymphedema: the "leaky lymph," weight loss resistance and the intestinal permeability connection. EC Nutr. 2017;11:233–43.
18. Szolnoky G, Nagy N, Kovacs RK, et al. Complex decongestive physiotherapy decreases capillary fragility in lipedema. Lymphology. 2008;41:161–6.
19. Szolnoky G. Lipedema. In: Bettany-Saltikov J, Paz-Lourido B, editors. Physical therapy perspectives in the 21st century: challenges and possibilities: BoD – Books on Demand. 2012.
20. Burger R, Jung M, Becker J, et al. Wirkung von Aqua-Cycling alsBewegungstherapiebei der Diagnose Lipödem. Phlebologie. 2019;48:182–6.
21. Deutsche Gesellschaft fürPhlebologie D: S1-Leitlinie Lipödem. AWMF 2015.
22. Baumgartner A, Hueppe M, Schmeller W. Long-term benefit of liposuction in patients with lipoedema: a follow-up study after an average of 4 and 8 years. Br J Dermatol. 2016;174:1061–7.
23. Schmeller W, Hueppe M, Meier-Vollrath I. Tumescent liposuction in lipoedema yields good long-term results. Br J Dermatol. 2012;166:161–8.
24. Dadras M, Mallinger P, Corterier C, Theodosiadi S, Ghods M. Liposuction in the treatment of lipedema: alongitudinal study. Arch Plast Surg. 2017;44:324–31.
25. Rapprich S, Dingler A, Podda M. Liposuction is an effective treatment for lipedema-results of a study with 25 patients. J Dtsch Dermatol Ges. 2011;9:33–40.
26. Wollina U, Heinig B, Schonlebe J, Nowak A. Debulking surgery for elephantiasis nostras with large ectaticpodoplanin-negative lymphatic vessels in patients with lipo-lymphedema. Eplasty. 2014;14:e11.
27. Peled AW, Slavin SA, Brorson H. Long-term outcome after surgical treatment of lipedema. Ann Plast Surg. 2012;68:303–7.
28. Cobos L, Herbst KL, Ussery C. Liposuction for Lipedema (persistent fat) in the US improves quality of life. J Endocr Soc. 2019,3(Suppl 1):MON-116.
29. Stutz JJ, Krahl D. Water jet-assisted liposuction for patients with lipoedema: histologic and immunohistologic analysis of the aspirates of 30 lipoedema patients. Aesthet Plast Surg. 2009,33.153–62.
30. Bertsch T, Erbacher G. Lipödem – Mythen und Fakten Teil 3. Phlebologie. 2018;47:188–98.
31. Wollina U, Heinig B. Treatment of lipedema by low-volume micro-cannular liposuction in tumescent anesthesia: results in 111 patients. Dermatol Ther. 2019:e12820.

Posttraumatic Lower Limb Edema 22

Ajit Singh

22.1 Background

Traumatic injuries of the musculoskeletal system are categorized as direct or indirect, ranging from simple abrasions, lacerations, tendon ruptures, avulsions to complex tissue crushing and fractures of various types.

Thrombosis and edema often complicate mechanical trauma to the soft tissues and bones of the lower limbs both at the site of the trauma and distally. Edema is a chronic disorder caused by the presence of extra fluid in the extracellular space. This complication affects almost all patients with fractures of the lower limbs, whether they undergo surgery or not. Posttraumatic lower limb edema (PTLLO) has a significant effect on the timing of surgical intervention. The risk of chronic wounds and infections can also increase [1]. PTLLO treatment can be demanding and prolonged and seldom leads to full healing. Neither the pathogenesis of posttraumatic edema has been completely elucidated, nor has the mechanism causing this disease to become chronic [2]. Inflammation and lymphatic obstruction at the trauma site and deep venous thrombosis (DVT) are likely to play a significant role [3]. This chapter discusses the etiopathogenesis of posttraumatic edema in lower limbs and a study of the related literature of the last few years, discussing the results of treatment and future treatment prospects.

22.2 Etiopathogenesis (Table 22.1)

The four cardinal signs of inflammation identified by Celsus, i.e., erythema, pain, raised local temperature and edema, are invariably associated with musculoskeletal injury. Edema (swelling) is mainly caused by extravasated blood, which increases

A. Singh (✉)
Institute of Medical Sciences, Banaras Hindu University, Varanasi, India

S. K. Tiwary (ed.), *Approach to Lower Limb Oedema*,
https://doi.org/10.1007/978-981-16-6206-5_22

Table 22.1 Common causes of PTLLO with underlying mechanism

Cause	Underlying mechanism
Secondary Lymphedema (surgery/trauma)	Lymphatic obstruction
Chronic venous insufficiency	Increased capillary permeability caused by local venous hypertension
Deep venous thrombosis	Increased capillary permeability
Complex regional pain syndrome (reflex sympathetic dystrophy)	Increased capillary permeability (neurogenically mediated)
Infection/cellulitis	Increased capillary permeability

the content of tissue compartments. An inflammatory response to the damaged tissues and extravasated blood is followed by this. The enhanced vascular endothelial permeability increases fluid filtration in extravascular and extracellular spaces. This results in more tissue volume enlargement and impaired perfusion of the affected tissue. The reduced supply of blood compromises circulation in the tissues and induces a deficiency of oxygen in the region. This oxygen deficiency disrupts cellular metabolism. As they do not have adequate energy for active transport across the cell membrane, hypoxic cells lose water. As a result, leakage of intracellular fluid further exacerbates edema. The increased distance between the capillary vessel and the cell reduces the availability of oxygen to cells that already have increased demand for it. The diffusion of oxygen decreases approximately three-fold for each unit of distance between the cell and the capillary vessel. Edema leads not only to cellular hypoxia but also to increased interstitial pressure, capillary constriction and impaired blood flow. Following the extravasation of blood or bone marrow into the surrounding tissues, most of the edema fluid is removed through venous vessels through resorption by the capillaries. However, cellular components and cell fragments as well as large molecular weight proteins are removed through lymphatics. First, they are taken up by capillary vessels that open into extravascular space. Subsequently, the lymph travels through the ascending vessels to the lymph nodes and through the descending vessels to the thoracic duct, which leads to the left venous angle. The lymphatic system has valves that prevent the lymph from moving backward. However, this is not to say that the lymphatic system functions in the same way as the vascular system. The lymphatic system is open, which means that the lymph can travel from distal to proximal locations, from subfascial to superficial vessels, but also in reverse direction [4]. Over the last years, resolution techniques superior to those of the "older" techniques of lymphoscintigraphy and lymphography have been used to depict the structure of lymphatic vessels during the posttraumatic edema of the lower limbs. Lohrmann et al. [5], who used magnetic resonance for lymphangiography in a group of patients with chronic posttraumatic edema, revealed lymphectasis up to 5 mm in diameter, increased lymphatic outflow and development of collateral vessels at calf level. Interestingly, collateral vessels developed for both suprafascial and subfascial (deep) lymph vessels [5]. Immobilization is one of the factors supporting posttraumatic edema. The effect can be explained both by the mechanism of the muscle pump, described by Le Dentu in the nineteenth century and by other independent mechanisms related to the loading of the limb, which most likely leads to the longitudinal stretching of venous vessels and thus emptying them [6]. On the other hand, recent studies have shown that the lymphatic system is solely responsible for the removal of fluid from extracellular space [7]. The roles of all "players" in the flow of blood, lymph and extracellular fluid in the human body have not been fully determined to date and further study of edema pathogenesis is required. Studies are currently underway on individual susceptibility to the edema of the lower limbs. The results by Sugisawa [8] show reduced pumping pressure in the lymphatic system as an independent risk factor for the development of the lower limb edema [8]. It is possible that idiosyncratically low pumping pressures in the venous system would predispose these individuals to more severe PTLLO. A significant proportion of posttraumatic edema patients have not shown signs of active or past thrombosis. In addition, the classical theory that emphasizes the role of extravasated blood as a factor that promotes lymphatic blockage has been largely negated by the results of newer studies by Szczesny and Olszewski and Lippi et al. [9, 10]. In addition, many patients with posttraumatic edema of the lower limbs have the classic signs of inflammation, which would be difficult to attribute solely to impaired venous or lymphatic outflow. The long-term activation of the inflammatory process involving numerous cells and transmitters is likely to occur in patients with PTLLO [11]. It is caused by the accumulation in tissues of protein-rich filtrate, which indicates an inflammatory reaction. In fact, Maisel et al. [12] have concluded that this contributes to fibrosis, weakened immunity and diminished healing abilities [12]. In some chronic cases, edema of the limb favors erysipelas infections due to insufficient venous and lymphatic circulation, while erysipelas becomes an aggravating factor for lymphedema as a consequence of relapsing outbreaks [13].

22.3 Assessment of PTLLO

22.3.1 History

The history should include the timing and mechanism of the injury, treatment received and progression of swelling and intensity of pain in acute cases. Swelling may be in the soft tissues, the joint or the bone. It is important to establish whether it followed an injury, whether it appeared rapidly (think of a hematoma or a hemarthrosis) or slowly (due to inflammation, a joint effusion or infection. In cases with delayed presentation, a suspicion of cellulitis, DVT (Fig. 22.1) and compartment syndrome should be kept in mind while elucidating history.

22.3.2 Physical Examination

The lower extremity inspection should focus on the medial malleolus, the bony part of the tibia, and the dorsum of the foot. Particular attention should be made to the skin condition, vascular inflow, and innervation. Acute changes in the skin from the injury include wounds (Fig. 22.2), hematomas, degloving injuries, ecchymoses, and blisters (Fig. 22.3) The zone of internal injury is often greatly underestimated by the

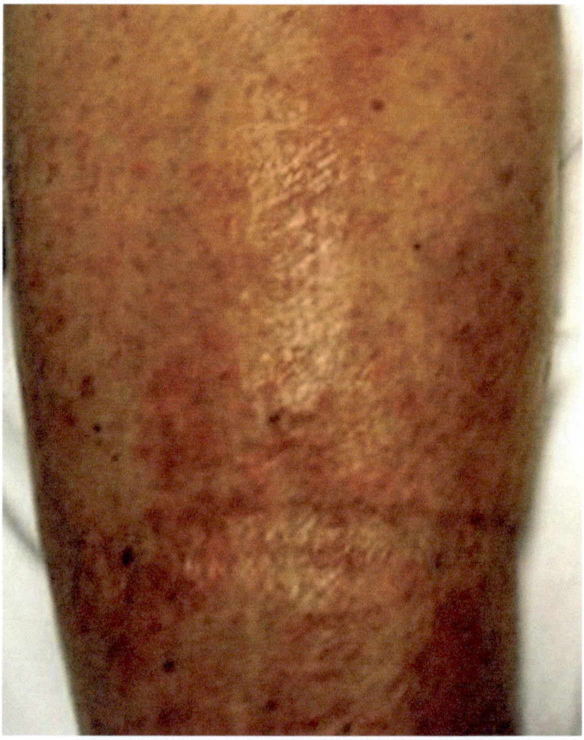

Fig. 22.1 Acute DVT with overlying cellulitis

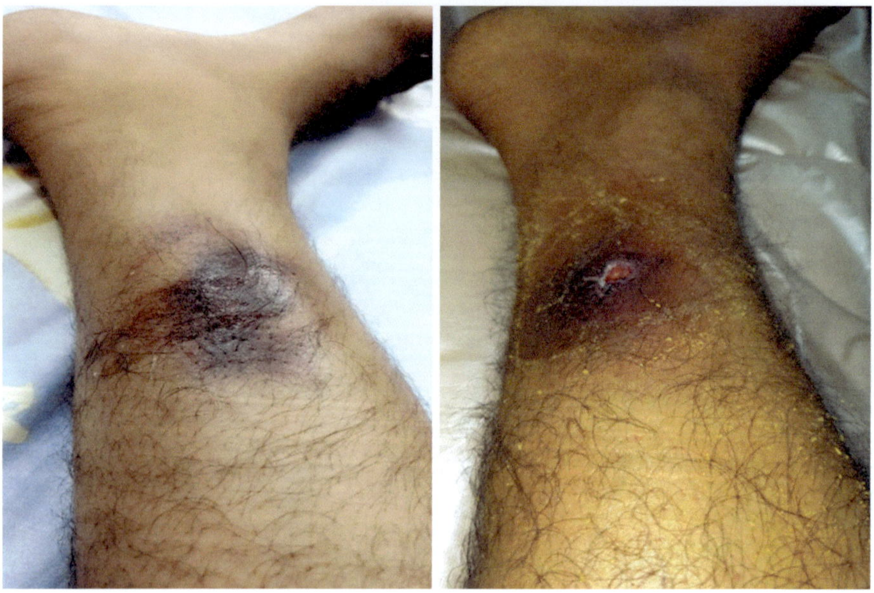

Fig. 22.2 Posttraumatic Cellulitis (right) later changing into abscess (left)

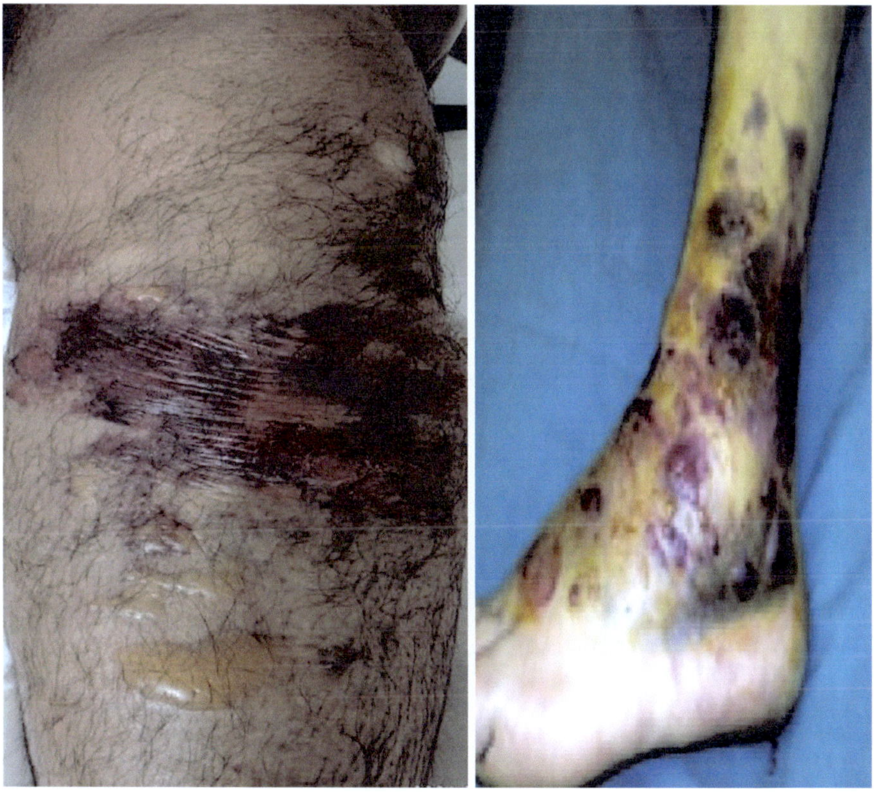

Fig. 22.3 Hemorrhagic blebs

Fig. 22.4 Non-hemorrhagic blebs with impending compartment syndrome

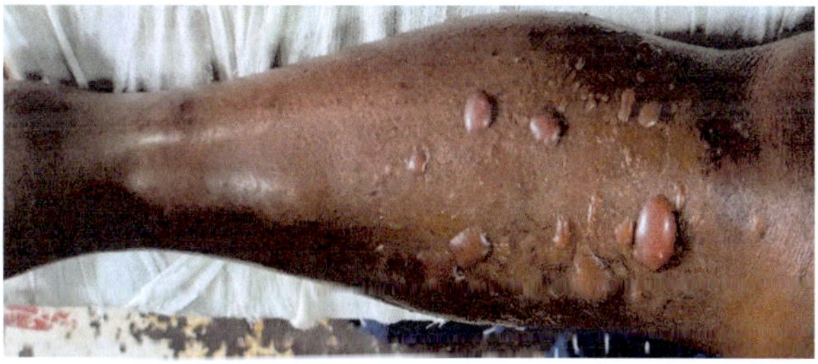

external appearance of the limb and actual extent will be revealed later on. An injury with an associated fracture can cause diffuse vascular damage to the bone, periosteum, and muscle. Acute interstitial swelling can proceed to the point where capillary pressure is overcome and can lead to compartment syndrome (Fig. 22.4). Two distinct blister types are sometimes seen after fractures: clear fluid-filled vesicles and blood-stained ones (Fig. 22.5). Both occur during limb swelling and are due to the elevation of the epidermal layer of skin from the dermis [14]. There is no

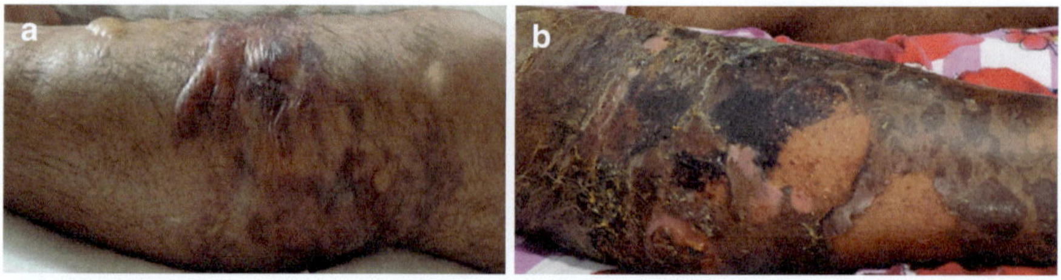

Fig. 22.5 Acute hemorrhagic blebs (**a**). See the true extent of soft tissue involvement which is revealed after 2–3 weeks post injury (**b**)

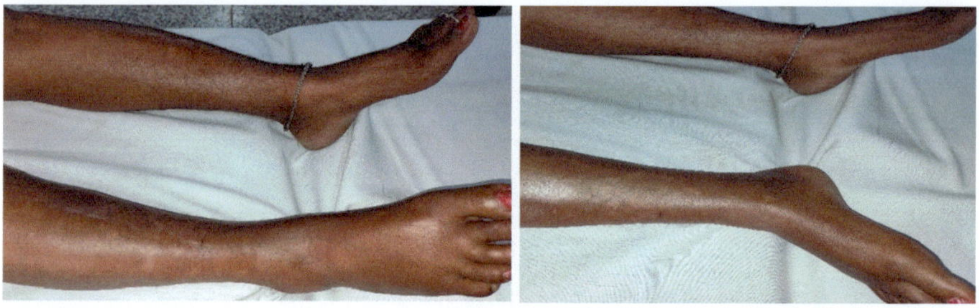

Fig. 22.6 Complex Regional Pain Syndrome (CRPS). (Note the shiny skin and trophic changes as compared to contralateral limb)

advantage to puncturing the blisters (it may even lead to increased local infection) and surgical incisions through blisters, while generally safe, should be undertaken only when limb swelling has decreased.

In cases presenting late, tenderness to palpation over the edematous area is consistent with DVT and complex regional pain syndrome type 1, i.e., reflex sympathetic dystrophy (Fig. 22.6). In comparison, lymphedema normally does not elicit tenderness. For example, acute cellulitis and DVT (Table 22.2) can cause increased local temperature and erythematous discoloration of the skin. The skin can look shiny with atrophic changes in the late stages of complex regional pain syndrome. In the early stages of lymphedema, the skin has a doughy texture, and in later stages, it becomes fibrotic, thickened, and verrucous.

Koban et al. [15] have shown that contralateral leg may be used to assess whether the affected leg is actually swollen by using a relatively simple normal tape measure although it is not a reliable technique [15]. Water displacement volumetry is a more accurate method that measures leg volume but is used mainly in research settings.

Chronic venous stasis disease can complicate both operative and nonoperative treatment methods. An incision through tortuous dilated veins leads to difficulty in hemostasis, bleeding, hematoma formation, and occasionally difficulty with wound healing. Varicosities predispose to venous stasis, especially in an immobilized limb. The risk of venous thrombosis and pulmonary embolism are increased.

Table 22.2 Common causes of PTLLO with their clinical presentation

Cause	Presentation	Examination
Secondary lymphedema (surgery/trauma)	Onset: Chronic; insidious; often following lymphatic obstruction from trauma or surgery	Early: Dough-like skin; pitting Late: Thickened, verrucous, fibrotic, hyperkeratotic skin, painless heaviness in extremity
Chronic venous insufficiency	Onset: Chronic	Soft, pitting edema with reddish-hued skin; predilection for medial ankle/calf, venous ulcerations over medial malleolus
Deep venous thrombosis	Onset: Acute	Pitting edema with tenderness, with or without erythema; positive Homans sign
Complex regional pain syndrome (reflex sympathetic dystrophy)	Onset: Chronic; following trauma	Soft tissue edema distal to traumatized part Associated findings: (early) warm, tender skin with diaphoresis; (late) thin, shiny skin with atrophic changes
Infection/cellulitis	Onset: Acute	Warmth, tender and erythema

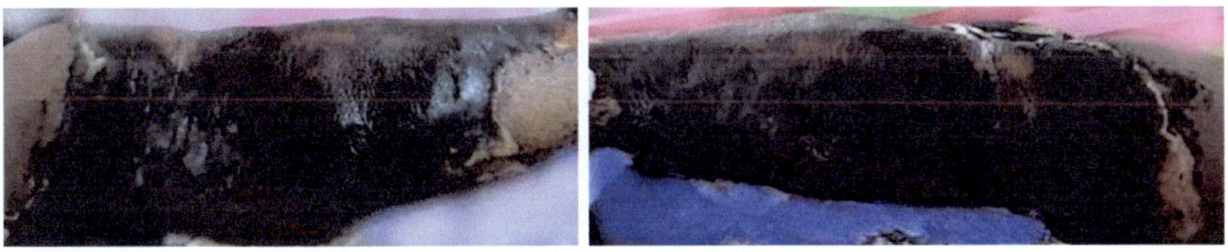

Fig. 22.7 Morel-Lavallée lesion of tibia without any fracture

Another entity, although rare is a Morel-Lavallée lesion (Fig. 22.7). This is a posttraumatic, closed degloving injury occurring deep to subcutaneous plane due to disruption of capillaries resulting in an effusion containing hemolymph and necrotic fat. MRI is the investigation of choice in the evaluation of the Morel-Lavallée lesion. Early diagnosis and management is a must as any delay or missed lesion will lead to infection of effusion and/or extensive skin necrosis.

22.3.3 Diagnostic Testing

In patients who present with acute onset of unilateral lower extremity swelling, a d-dimer enzyme-linked immunosorbent assay can rule out DVT in low risk patients. However, as per the latest ACR guidelines, this test has a low specificity, and d-dimer levels may be increased even in the absence of thrombosis [16].

22.3.4 Ultrasonography

Venous ultrasonography is the imaging modality of choice in the evaluation of suspected DVT [16]. Duplex ultrasonography can also be used to confirm the diagnosis of chronic venous insufficiency.

22.3.5 Lymphoscintigraphy

USG cannot detect lymph flow, therefore, indirect radionuclide lymphoscintigraphy, which shows absent or delayed filling of lymphatic channels, is the diagnostic modality for lymphedema when clinical diagnosis is doubtful. T1-weighted MR lymphangiography can be used to directly visualize the lymphatic channels in suspected lymphedema cases.

22.3.6 Magnetic Resonance Imaging

Patients with unilateral PTLLO, who are negative for DVT on duplex ultrasonography certainly require additional imaging to detect the cause of edema (Table 22.3). MR angiography with venography of the lower limb is used to evaluate for intrinsic or extrinsic pelvic or thigh DVT [16]. Magnetic resonance imaging may aid in the diagnosis of other musculoskeletal pathologies, such as a gastrocnemius muscle tear or ruptured popliteal cyst.

Table 22.3 Common causes of PTLLO along with common diagnostic modalities and management strategies

Cause	Diagnosis	Management
Secondary lymphedema (surgery/trauma)	Mainly clinical diagnosis Lymphoscintigraphy T1-weighted magnetic resonance lymphangiography	Manual decongestive physiotherapy with Compression stockings and adjuvant pneumatic compression
Chronic venous insufficiency	Duplex ultrasonography Ankle-brachial index to evaluate for arterial insufficiency	Compression stockings or Pneumatic compression device
Deep venous thrombosis	D-dimer assay Duplex ultrasonography MR venography to rule out pelvic or thigh DVT	Anticoagulation therapy Compression stockings Thrombolysis in select patients
Complex regional pain syndrome (reflex sympathetic dystrophy)	Clinical mainly Radiography Three-phase bone scintigraphy Magnetic resonance imaging	Physical therapy Tricyclic antidepressants Calcium channel blockers Ganglionic blocks Systemic steroids

22.4 Therapy of PTLLO in View of the Latest Studies

Swelling is almost inevitable after a fracture and may cause skin stretching and blisters. Persistent edema is an important cause of joint stiffness and therefore it should be prevented if possible and treated energetically if it is already present, by a combination of elevation and exercise and stabilization of fractures. An injured limb usually needs to be elevated; after reduction of a leg fracture the foot of the bed is raised and exercises are begun. Active movement helps to pump away edema fluid, stimulates the circulation, prevents soft-tissue adhesion and promotes fracture healing. A limb encased in plaster is still capable of static muscle contraction and the patient should be taught how to do this.

22.4.1 Lifestyle Programs

Patients of PTLLO are recommended to maintain a healthy body mass Index, as obesity itself results in edema [17].

22.4.2 Elevation

Elevation is a simple, effective and popular treatment method, particularly immediately following an injury. However, the need to immobilize the patient is associated with it, which may give rise to more complications.

22.4.3 Cryotherapy Facilities

In continuous cryotherapy, ice water circulates between icebox and cold pad applied to the patient with a daily change of ice water. In standard cryotherapy, the injured limb is treated with ice packs which are usually changed 4 times a day or as tolerated by the patient. The 24-hour circumferential reduction in PTLLO is around 16% after standard cryotherapy and 32% after continuous cryotherapy. The efficacy of cryotherapy has not yet been reliably investigated in posttraumatic edema [18]. At the same time, according to Hohenauer et al. [19] the reduction of edema by cryotherapy is most likely not due to a simple reduction in vascularization due to decreased vessel contraction, but also because of a decrease in leukocyte adhesion [19].

22.4.4 Compression

Compression therapy increases the outflow of venous and lymphatic fluids, prevents fluid retention in extracellular space and allows for virtually unrestricted activity. The use of personalized stockings prepared to accommodate the patient's leg size is included in the guidelines for the treatment of chronic conditions given by the Executive Committee of the International Society of Lymphology in 2020 [20]. It is recommended that elastic bandages be used alone or alternately with layers of compressed cotton wool in the treatment of acute cases. Rohner-Spengler et al. [1] compared three treatment regimens for posttraumatic edema in the lower limbs immediately before and after surgery in a randomized clinical trial with a strict protocol. Patients of the unilateral ankle or hindfoot fractures were split into three categories treated with (1) ice compresses and limb raising, (2) multilayer compression with elastic bandage or (3) intermittent pneumatic compression. Compression bandaging with elevation was found to be most effective in reducing posttraumatic edema in both pre- and post-surgery cases [1]. Mechanical therapies, including leg elevation and compression stockings, are recommended [21]. Compression therapy is contraindicated in patients with peripheral arterial disease.

22.4.5 Physical Therapy

According to the latest opinion of the International Society of Lymphology, as a stand-alone procedure, lymphatic drainage, used in some centers, is ineffective [20]. As per Cohen [22], combination of manual treatment, *skin care*, and compression bandaging are very effective in complicated decongestive therapy, but it requires high costs and is time-consuming [22]. To date, no definitive findings have been used in trials affecting large numbers of patients; this approach is, therefore, not approved for general use in the literature. If this procedure is taken into consideration, it must be borne in mind that the effectiveness of therapy relies on daily treatment by a trained physiotherapist who massages the proximal and then distal parts of the limb in order to stop an uncontrolled rise of pressure in the soft tissues [23].

The supporters of Kinesio Taping say that it promotes the drainage of interstitial edema into lymph vessels [24]. There is some evidence for the efficacy of Kinesio taping for the treatment of postoperative edema. This evidence is, however, not yet convincing given the limitations of the published trials [24].

22.4.6 Heat Therapy

Heat treatment, which involves warm saline water immersion, laser, and electromagnetic irradiation, is effective in chronic situations. To decrease leg volume and enhance skin tonometry, microwave heat treatment was paired with compression stockings, wet saline water immersion, and benzopyrones [25]. This method of therapy is widely used because it has no side effects before or after treatment and assists in the regaining of joint mobility.

The mechanism of action of thermal treatment is not fully known. One recent review concluded that electromagnetic radiation heat reduces edema by decreasing inflammation rather than by improving lymphatic flow. However, the biggest weakness of this study was that it was done on normal healthy volunteers rather than patients with lymphedema, and heat may produce different effects in the two groups [26]. Histologically, the skin after heat treatment for lymphedema shows a near resolution of perivascular cellular infiltration, disappearance of the so-called lymph lakes, and dilatation of blood capillaries.

22.4.7 Pharmacotherapy Programs

Currently, diuretic medications, traditionally recommended for acute edema reduction, are not advised for the care of PTLLO patients. Water and electrolyte balance are disrupted, edema returns soon after discontinuation of drug administration and, most importantly, protein content in the extracellular space can increase [17].

22.4.8 Micronized Purified Flavonoid Fraction (MPFF)

Micronized distilled flavonoid fractions are well-known venoactive drugs. They play an important role in the management of edema in the lower limbs caused by chronic venous and lymphatic insufficiency. The medication's numerous beneficial effects, such as enhancing lymphatic pump efficiency, reducing capillary filtration, and suppressing the involvement of enzymes involved in the synthesis of inflammatory mediators, have all been well established in previous studies [27].

However, Fotiadis et al. [28] found that venoactive agents (a combination of diosmin and hesperidin) have been not effective in posttraumatic edema and the agents have not diminished edema or pain [28].

For the prevention of posttraumatic edema, proteolytic enzymes combined with other medications have also been used. PTLLO after ankle sprains was not minimized by phlogenzyme, a mixture of trypsin, bromelain, and rutin [29].

22.4.9 Benzopyrones

Benzopyrenes help to treat lymphedema by eliminating edema fluid, increasing limb softness, and decreasing raised local temperatures. Benzopyrones function by increasing the number of macrophages in the body, which improves proteolysis and, as a result, protein and edema removal. Furthermore, excess protein reduces inflammatory and fibrotic processes, as protein which is a good culture medium for bacterial growth is eliminated, resulting in significantly fewer secondary infections. Low toxicity, oral or topical application, and the lack of need for compression therapy were all listed as benefits of benzopyrones, which is especially advantageous for patients who cannot tolerate high-pressure treatment [30].

22.5 Other Causes

Complex Regional Pain Syndrome (CRPS) is a chronic pain condition that occurs due to posttraumatic tissue injury of the lower extremities. A clear pathophysiological mechanism has not been established yet and different mechanisms are considered to play a role in the etiopathogenesis of CRPS [31]. Complex regional pain syndrome is treated with physical therapy in combination with ganglionic blocks and medications such as systemic steroids and tricyclic antidepressants [32].

22.5.1 Future Prospects

There are results based on animal tests, showing the feasibility of treatment with saturated physiological saline solutions which enforce osmosis across the skin. In these studies, the skin is viewed as a semipermeable membrane through which osmosis can occur. No human trials of this approach have been published.

Sports centers employ different devices to incorporate cryotherapy with intermittent pneumatic compression (e.g., Powerplay). According to the hypothesis, muscle temperature drops more rapidly in the midst of simultaneous compression. More research is needed to evaluate the effect of compression on physical activity, which is calculated as the same as exercise, as well as the efficacy of such therapies [33].

Sulodexide facilitates the healing of venous ulcers and is frequently used in patients to prevent a recurrence. In a metanalysis, it was found that sulodexide was a beneficial venoactive with a positive effect on the major signs and symptoms of chronic venous disease including reduction of edema [34]. It is also likely to exert a systemic effect on the course of chronic venous disease by interfering with inflammatory chemokines. But to date, there have been no studies of sulodexide in PTTLO.

Indocyanine green fluorescence lymphography is a novel, real-time imaging technique for superficial lymphatic mapping [35]. van Zanten et al. [4] used this technique to image the superficial lymphatic vessels of the lower limbs in patients with severe compound tibial fracture and also to evaluate the length of the maximum regeneration of lymphatic function in these patients after reconstructive plastic surgical procedures [4]. None of the free flaps demonstrated any functional lymphatic vessels; the fasciocutaneous flaps and the skin graft demonstrated impaired lymphatic vessel function and dermal backflow pattern similar to that in lymphedema. Local flaps demonstrated lymphatic blockage at the scar edge.

Hu and Pan [36] have discussed in a recent review about the potential of Adipose-derived stem cells (ADSCs) therapy as a promising approach for lymphedema [36]. Lin et al. [37] concluded that prophylactic ciNPT (closed incision negative pressure therapy) use in the trauma area after surgery reduced postoperative swelling and pain resulting in the improved early range of motion [37].

Further clinical trials are also needed to find the early and vigilant treatment of soft tissue and bone fractures that facilitate quicker recovery of natural circulation in the vascular and lymphatic beds.

22.6 Summary

Treatment of posttraumatic edema in the lower limbs can be difficult and lengthy and seldom leads to full healing. Posttraumatic edema pathogenesis has not been fully explained. Most of the work in this field has been done by Szczęsny and Olszewski [9, 38, 39]. They have studied the primary role of immune response and lymphatic obstruction in the development of PTLLO. The extravagated blood had little effect on the skin, subcutaneous tissue, or lymphatics, although it activates lymphocytes in the LN. The BMC and saprophyte bacteria triggered a significant inflammatory reaction in the local area and lymph nodes. All of these factors can contribute to local edema during the early stages of traumatized tissue healing. Although the fracture or wounded tissues are clinically healed, the local inflammatory response at the injury site continues, and cytokine signals are transmitted to the regional lymph nodes (Szczęsny and Olszewski 2000–2012) [9]. Isotope lymphography was used to assess the immune and lymphatic system responses of trauma patients with closed lower limb fractures and soft tissue injuries. All had dilated lymphatics in the limb, and swollen inguinal lymph nodes in 62% of the cases while only 24% of the patients had venous thrombosis [39]. The role of the immune system in the development of CRPS has been documented in several studies.

Hörmann et al. [24] have concluded in a recent systemic review that, there is some evidence for the efficacy of Kinesio taping for the treatment of postoperative edema [19]. Multilayer compression therapy results in a faster reduction of ankle and hindfoot edema and was an effective treatment of PTTLO in patients with ankle and hindfoot fractures [1].

References

1. Rohner-Spengler M, Frotzler A, Honigmann P, Babst R. Effective treatment of posttraumatic and postoperative edema in patients with ankle and hindfoot fractures: a randomized controlled trial comparing multilayer compression therapy and intermittent impulse compression with the standard treatment with ice. JBJS. 2014;96(15):1263–71.
2. Aydogan E, Langer S, Josten C, Fakler JK, Henkelmann R. Outcomes of tissue reconstruction in distal lower leg fractures: a retrospective cohort study. BMC Musculoskelet Disord. 2020 Dec;21(1):1–6.
3. Zhu Y, Chen W, Li J, Zhao K, Zhang J, Meng H, Zhang Y, Zhang Q. Incidence and locations of preoperative deep venous thrombosis (DVT) of lower extremity following tibial plateau fractures: a prospective cohort study. J Orthop Surg Res. 2021;16(1):1–8.
4. van Zanten MC, Mistry RM, Suami H, Campbell-Lloyd A, Finkemeyer JP, Piller NB, Caplash Y. The lymphatic response to injury with soft-tissue reconstruction in high-energy open tibial fractures of the lower extremity. Plast Reconstr Surg. 2017 Feb 1;139(2):483–91.
5. Lohrmann C, Pache G, Felmerer G, Foeldi E, Schaefer O, Langer M. Posttraumatic edema of the lower extremities: evaluation of the lymphatic vessels with magnetic resonance lymphangiography. J Vasc Surg. 2009 Feb 1;49(2):417–23.
6. Klit T, Dahl M, Houlind KC, Ravn H. Effect of impulsive compression treatment on postoperative complications after open peripheral vascular revascularization (in situ): protocol for a randomized control trial. JMIR Res Protocols. 2018;7(2):e58.

7. Michel CC, Woodcock TE, Curry FR. Understanding and extending the Starling principle. Acta Anaesthesiol Scand. 2020 Sept;64(8):1032–7.
8. Sugisawa R, Unno N, Saito T, Yamamoto N, Inuzuka K, Tanaka H, Sano M, Katahashi K, Uranaka H, Marumo T, Konno H. Effects of compression stockings on elevation of leg lymph pumping pressure and improvement of quality of life in healthy female volunteers: a randomized controlled trial. Lymphat Res Biol. 2016 Jun 1;14(2):95–103.
9. Szczesny G, Olszewski WL. The pathomechanism of posttraumatic edema of lower limbs: I. The effect of extravasated blood, bone marrow cells, and bacterial colonization on tissues, lymphatics, and lymph nodes. J Trauma Acute Care Surg. 2002;52(2):315–22.
10. Lippi G, Favaloro EJ, Cervellin G. Hemostatic properties of the lymph: relationships with occlusion and thrombosis. In: Seminars in thrombosis and hemostasis 2012 38, 2, pp. 213–221). Thieme Medical Publishers.
11. Jiang X, Nicolls MR, Tian W, Rockson SG. Lymphatic dysfunction, leukotrienes, and lymphedema. Annu Rev Physiol. 2018 Feb 10;80:49–70.
12. Maisel K, Sasso MS, Potin L, Swartz MA. Exploiting lymphatic vessels for immunomodulation: rationale, opportunities, and challenges. Adv Drug Deliv Rev. 2017;114:43–59.
13. Pereira de Godoy AC, Ocampos Troitino R, de Fátima Guerreiro Godoy M, Pereira de Godoy JM. Lymph drainage of posttraumatic edema of lower limbs. Case reports in orthopedics. 2018 Mar 5;2018.
14. Giordano CP, Koval KJ, Zuckerman JD, Desai P. Fracture blisters. Clin Orthop Relat Res. 1994;307:214–21.
15. Koban KC, Titze V, Etzel L, Frank K, Schenck T, Giunta R. Quantitative volumetrische Analyse der unteren Extremität: ValidierunggegenüberetablierterMaßbandmessung und Wasserverdrängung. Handchirurgie·Mikrochirurgie· Plastische. Chirurgie. 2018;50(06):393–9.
16. Hanley M, Steigner ML, Ahmed O, Azene EM, Bennett SJ, Chandra A, Desjardins B, Gage KL, Ginsburg M, Mauro DM, Oliva IB. ACR appropriateness criteria® suspected lower extremity deep vein thrombosis. J Am Coll Radiol. 2018;15(11):S413–7.
17. Kataru RP, Park HJ, Baik JE, Li C, Shin J, Mehrara BJ. Regulation of lymphatic function in obesity. Front Physiol. 2020;11
18. Halabchi F, Hassabi M. Acute ankle sprain in athletes: clinical aspects and algorithmic approach. World J Orthop. 2020;11(12):534.
19. Hohenauer E, Taeymans J, Baeyens JP, Clarys P, Clijsen R. The effect of post-exercise cryotherapy on recovery characteristics: a systematic review and meta-analysis. PLoS One. 2015;10(9):e0139028.
20. Executive Committee. The diagnosis and treatment of peripheral lymphedema: 2016 consensus document of the International Society of Lymphology. Lymphology. 2016;49(4):170–84.
21. Berszakiewicz A, Sieroń A, Krasiński Z, Cholewka A, Stanek A. Compression therapy in venous diseases: current forms of compression materials and techniques. Adv Dermatol Allergol/PostępyDermatologiiiAlergologii. 2020;37(6):836.
22. Cohen MD. Complete decongestive physical therapy in a patient with secondary lymphedema due to orthopedic trauma and surgery of the lower extremity. Phys Ther. 2011;91(11):1618–26.
23. Majewski-Schrage T, Snyder K. The effectiveness of manual lymphatic drainage in patients with orthopedic injuries. J Sport Rehabil. 2016;25(1):91–7.
24. Hörmann J, Vach W, Jakob M, Seghers S, Saxer F. Kinesiotaping for postoperative oedema–what is the evidence? A systematic review. BMC Sports Sci Med Rehabil. 2020;12(1):1–4.
25. Chang TS, Gan JL, Fu KD, Huang WY. The use of 5, 6 benzo-[α]-pyrone (coumarin) and heating by microwaves in the treatment of chronic lymphedema of the legs. Lymphology. 1996;29(3):106–11.
26. van der Veen P, Kempenaers F, Vermijlen S, Van Waeyenberghe C, Kerckhofs E, Bossuyt A, Van den Brande P, Lievens P. Electromagnetic diathermia: a lymphoscintigraphic and light reflection rheographic study of leg lymphatic and venous dynamics in healthy subjects. Lymphology. 2000;33(1):12–8.
27. Kakkos SK, Nicolaides AN. Efficacy of micronized purified flavonoid fraction (Daflon®) on improving individual symptoms, signs and quality of life in patients with chronic venous dis-

ease: a systematic review and meta-analysis of randomized double-blind placebo-controlled trials. Int Angiol. 2018;37(2):143–54.
28. Fotiadis E, Kenanidis E, Samoladas E, Chytas A, Lyrtzis C, Koimtzis M, Chalidis B. Are venotonic drugs effective for decreasing acute posttraumatic oedema following ankle sprain? A prospective randomized clinical trial. Arch Orthop Trauma Surg. 2011;131(3):389–92.
29. Kerkhoffs GM, Struijs PA, de Wit C, Rahlfs VW, Zwipp H, van Dijk CN. A double blind, randomised, parallel group study on the efficacy and safety of treating acute lateral ankle sprain with oral hydrolytic enzymes. Br J Sports Med. 2004;38(4):431–5.
30. Badger CM, Preston NJ, Seers K, Mortimer PS. Benzo-pyrones for reducing and controlling lymphoedema of the limbs. Cochrane Database Syst Rev. 2004;2
31. Ratti C, Nordio A, Resmini G, Murena L. Post-traumatic complex regional pain syndrome: clinical features and epidemiology. Clin Cases Miner Bone Metab. 2015;12(Suppl 1):11.
32. O'Connell NE, Wand BM, McAuley JH, Marston L, Moseley GL. Interventions for treating pain and disability in adults with complex regional pain syndrome-an overview of systematic reviews. Cochrane Database Syst Rev. 2013;4
33. Ostrowski J, Purchio A, Beck M, Leisinger J, Tucker M, Hurst S. Examination of intramuscular and skin temperature decreases produced by the power play intermittent compression cryotherapy. J Sport Rehabil. 2018;27(3):244–8.
34. Bignamini AA, Matuška J. Sulodexide for the symptoms and signs of chronic venous disease: a systematic review and meta analysis. Adv Ther. 2020;37(3):1013–33
35. Ito T, Saito T, Ishiura R, Yamamoto T. Diagnosis of trauma-induced lymphedema using indocyanine green lymphography. J Plast Reconstr Aesthet Surg. 2015;68(11):e177–8.
36. Hu LR, Pan J. Adipose-derived stem cell therapy shows promising results for secondary lymphedema. World J Stem Cells. 2020;12(7):612.
37. Lin KC, Li YS, Tarng YW. Safety and efficacy of prophylactic closed incision negative pressure therapy after acute fracture surgery. Injury. 2020;51(8):1805–11.
38. Szczesny G, Olszewski WL. The pathomechanism of posttraumatic edema of the lower limbs: II—changes in the lymphatic system. J Trauma Acute Care Surg. 2003;55(2):350–4.
39. Szczęšsny G, Olszewski WL, Zaleska M. Limb lymph node response to bone fracture. Lymphat Res Biol 2004 Dec 1;2(4):155–164.

23 Quality of Life in Lower Limb Lymphoedema Patients

Matthew K. H. Tan and Alun H Davies

23.1 Introduction

Lymphoedema is estimated to affect up to 15% of the global population [1] and at least 100,000 people in the United Kingdom (UK). Referring to the accumulation of lymphatic fluid resulting in swelling of part of the body, this can be broadly divided into primary or secondary types. While primary lymphoedema is rare, with prevalence estimated at 0.17 per thousand [2], secondary lymphoedema, which is mostly oncology-related (such as in breast cancer), is significantly more common [3]. Due to the variable patient description of lymphoedema and diagnostic uncertainty even after clinical assessment, studies have shown that patients with this "forgotten vascular disease" [4] receive varying treatments depending on aetiology [5] and often failing to receive the complex comprehensive multidisciplinary care they need [6]. Additionally, insufficiently untreated lymphoedema tends to worsen over time [7], leading to further reduced health-related quality of life (HRQoL).

HRQoL is defined by the World Health Organisation as an "individuals' perception of their position in life in the context of the culture and value systems in which they live and in relation to their goals, expectations, standards and concerns" [8]. Lymphoedema notwithstanding, increased emphasis on HRQoL has been seen in all fields of medicine, being seen as a more holistic view of patients' experience of disease. From a healthcare provision perspective, economic analysis determining cost-effectiveness of specific treatments or procedures are also calculated based on HRQoL, with quality-adjusted life-years determined using HRQoL gains or losses [9].

M. K. H. Tan · A. H. Davies (✉)
Academic Section of Vascular Surgery, Division of Surgery, Department of Surgery and Cancer, Imperial College London, Charing Cross Hospital, London, UK
e-mail: a.h.davies@imperial.ac.uk

S. K. Tiwary (ed.), *Approach to Lower Limb Oedema*,
https://doi.org/10.1007/978-981-16-6206-5_23

There are multiple tools for measuring changes in HRQoL. Generic instruments, such as the Short Form-36 or -12 (SF-36, SF-12) or the EuroQoL-5D, include multidimensional questions which focus on patients' biopsychosocial functioning together with their perceptions of health. These tools are useful to assess various disease, but their nature prevents condition-specific traits that may adversely affect HRQoL. To overcome this, disease-specific instruments may be employed to explore disease-specific issues; commonly used lymphoedema-specific tools include the Lymphoedema Quality of Life Inventory (LyQLI) [10] and the Lymphoedema Quality of Life Questionnaire (LYMQoL) [11].

This chapter focuses on the literature in the last 10 years surrounding the impact of lower limb lymphoedema on patients' HRQoL. It will first discuss the level of HRQoL impairment in both primary and secondary lymphoedema, collating the observational evidence currently available. This will then be followed by a discussion of how HRQoL may be improved by the various non-surgical and surgical treatment options that are widely used in the treatment of lower limb lymphoedema.

23.2 Health-Related Quality of Life in Lymphoedema

While there is increasing focus on lymphoedema as a research subject, the quality of the literature available over the last 10 years is variable at best, reflecting its previous position in the hierarchy of vascular diseases. This is even more so on the specific topic of HRQoL in lymphoedema patients, with most of the current literature falling into the lower tiers of evidence levels and a greater focus on secondary lymphoedema with paucity of literature on HRQoL in patients living with the primary types. However, based on the papers reviewed, it is likely that lymphoedema in general, including both primary and secondary types, has a significant negative impact on HRQoL.

23.2.1 Physical and Functional Health-Related Quality of Life

Lymphoedema of the lower limb is characterised by aching and feeling of heaviness in the affected limb, with resulting difficulty in movement and impairment of physical health and function (1). Since lower limbs are directly related to physical activity, lower limb lymphoedema affects patients' mobility, daily and professional activities, and therefore contributes greatly to the impairment of patients' functional independence. For example, lower limb lymphoedema has been shown to have significantly worse practical scores on the LyQLI when compared to upper limb, as well as head and neck lymphoedema [12].

Studies largely agreed that physical function was affected by the presence of lymphoedema, with quantifiable effects on both generic and disease-specific HRQoL instruments. In a cross-sectional study of 418 patients who attended wound management and vascular clinics, only 11 were diagnosed with lymphoedema (2.6%). This study showed that the SF-36 physical functioning domain was most affected by lymphoedema [13]. This has been reflected in other cross-sectional studies; one showed that lymphoedema had the greatest negative impact on physical and functional capacity domains on the SF-36 [14]. In addition, while another study reported significantly lower physical functioning and role physical scores in secondary lymphoedema patients when compared to population norms, this was not reflected in primary lymphoedema patients. Primary lymphoedema patients had higher SF-36 scores when compared to secondary lymphoedema patients, with better physical function and role physical scores, which were not significantly different from population norms [15]. This comparable physical HRQoL was also seen in a study that focused on primary lymphoedema patients, with the mean SF-36 physical component score (PCS) not significantly different from the Japanese population norms [16].

As a recognised post-operative complication of oncological procedures that involve the pelvis or lower limb, lower limb lymphoedema, together with the impact of cancers themselves, contributes to the HRQoL impairments that oncological patients experience. HRQoL in lymphoedema secondary to cancers has largely been studied in gynaecological cancers, as discussed below.

An isolated study showed that post-operative presence of lymphoedema did not have any significant impact on HRQoL scores as measured using the Functional Assessment of Cancer Therapy: General (FACT-G) tool. This cohort study, which looked at 97 patients after minimally invasive staging surgery for endometrial cancer, showed that HRQoL was not impaired at any measured timepoint up to 18-months post-operatively [17]. This is, however, in contrast to the findings of all other studies that were identified during the literature review. Poor physical function [18–21], decreased sexual function [19], increased fatigue [20], functional impairments [22], worsening pain [19, 20] and other symptoms such as limb heaviness and swelling [23] have been reported in multiple studies following surgical treatment for gynaecological cancers. One study also showed that the odds of reporting poor physical function on the SF-12 to be raised by 5.25 times in the presence of lymphoedema [18]. Physical well-being was also shown to be significantly affected by the presence of lymphoedema [24], with physical role limitations reported as well [21].

In a study reporting specifically on HRQoL in patients with lower limb lymphoedema post-melanoma surgery, limb volume changes (LVC) of <10% were associated with improved FACT: Melanoma (FACT-M) scores and declining scores if LVC was >10%. Therapeutic lymph node dissection was also shown to have a worse impact on HRQoL when compared to sentinel lymph node biopsy surgery [25].

23.3 Emotional and Mental Health-Related Quality of Life

This impact on physical and functional health in turn leads to effects on patients' emotional and mental health. Losing functional independence results in inability to perform activities of daily living, social activities, and professional duties, and together with changes in physical appearance, may have direct or indirect significant effects on patients' self-worth, feelings, and mental status.

In the current literature, less comments have been made regarding this psychological aspect of HRQoL in lower limb lymphoedema patients, with mixed observations reported by the various cross-sectional studies included. Interestingly, a small cross-sectional study of 25 patients in Brazil reported lymphoedema to have a greater impact on emotional HRQoL than physical health [14], but this was not corroborated by another small study which found that SF-36 emotional functioning scores were least affected in this patient population in a cohort of 11 patients [13]. Patients with secondary lower limb lymphoedema were shown to have significantly lower role emotional scores when compared to the normal population. Both primary and secondary lymphoedema patients show a trend towards better mental health and less pain compared to population norms, but this was not statistically significant. When considered independently, primary lymphoedema patients also had no significant scoring differences in the SF-36 domains concerning emotional and mental HRQoL [15]. This was further supported by a Japanese study which showed no significant differences in the mean mental component score (MCS) when compared to the normal population [16].

More consistency was noted in patients with lymphoedema post-gynaecological cancer surgery. One cohort study showed that emotional well-being at 3- and 6-months post-surgery was significantly affected if lymphoedema was present post-treatment [24]. Severity of lymphoedema was directly correlated to its impact on emotional as well as social HRQoL [25].

23.4 Relationship to Socio-Clinico-Demographic Factors

One of the largest international multicentre cross-sectional studies included 1094 participants in six countries (Canada, Denmark, France, Ireland, Japan, and Turkey). The LIMPRINT study, designed to assess the HRQoL of patients living with chronic primary and secondary lymphoedema, correlated LYMQoL VAS and EQ-5D VAS to various clinical, social, and demographic characteristics. While the LYMQoL VAS was not associated with any socio-demographic characteristics (and only related to LYMQoL function and mood domains), higher EQ-5D VAS was independently associated with younger age and male gender [26]. This study also showed non-obesity to be related to higher HRQoL as measured using the EQ-5D VAS. This was also shown in another cross-sectional study of 591 patients with secondary lymphoedema, which reported the worst level of HRQoL in patients who were affected by both obesity and lymphoedema [27]. However, this study also shown that lymphoedema played a bigger role in impacting HRQoL than obesity when measured using European Organisation for Research and Treatment of Cancer (EORTC) tools (QLQ-C30 and EN24) [27].

One of the more commonly used staging systems used to obesity when determining the progression and severity of disease is the International Society of Lymphoedema (ISL) staging system (1). Associations between HRQoL and ISL stage have been studied in two cross-sectional studies. In a 2013 study that looked specifically at Japanese population of primary lymphoedema patients, higher ISL stage was shown to be associated with a lower SF-36 PCS but not MCS [16]. This study also found lower EQ-5D to be associated with higher ISL stage ($p = 0.010$). Conversely, a small cross-sectional study of 54 Australian patients showed no relationship between ISL staging and LYMQoL domains or overall HRQoL [28].

23.5 Post-Treatment Quality of Life

These physical and psychological deficiencies in HRQoL may be corrected by both non-surgical and surgical means, ranging from manual lymphatic drainage and compression therapies to microsurgical approaches such as vascularised lymph node transfers and lymph venous anastomoses. While these techniques have all been shown to have an impact to varying extents, it is still unclear on which the most effective treatment modality is for lymphoedema, especially with regards to patients' HRQoL.

23.5.1 Complex Decongestive Physiotherapy

The current standard for care in lymphoedema is complex decongestive physiotherapy (CDP) [1] which involves a combination of manual lymphatic drainage performed by a trained physiotherapist, lymphatic massages, compression therapy (bandages or stockings), exercise, and skincare. This therapy focuses on reducing limb volume and maintaining healthy skin and has been shown to improve HRQoL in patients with lower limb lymphoedema.

In the current literature, most studies agree that CDP has a significant positive impact on patients' HRQoL. Measured using the LYMQoL instrument, a cohort study from Turkey showed HRQoL to be improved significantly with isolated use of CDP [29]. However, a randomised controlled trial (RCT) from South Korea, which looked at HRQoL in lower limb lymphoedema post-gynaecological cancer surgery, found that while isolated CDP resulted in improvement in EORTC QLQ-C30 fatigue and pain scores, patients' physical functioning was only improved when this therapy was complemented with a rehabilitation exercise programme. This consisted of stretching, strengthening, core stability, and aerobic exercises [30]. The benefits of combining CDP and rehabilitation exercise programmes were reflected in another RCT from China which also investigated lower limb lymphoedema post-gynaecological cancer surgeries. This study found significantly higher general health and function scale, and lower symptoms scale in patients undergoing CDP and rehabilitation exercises when compared to controls (who received only nursing care) [31]. Finally, in the most recent RCT at the time of writing, a small study of 49 patients compared isolated CDP to CDP with platelet-rich plasma therapy or low-level laser therapy. Isolated CDP showed significant improvement in LYMQoL scores, and while adding on platelet-rich plasma therapy had the largest effect size, no significant difference in improvements was seen when the three groups were compared [32].

23.5.2 Rehabilitation Exercise

As covered previously, rehabilitation exercises can be used in conjunction with other therapies, with significant benefit over isolated CDP or routine nursing care shown [30, 31]. In isolation, these exercises have been shown to result in physical function and vitality improvements [33], with this specific added benefit of physical function improvement also seen when added to CDP [30].

23.5.3 Intermittent Pneumatic Compression

Another treatment modality for the treatment of lower limb lymphoedema is the application of intermittent pneumatic compression (IPC). This therapy is delivered through devices that use air to fill cuffs and apply pressure onto the lower limbs sporadically, mimicking the effects of the normal musculo-venous pumps to return venous blood and lymphatic fluid back to the central circulation. While studies have shown the clinical effectiveness of this treatment [34, 35], the use of these devices is largely limited by the costs involved and the data is limited on HRQoL improvements with them. In a cohort study from the United States of America (USA), 128 patients were provided with IPCs and followed up at 3-month and 1-year intervals. SF-36 score improvements were seen in all domains except role limitations due to emotional problems at the 3-month timepoint, with these improvements persisting till the end of the study [36]. An RCT comparing IPC and a novel pulsating suit found that both methods resulted in improvements in HRQoL as measured using the SF-36, with no significant difference between the two modalities studied [37].

23.5.4 Vascularised Lymph Node Transfer

Vascularised lymph node transfer (VLNT) involves the microsurgical transfer of tissue which contains one or more lymph nodes to a lymphoedematous limb, allowing drainage of lymphatic fluid from the limb into the venous system via the newly transferred lymph node. Multiple cohort studies have observed the impact of VLNT on patients' HRQoL, with all studies agreeing that VLNT significantly improves HRQoL as measured using the LYMQoL overall score [38–40] and individual domain scores [38, 39]. Lymph vessel transplantation was also found to improve physiological and psychological SF-12 scores in a large cohort study of 107 lower limb lymphoedema patients in Germany [41].

In particular, VLNT was compared against another surgical technique known as lymphovenous anastomosis (LVA), which is discussed later in this chapter. In this cohort study from Taiwan, patients underwent VLNT or LVA, and while both groups showed improvements in both LYMQoL overall and individual domain scores, this was not significant in the LVA group [38]. In another study, VLNT was combined with modified radical reduction with preservation of perforators which involves the debulking of lymphoedematous skin and subcutaneous tissue. This combined approach also improved both the LYMQoL overall score and individual domain scores [42].

23.5.5 Lymphovenous Anastomosis

LVA involves the joining of a lymphatic channel to a subdermal venule, creating a new channel through which lymphatic fluid can return to the venous circulation. As mentioned previously, this technique was not found to result in significant improvements on LYMQoL overall and individual domain scores in a cohort study from Taiwan [38]. However, two other cohort studies found a positive HRQoL impact in patients undergoing LVA.

In a study from Italy that observed 26 patients with lower limb lymphoedema (together with 44 patients with upper limb lymphoedema), significant improvement in LYMQoL overall and individual domain scores were seen post-LVA. This improvement was greater in patients with lower limb lymphoedema when compared to those with upper limb lymphoedema [43]. A cohort study from the UK who underwent LVA found that 24 out of 29 patients showed improved HRQoL post-operatively, with median LYMQoL overall score improving from 72 to 90 points. Interestingly though, no association between limb volume reduction and HRQoL improvements were seen [44].

23.6 Discussion

Lymphoedema is a debilitating chronic condition characterised by excessive accumulation of fluid in the interstitium of soft tissues secondary to impaired lymphatic drainage. While initially presenting with swelling, heaviness, and pain in the affected limb(s), skin and subcutaneous changes soon follow if left untreated, leading to skin fibrosis and fat accumulation [45]. HRQoL is well documented to be significantly affected in patients living with chronic conditions [46–48], and lymphoedema is no different.

Clearly, the impact of lower limb lymphoedema on patients' HRQoL can only be a negative one. With lymphoedema eventually leading to extremity disability, recurrent skin infections, breakdown and ulceration, and even malignant transformation (e.g., lymphangiosarcoma), the impact on physical health only compounds with time. Quantifiable decreases in HRQoL have been recorded in all the studies that have been included in this literature review, with statistically significant impacts noted on both generic and disease-specific instruments. What is interesting to note is that patients with primary lymphoedema appear to have physical HRQoL impairments that are less severe compared to those with secondary lymphoedema [15], and physical HRQoL levels in this population is also comparable to population norms [15, 16].

Psychological and emotional HRQoL may, on the other hand, be related to how well patients cope with the disease and the ability to which they are able to adjust to the complications that arise from lymphoedema. The literature is less clear-cut with regards to the impact of lymphoedema on these HRQoL domains—this may be dependent on the specific patient population in question. It appears that primary lymphoedema patients once again have an advantage over their secondary lymphoedema peers, with no significant differences in psychological scores were seen from population norms, while secondary lymphoedema patients exhibited worse scores. It has been speculated that this could be due to primary lymphoedema patients having developed better coping strategies for their disease, having lived with the condition for longer than those with secondary lymphoedema. This level of resilience may also differ from patient to patient, leading to a less direct correlation between disease and the mental state of patients.

However, in lymphoedema research, defining the target population is further complicated by two-tiered system, with a greater focus on secondary lymphoedema related to cancer (specifically breast cancer and thus upper limb lymphoedema) and HRQoL studies and treatment provision are therefore often restricted to these patients [49]. Patients suffering from lymphoedema of other causes are oft neglected [50]. For example, a systematic review that considered treatment gaps in lymphoedema found that 94% of breast cancer-related lymphoedema patients received treatment for limb swelling, while only 82% of venous leg ulcer patients with phlebolymphoedema were treated [50]. Interestingly, the current literature review has highlighted a paucity of research into HRQoL for non-gynaecological cancer-related lymphoedema (including melanomas, prostate, etc.), suggesting that the greater focus in gynaecological cancers may be in part due to lower limb lymphoedema being a better recognised complication by both physicians and patients. Furthermore, few studies also looked at primary lymphoedemas independently, which particularly in HRQoL research may be problematic due to the issues raised in the previous paragraphs.

With regards to treatment for lower limb lymphoedema, CDP is currently considered the optimal treatment and is recommended as the first line for the management of lymphoedema [1]. This is not surprising given the proven clinical effectiveness of CDP, but this evidence is largely based on the reduction of limb volume and oedema [51–53]. However, the evidence is less clear on the impact of isolated on CDP on HRQoL improvements, with recent studies combining this therapy with longer term rehabilitation exercises with resulting improvements in patients' physical function. Clinical endpoints mean less to patients than to clinicians, and preserving physical function would likely be of greater importance to the patient than limb volume measurements.

While surgical intervention appears to improve HRQoL in lower limb lymphoedema, where it fits into the picture is currently unclear. This may be in part be due to the novelty of this approach, and as a result, while increasing in popularity, small numbers of operations have been performed. Indeed, within this literature review, the largest patient cohort of 107 lower limb lymphoedema patients undergoing VLNT was only achieved after 24 years of recruitment (1983 to 2007) [41], with other studies recruiting smaller cohorts of between 10 to 29 patients after 2 to 8 years of recruitment. This leads to difficulty when comparing surgical approaches (for e.g., LVA versus VLNT) and conservative methods. Further trials are indeed required to compare the impact of conservative, pharmacological, and surgical interventions on lymphoedema patients' both from a clinical effectiveness and HRQoL point of view. These trials should also focus on if and how treatment outcomes relate to HRQoL changes—limb volume changes may not be sufficient as a clinical endpoint in future studies. It would also be important to determine the right treatments for the right populations; with HRQoL impacted differently between primary and secondary lymphoedema patients, this may necessitate different treatment regimens for these disparate populations.

23.7 Conclusions

In the most recent 10 years of literature, studies largely agree that lower limb lymphoedema is a chronic, debilitating condition that has a negative impact on patients' HRQoL, with consequences on both physical and psychological HRQoL. The body of evidence is not yet completely clear regarding the actual domains and degree of impact, with differential impact stratified based on the primary and secondary lymphoedema populations. Further trials are required to compare the impact of conservative and surgical interventions on patients' HRQoL. Further work is required to determine the target populations for specific interventions to maximise HRQoL benefits.

References

1. Executive Committee of the International Society of Lymphology. The diagnosis and treatment of peripheral lymphedema: 2020 consensus document of the International Society of Lymphology. Lymphology. 2020;53(1):3–19.
2. Lymphoedema [Internet]. nhs.uk. 2017 [cited 2019 Nov 27]. Available from: https://www.nhs.uk/conditions/lymphoedema/
3. Kissin MW, Querci della Rovere G, Easton D, Westbury G. Risk of lymphoedema following the treatment of breast cancer. Br J Surg. 1986;73(7):580–4.
4. Adamczyk LA, Gordon K, Kholová I, Meijer-Jorna LB, Telinius N, Gallagher PJ, et al. Lymph vessels: the forgotten second circulation in health and disease. Virchows Arch. 2016;469(1):3–17.
5. Son A, O'Donnell TF, Izhakoff J, Gaebler JA, Niecko T, Iafrati MA. Lymphedema-associated comorbidities and treatment gap. J Vasc Surg Venous Lymphat Disord. 2019;7(5):724–30.
6. Rockson SG, Rivera KK. Estimating the population burden of lymphedema. Ann N Y Acad Sci. 2008;1131:147–54.
7. Casley-Smith JR. Alterations of untreated lymphedema and it grade over time. Lymphology. 1995;28(4):174–85.
8. WHO. WHOQOL: Measuring quality of life [Internet]. World Health Organisation; 1997 [cited 2020 Aug 23]. Available from: https://www.who.int/mental_health/media/68.pdf
9. Whitehead SJ, Ali S. Health outcomes in economic evaluation: the QALY and utilities. Br Med Bull. 2010;96(1):5–21.

10. Klernäs P, Johnsson A, Horstmann V, Kristjanson LJ, Johansson K. Lymphedema quality of life inventory (LyQLI)-development and investigation of validity and reliability. Qual Life Res. 2015;24(2):427–39.
11. Keeley V, Crooks S, Locke J, Veigas D, Riches K, Hilliam R. A quality-of-life measure for limb lymphoedema (LYMQOL). J Lymphoedema. 2010;5(1):26–37.
12. Klernäs P, Johnsson A, Horstmann V, Johansson K. Health-related quality of life in patients with lymphoedema - a cross-sectional study. Scand J Caring Sci. 2018;32(2):634–44.
13. Gethin G, Byrne D, Tierney S, Strapp H, Cowman S. Prevalence of lymphoedema and quality of life among patients attending a hospital-based wound management and vascular clinic. Int Wound J. 2012;9(2):120–5.
14. Pedrosa BC de S, Maia JN, Ferreira AP de L, de Araújo M das GR, Montenegro EJN, da Silva FL, et al. Functionality and quality of life of patients with unilateral lymphedema of a lower limb: a cross-sectional study. J Vasc Bras 2019;18:e20180066.
15. Huggenberger K, Wagner S, Lehmann S, Aeschlimann A, Amann-Vesti B, Angst F. Health and quality of life in patients with primary and secondary lymphedema of the lower extremity. VASA Z Gefasskrankheiten. 2015;44(2):129–37.
16. Okajima S, Hirota A, Kimura E, Inagaki M, Tamai N, Iizaka S, et al. Health-related quality of life and associated factors in patients with primary lymphedema. Jpn J Nurs Sci JJNS. 2013;10(2):202–11.
17. Watson CH, Lopez-Acevedo M, Broadwater G, Kim AH, Ehrisman J, Davidson BA, et al. A pilot study of lower extremity lymphedema, lower extremity function, and quality of life in women after minimally invasive endometrial cancer staging surgery. Gynecol Oncol. 2019;153(2):399–404.
18. Brown JC, Lin LL, Segal S, Chu CS, Haggerty AE, Ko EM, et al. Physical activity, daily walking, and lower limb lymphedema associate with physical function among uterine cancer survivors. Support Care Cancer Off J Multinatl Assoc Support Care Cancer. 2014;22(11):3017–25.
19. Farrell R, Gebski V, Hacker NF. Quality of life after complete lymphadenectomy for vulvar cancer: do women prefer sentinel lymph node biopsy? Int J Gynecol Cancer Off J Int Gynecol Cancer Soc. 2014;24(4):813–9.
20. de Melo Ferreira AP, de Figueiredo EM, Lima RA, Cândido EB, de Castro Monteiro MV, de Figueiredo Franco TMR, et al. Quality of life in women with vulvar cancer submitted to surgical treatment: a comparative study. Eur J Obstet Gynecol Reprod Biol. 2012;165(1):91–5.
21. Rowlands IJ, Beesley VL, Janda M, Hayes SC, Obermair A, Quinn MA, et al. Quality of life of women with lower limb swelling or lymphedema 3-5 years following endometrial cancer. Gynecol Oncol. 2014;133(2):314–8.
22. Trott S, Höckel M, Dornhöfer N, Geue K, Aktas B, Wolf B. Quality of life and associated factors after surgical treatment of vulvar cancer by vulvar field resection (VFR). Arch Gynecol Obstet. 2020;302(1):191–201.
23. Kim SI, Lim MC, Lee JS, Lee Y, Park K, Joo J, et al. Impact of lower limb lymphedema on quality of life in gynecologic cancer survivors after pelvic lymph node dissection. Eur J Obstet Gynecol Reprod Biol. 2015;192:31–6.
24. Omichi C, Nakamura K, Haraga J, Ida N, Saijo M, Nishida T, et al. The influence of adverse effects on quality of life of survivors of Gynecologic cancer. Int J Gynecol Cancer Off J Int Gynecol Cancer Soc. 2017;27(9):2014–9.
25. Cromwell KD, Chiang YJ, Armer J, Heppner PP, Mungovan K, Ross MI, et al. Is surviving enough? Coping and impact on activities of daily living among melanoma patients with lymphoedema. Eur J Cancer Care (Engl). 2015;24(5):724–33.
26. Mercier G, Pastor J, Moffatt C, Franks P, Quéré I. LIMPRINT: health-related quality of life in adult patients with chronic Edema. Lymphat Res Biol. 2019;17(2):163–7.
27. Yost KJ, Cheville AL, Al-Hilli MM, Mariani A, Barrette BA, McGree ME, et al. Lymphedema after surgery for endometrial cancer: prevalence, risk factors, and quality of life. Obstet Gynecol. 2014;124(2 Pt 1):307–15.
28. Lee TS, Morris CM, Czerniec SA, Mangion AJ. Does lymphedema severity affect quality of life? Simple question. Challenging answers. Lymphat Res Biol. 2018;16(1):85–91.

29. Tugral A, Viren T, Bakar Y. Tissue dielectric constant and circumference measurement in the follow-up of treatment-related changes in lower-limb lymphedema. Int Angiol J Int Union Angiol. 2018;37(1):26–31.
30. Do JH, Choi KH, Ahn JS, Jeon JY. Effects of a complex rehabilitation program on edema status, physical function, and quality of life in lower-limb lymphedema after gynecological cancer surgery. Gynecol Oncol. 2017;147(2):450–5.
31. Wu X, Liu Y, Zhu D, Wang F, Ji J, Yan H. Early prevention of complex decongestive therapy and rehabilitation exercise for prevention of lower extremity lymphedema after operation of gynecologic cancer. Asian J Surg. 2020 May 10.
32. Akgul A, Tarakci E, Arman N, Civi T, Irmak S. A randomized controlled trial comparing platelet-rich plasma, low-level laser therapy, and complex decongestive physiotherapy in patients with lower limb lymphedema. Lymphat Res Biol. 2020 Feb 19.
33. Ergin G, Karadibak D, Sener HO, Gurpinar B. Effects of aqua-lymphatic therapy on lower extremity lymphedema: a randomized controlled study. Lymphat Res Biol. 2017;15(3):284–91.
34. Blumberg SN, Berland T, Rockman C, Mussa F, Brooks A, Cayne N, et al. Pneumatic compression improves quality of life in patients with lower-extremity lymphedema. Ann Vasc Surg. 2016;30:40–4.
35. Uzkeser H, Karatay S, Erdemci B, Koc M, Senel K. Efficacy of manual lymphatic drainage and intermittent pneumatic compression pump use in the treatment of lymphedema after mastectomy: a randomized controlled trial. Breast Cancer. 2015;22(3):300–7.
36. Desai SS, Shao M. Vascular outcomes collaborative. Superior clinical, quality of life, functional, and health economic outcomes with pneumatic compression therapy for lymphedema. Ann Vasc Surg. 2020;63:298–306.
37. Jonas P, Charlois S, Chevalerias M, Delmas D, Kerihuel J-C, Blanchemaison P. Efficacy of the Stendo pulsating suit in patients with leg lymphedema: a pilot randomized study. Eur J Dermatol EJD. 2016;26(1):82–9.
38. Cheng M-H, Loh CYY, Lin C-Y. Outcomes of vascularized lymph node transfer and Lymphovenous anastomosis for treatment of primary lymphedema. Plast Reconstr Surg Glob Open. 2018;6(12):e2056.
39. Patel KM, Lin C-Y, Cheng M-H. A prospective evaluation of lymphedema-specific quality-of-life outcomes following vascularized lymph node transfer. Ann Surg Oncol. 2015;22(7):2424–30.
40. Maruccia M, Pezzolla A, Nacchiero E, Dicillo P, Macchia L, Fiore P, et al. Efficacy and early results after combining laparoscopic harvest of double gastroepiploic lymph node flap and active physiotherapy for lower extremity lymphedema. Microsurgery. 2019;39(8):679–87.
41. Springer S, Koller M, Baumeister RGH, Frick A. Changes in quality of life of patients with lymphedema after lymphatic vessel transplantation. Lymphology. 2011;44(2):65–71.
42. Ciudad P, Manrique OJ, Adabi K, Huang TC-T, Agko M, Trignano E, et al. Combined double vascularized lymph node transfers and modified radical reduction with preservation of perforators for advanced stages of lymphedema. J Surg Oncol. 2019;119(4):439–48.
43. Salgarello M, Mangialardi ML, Pino V, Gentileschi S, Visconti G. A prospective evaluation of health-related quality of life following Lymphaticovenular anastomosis for upper and lower extremities lymphedema. J Reconstr Microsurg. 2018;34(9):701–7.
44. Phillips GSA, Gore S, Ramsden A, Furniss D. Lymphaticovenular anastomosis in the treatment of secondary lymphoedema of the legs after cancer treatment. J Plast Reconstr Aesthetic Surg JPRAS. 2019;72(7):1184–92.
45. Di S, Ziyou Y, Liu N-F. Pathological changes of Lymphedematous skin: increased mast cells, related proteases, and activated transforming growth factor-β1. Lymphat Res Biol. 2016;14(3):162–71.
46. Dracup K, Walden JA, Stevenson LW, Brecht ML. Quality of life in patients with advanced heart failure. J Heart Lung Transplant. 1992;11(2 Pt 1):273–9.
47. Ståhl E, Lindberg A, Jansson S-A, Rönmark E, Svensson K, Andersson F, et al. Health-related quality of life is related to COPD disease severity. Health Qual Life Outcomes. 2005;3(1):56.

48. Lönnfors S, Vermeire S, Avedano L. IBD and health-related quality of life — discovering the true impact. J Crohns Colitis. 2014;8(10):1281–6.
49. Calman KC, Hine D. A policy framework for commissioning cancer services. A report by the expert advisory group on cancer to the chief medical officers of England and Wales: guidance for purchasers and providers of cancer services. Department of Health; 1995.
50. Moffatt CJ, Franks PJ, Doherty DC, Williams AF, Badger C, Jeffs E, et al. Lymphoedema: an underestimated health problem. QJM Mon J Assoc Physicians. 2003;96(10):731–8.
51. Liao S-F, Li S-H, Huang H-Y. The efficacy of complex decongestive physiotherapy (CDP) and predictive factors of response to CDP in lower limb lymphedema (LLL) after pelvic cancer treatment. Gynecol Oncol. 2012;125(3):712–5.
52. Yamamoto R, Yamamoto T. Effectiveness of the treatment-phase of two-phase complex decongestive physiotherapy for the treatment of extremity lymphedema. Int J Clin Oncol. 2007;12(6):463–8.
53. Hinrichs CS, Gibbs JF, Driscoll D, Kepner JL, Wilkinson NW, Edge SB, et al. The effectiveness of complete decongestive physiotherapy for the treatment of lymphedema following groin dissection for melanoma. J Surg Oncol. 2004;85(4):187–92.

MIX
Papier aus verantwortungsvollen Quellen
Paper from responsible sources
FSC® C105338

If you have any concerns about our products,
you can contact us on
ProductSafety@springernature.com

In case Publisher is established outside the EU,
the EU authorized representative is:
Springer Nature Customer Service Center GmbH
Europaplatz 3, 69115 Heidelberg, Germany

Printed by Libri Plureos GmbH
in Hamburg, Germany